Emerging Cancer Therapeutics

Jame Abraham, MD, FACP

Editor-in-Chief

Bonnie Wells Wilson Distinguished Professor and Eminent Scholar
Chief, Section of Hematology-Oncology
Medical Director, Mary Babb Randolph Cancer Center
West Virginia University
Morgantown, West Virginia

Editorial Board

Forthcoming Issues

Lymphoma
John Sweetenham, MD
Cleveland Clinic, Cleveland, Ohio

Melanoma
William H. Sharfman, MD
Johns Hopkins Medicine, Lutherville, Maryland

Emerging Cancer Therapeutics

VOLUME 3, ISSUE 1

Lung Cancer

Athanassios Argiris, MD, FACP
Guest Editor

A.B. Alexander Distinguished Chair in Oncology
Professor and Chief, Division of Hematology/Oncology
Associate Director for Clinical Research
Cancer Therapy & Research Center
UT Health Science Center at San Antonio
San Antonio, Texas

demosMEDICAL
New York

Acquisitions Editor: Richard Winters
Cover Design: Joe Tenerelli
Compositor: Newgen Imaging
Printer: Bradford & Bigelow

Visit our website at www.demosmedpub.com

Emerging Cancer Therapeutics is published three times a year by Demos Medical Publishing.

Business Office. All business correspondence including subscriptions, renewals, and address changes should be sent to Demos Medical Publishing, 11 West 42nd Street, 15th Floor, New York, NY, 10036.

ISSN: 2151-4194
ISBN: 978-1-936287-52-9
E-ISBN: 978-1-617050-97-8

Library of Congress Cataloging-in-Publication Data

Lung cancer / Athanassios Argiris, guest editor.
p. ; cm. — (Emerging cancer therapeutics, ISSN 2151-4194 ; v. 3, issue 1)
Includes bibliographical references and index.
ISBN 978-1-936287-52-9 — ISBN 978-1-61705-097-8 (e-ISBN)
I. Argiris, Athanassios. II. Series: Emerging cancer therapeutics ; v. 3, issue 1. 2151-4194
[DNLM: 1. Lung Neoplasms. WF 658]

616.99'424--dc23 2012011566

Reprints. For copies of 100 or more of articles in this publication, please contact Reina Santana, Special Sales Manager.

Special discounts on bulk quantities of Demos Medical Publishing books are available to corporations, professional associations, pharmaceutical companies, health care organizations, and other qualifying groups. For details, please contact:

Reina Santana, Special Sales Manager
Demos Medical Publishing LLC
11 W. 42nd Street
New York, NY 10036
Phone: 800-532-8663 or 212-683-0072
Fax: 212-941-7842
E-mail: rsantana@demosmedpub.com

Printed in the United States of America
12 13 14 15 5 4 3 2 1

Contents

Foreword

Cancer treatment is one of the fastest growing specialties in modern medicine, with better understanding of the disease, improved diagnostic tools, better prognostic information, and ever-changing management options. The most important tool a clinician can have in the fight against cancer is access to current information.

The Emerging Cancer Therapeutics (ECAT) series will provide a thorough analysis of key clinical research related to cancer therapeutics, including a discussion and assessment of current evidence, current clinical best practice, and likely near-future developments. The content will be in the form of review articles, but the volume format will allow for much more in-depth discussion than the typical journal review article. The goal will be to provide for the practicing clinician a source of thorough, ongoing analysis and translational assessment of "hot topics" and areas of rapidly emerging new data in cancer therapeutics with significant implications for clinical care.

The ECAT will be a valuable tool for practicing cancer specialists of all disciplines. This will provide the most comprehensive evidence-based review of pathology, radiology, pharmacology, surgical oncology, radiation oncology, and medical oncology of the topic.

The *Lung Cancer* volume provides a comprehensive approach to the pathophysiology, epidemiology, clinical features, diagnostic modalities, and current and future treatment options. Experts from around the country have contributed to this volume. This will be a valuable tool for any clinician, researcher, or student of oncology.

Jame Abraham, MD, FACP
Editor-in-Chief

Bonnie Wells Wilson Distinguished Professor and Eminent Scholar
Chief, Section of Hematology-Oncology
Medical Director, Mary Babb Randolph Cancer Center
West Virginia University
Morgantown, West Virginia

Preface

Lung cancer outcomes have marginally changed over the past four decades, a grim outlook that puts an enormous responsibility on those involved in the evaluation and treatment of patients with this disease. As key developments are reshaping the landscape of oncology, we are gradually changing the ways we approach lung cancer management. It has become apparent that lung tumors are widely heterogeneous at a molecular level, which can be exploited for therapeutic purposes. Mutations in epidermal growth factor receptor and the EML4-anaplastic lymphoma kinase translocation are among the first examples of validated molecular targets.

To cover breakthrough discoveries and state-of-the-art treatment of lung cancer, an extraordinary panel of experts has contributed to this volume of the Emerging Cancer Therapeutic series. Drs. Nwizu and Salgia review the molecular biology of lung cancer as it relates to the development of novel therapies, Drs. Pillai and Owonikoko comment on promising upcoming targeted agents, Drs. Vallabhaneni and Ramalingam focus on the use of anti-angiogenesis drugs, and Drs. Deming and Traynor assess the emerging applications of epidermal growth factor receptor tyrosine-kinase inhibitors in first-line therapy. Drs. Pallis, Georgoulias, and Agelaki evaluate the expanding armamentarium of chemotherapy regimens for advanced non-small cell lung cancer. Drs. Kotsakis, Kontopodis, and Georgoulias analyze the emerging role of maintenance therapy, an attractive option due to the availability of newer active agents with tolerable cumulative toxicities. The challenging field of small cell lung cancer treatment is reviewed by Drs. Lu, Giannatempo, and O'Brien. Dr. Rossi brings our attention to the special considerations and needs of the growing elderly population with lung cancer. Dr. Landreneau contributes an insightful update on surgical considerations for early-stage lung cancer. The impact of adjuvant chemotherapy for resected non-small cell lung cancer is addressed by Drs. Patel and Wakelee, whereas the complexity of radiotherapy to the chest and advances in technology are covered in detail by Drs. Amin, Raben, and Gaspar.

I anticipate that the material of this textbook will serve as a reference for up-to-date information that applies to clinical practice and will be useful to practicing oncologists, researchers, and trainees. With a fresh perspective on lung cancer therapeutics, we will hopefully be able to benefit more patients and save more lives.

Athanassios Argiris, MD, FACP

A.B. Alexander Distinguished Chair in Oncology
Professor and Chief, Division of Hematology/Oncology
Associate Director for Clinical Research
Cancer Therapy & Research Center
UT Health Science Center at San Antonio
San Antonio, Texas

Contributors

Sophia Agelaki, MD, PhD
Assistant Professor of Medical Oncology
Department of Medical Oncology
University Hospital of Heraklion
Heraklion, Greece

Neha P. Amin, MD
Department of Radiation Oncology
University of Colorado
Aurora, CO

Dustin A. Deming, MD
Oncology Fellow
Division of Hematology/Oncology
University of Wisconsin, Department of Medicine
University of Wisconsin Carbone Cancer Center
Madison, WI

Laurie E. Gaspar, MD, MBA
Department of Radiation Oncology
University of Colorado
Aurora, CO

Vassilis Georgoulias, MD, PhD
Professor of Medical Oncology
Department of Medical Oncology
University Hospital of Heraklion
Heraklion, Greece

Patrizia Giannatempo, MD
Oncology Fellow
Department of Medical Oncology
Fondazione IRCCS Istituto Tumori
University of Milan
Milan, Italy

Emmanouil Kontopodis, MD
Medical Oncologist, Research Fellow
Department of Medical Oncology
University Hospital of Heraklion
Heraklion, Greece

Athanasios Kotsakis, MD, PhD
Instructor of Medical Oncology
Department of Medical Oncology
University Hospital of Heraklion
Heraklion, Greece

Rodney J. Landreneau, MD
Professor of Surgery
Department of Cardio-Thoracic Surgery
University of Pittsburgh
Pennsylvania, PA

Shir Kiong Lu, MBChB, MRCP
Oncology Registrar
Department of Medical Oncology
Royal Marsden NHS Foundation Trust
London, UK

Tobenna Nwizu, MD
Fellow in Medical Oncology
Section of Hematology/Oncology, Department of Medicine
University of Chicago
Chicago, IL

Mary O'Brien, MD, FRCP
Consultant Medical Oncologist
Department of Oncology
Royal Marsden NHS Foundation Trust
Sutton, UK

Taofeek K. Owonikoko, MD, PhD
Assistant Professor
Department of Hematology and Medical Oncology
Emory University
Atlanta, GA

Athanasios G. Pallis, MD, PhD
Medical Oncologist
Department of Medical Oncology
University Hospital of Heraklion
Heraklion, Greece

Manali I. Patel, MD, MPH
Post-doctoral Fellow
Department of Oncology
Stanford University
Stanford, CA

Rathi N. Pillai, MD
Fellow
Department of Hematology and Medical Oncology
Emory University
Atlanta, GA

David Raben, MD
Department of Radiation Oncology
University of Colorado
Aurora, CO

Suresh Ramalingam, MD
Associate Professor
Department of Hematology and Medical Oncology
Winship Cancer Institute of Emory University
Atlanta, GA

Antonio Rossi, MD
Division of Medical Oncology
"S.G. Moscati" Hospital
Avellino, Italy

Ravi Salgia, MD, PhD
Professor of Medicine, Director of Thoracic Oncology Program
Section of Hematology/Oncology, Department of Medicine
University of Chicago
Chicago, IL

Anne M. Traynor, MD
Associate Professor
Division of Hematology/Oncology
University of Wisconsin, Department of Medicine
University of Wisconsin Carbone Cancer Center
Madison, WI

Geetha Vallabhaneni, MD
Fellow
Department of Hematology and Medical Oncology
Winship Cancer Institute of Emory University
Atlanta, GA

Heather Wakelee, MD
Assistant Professor
Department of Oncology
Stanford University
Stanford, CA

Emerging Cancer Therapeutics

VOLUME 3, ISSUE 1

Lung Cancer

demos MEDICAL

ECAT Emerging Cancer Therapeutics

Molecular Biology of Lung Cancer and Therapeutic Implications

Tobenna Nwizu and Ravi Salgia*

Section of Hematology/Oncology, Department of Medicine, University of Chicago, Chicago, IL

■ ABSTRACT

The emergence of new genomic and proteomic techniques has revealed that lung cancer is a heterogeneous disease with a wide variety of molecular aberrations, which are potential therapeutic targets. Recently, we have seen the emergence of targeted therapies in lung cancer that have shown promising results and improved overall survival. Molecular aberrations with therapeutic implications in lung cancer include the epidermal growth factor receptor (EGFR), echinoderm microtubule-associated protein-like 4-anaplastic lymphoma kinase fusion gene (EML4-ALK), KRAS, MET, ROS, and B-RAF, among others. EGFR is a member of the ErbB family of receptors and occurs more commonly in the adenocarcinoma variety of lung cancer, in females, and in nonsmokers. The tyrosine kinase inhibitors (TKI) gefitinib and erlotinib target EGFR, and clinical trials have shown superior outcomes with these TKIs as compared to standard cytotoxic chemotherapy in patients with EGFR mutations. On the other hand, KRAS mutation is seen to be more prevalent in smokers, and studies have shown that patients with KRAS mutations do not respond to the EGFR TKIs. More recently, the Food and Drug Administration approved crizotinib for the treatment of patients with lung cancer who harbor the EML4-ALK translocation. These patients are typically younger age and light-to-never smokers. Other molecular aberrations such as MET, ROS, and B-RAF are under clinical investigation as potential targets.

Keywords: epidermal growth factor receptor, anaplastic lymphoma kinase, MET, targeted therapy

*Corresponding author, 5841 S. Maryland Avenue, University of Chicago, MC2115, Chicago, IL 60637

E-mail address: rsalgia@medicine.bsd.uchicago.edu

Emerging Cancer Therapeutics 3:1 (2012) 1–10.

DOI: 10.5003/2151–4194.3.1.1

■ INTRODUCTION

Lung cancer is the second most common cancer and the leading cause of cancer mortality in the United States (1). The mortality rate from lung cancer has seen a decline from the 1990s in part due to earlier detection and recent advances in our understanding of the molecular basis of cancer. The recent emergence of targeted therapies in the field of lung cancer has lead to very promising results and improved overall survival. Lung cancer is a heterogeneous disease histologically and with a variety of molecular aberrations. With the development of new genomic and proteomic techniques like gene expression profiling, several molecular genetic abnormalities in lung cancer have been identified, which could be potential therapeutic targets. Examples of molecular genetic abnormalities include chromosomal aberrations, overexpression of oncogenes, deletion and/or mutations in tumor suppressor genes, and telomerase activity. As more molecular signatures are identified, we are likely to see the emergence of increasing number of highly targeted therapeutics in lung and other cancers, which will hopefully lead to better survival and higher cure rates.

Described are some of the molecular abnormalities that can occur in lung cancer (especially non-small cell lung cancer [NSCLC]) that have been targeted therapeutically.

■ EPIDERMAL GROWTH FACTOR RECEPTOR

Epidermal growth factor receptor (EGFR) is a member of the ErbB family of receptors, and is the cell surface receptor for members of the epidermal growth factor family of extracellular protein ligands. The ErbB family of receptors consists of four closely related receptor tyrosine kinases: EGFR/ERBB1/HER1, ERBB2/HER2, ERBB3/HER3, and ERBB4/HER4 (2).

The EGFR gene is located on chromosome 7p 12–13. EGFR was the first member of the HER family of receptors to be discovered, and has an essential role in both normal physiological and cancerous conditions by playing a key role in signal transduction processes by regulating major cellular functions such as survival, apoptosis, and proliferation. It is a 170-kDa receptor tyrosine kinase that exists on the cell surface and is activated by binding of its specific ligands, which include epidermal growth factor (EGF), transforming growth factor α (TGFα), betacellulin, and epiregulin.

EGF was first isolated by Stanley Cohen in 1962 as a protein extracted from the mouse submaxillary gland that accelerated incisor eruption and eyelid opening in the newborn animal, and hence was originally called tooth-lid factor (3), but it was later renamed EGF because it stimulated the proliferation of epithelial cells (4,5).

EGFR like all ErbB proteins has four functional domains: an extracellular ligand-binding domain, a transmembrane domain, an intracellular tyrosine kinase domain, and a C-terminal regulatory domain (6,7). The extracellular domain is further subdivided into four domains. The intracellular tyrosine kinase domain consists of an N-lobe and a C-lobe, and adenosine triphosphate (ATP) binds to the cleft formed between these two lobes. The C-terminal regulatory domain has several tyrosine kinase (TK) domains that are phosphorylated specifically in ligand binding. Upon binding its ligand, dynamic conformational changes occur in both extracellular and intracellular domains of the receptor kinase leading to transphosphorylations of tyrosine residues in the C-terminal regulatory domain. These provide docking sites for downstream molecules, which lead to activation of multiple signaling pathways including mitogen-activated protein kinase (MAPK), phosphatidylinositol 3-kinase/AKT, and the signal transducer and activator of transcriptions (STAT) 3 and STAT5 pathways. Activation of these pathways leads to the evasion of apoptosis, proliferation, invasion, and metastasis, all of which are important for the cancer phenotype.

EGFR was the first cell surface receptor to be linked directly with cancer when Stanley Cohen et al. described the downregulation of EGFR in fibroblasts infected with oncogenic viruses (8).

The oncogenic effect of EGFR was first demonstrated by the overexpression of the receptor in NIH3T3 cells and the stimulation by EGF leading to the formation of tumors in nude mice bearing the transformed NIH3T3 cells. Abnormalities in EGFR can include either overexpression or molecular alterations in the TK domain.

EGFR aberrations are seen in multiple malignancies that include lung, colon, head and neck, pancreas, ovary, bladder, breast, kidney, and gliomas. EGFR mutations in the TK domain are however seen almost exclusively in lung cancer. EGFR overexpression is seen in more than 60% of NSCLC but no to minimal expression is seen in small cell lung cancer (SCLC) (9). Some studies have reported the incidence of EGFR mutation to be 47% in lung cancer (10). There are reports that EGFR can be mutated in peritoneal mesothelioma (11).

EGFR mutations in lung cancer typically occur more frequently in the adenocarcinoma variety, more in well to moderately differentiated than poorly differentiated adenocarcinoma. EGFR mutation has also been found to be more prevalent in females, and in nonsmokers with the frequency inversely associated with the amount of tobacco smoked (10). EGFR mutations were actually the first molecular aberrations found in lung cancer that are more frequent among patients without a smoking history than among those with one (6). Heavy smoking however does not indicate that a patient cannot have the EGFR mutations, as this mutation is seen in more than 20% of heavy smokers (10).

Multivariate analysis of a study by Kosaka et al. suggested that nonsmoking status and adenocarcinoma histology independently contributed to EGFR mutations, but female gender did not (10). Premenopausal women were found not to have a higher incidence of EGFR mutation indicating that the difference in male and female incidence was caused by difference in lifestyle including smoking habits, rather than gender difference. EGFR mutations were also found not to be associated with the stage of disease, suggesting that the EGFR mutations occur early in the clinical course and so were associated with pathogenesis rather than progression. Most of the EGFR mutations found were in the TK domain with more than 90% of the mutation being either deletions around codons 746 to 750 in exons 19 or missense mutations resulting in a substitution of leucine with arginine at codon 858 (L858R) in exon 21. These all flank the ATP binding pocket, which is important for TK activity (10). There is also an ancestral variation of EGFR mutation found more commonly in Asian population.

EGFR mutations implicated in the pathogenesis of lung cancer are strictly mutually exclusive of KRAS mutations. There are more than 20 variant types of deletion, including larger deletions, deletions plus point mutations, and deletions plus insertions.

Exon 19 deletional mutation and L858R result in increased and substantial phosphorylation of EGFR and other ERBB family proteins without ligand stimulation. Mutant EGFR selectively activates the AKT and STAT signaling pathways that promote cell survival, but has no effect on the MAPK pathway that induces cell proliferation (6).

Patients with EGFR mutations are more responsive to treatment with EGFR tyrosine kinase inhibitors (TKI). Gefitinib and erlotinib are the two EGFR TKIs presently on the market. In 2004, it was discovered that patients who had response to gefitinib had activating mutations of the EGFR gene. One study found that somatic mutations were identified in the TK domain of the EGFR gene in eight of nine patients with gefitinib-responsive lung cancer, as compared with none of the seven patients with no response ($P < .001$). Mutations found in this study were either small in frame deletions or amino acid substitutions clustered around the ATP-binding pocket of the TK domain (12). Other studies also confirmed that mutations in the EGFR gene were found in lung cancer samples from patients who had responded to gefitinib or erlotinib but not in gefitinib-insensitive tumors or cell lines (13, 14). This discovery helped explain why female, nonsmoking, adenocarcinoma patients of East Asian origin with lung cancer had a higher response rate to EGFR TKIs. Some studies have shown that the response rate to EGFR TKIs is highest in exon 19 deletions followed by L858R (15).

A Phase III clinical trial showed that patients with EGFR mutated NSCLC had superior outcomes with gefitinib as compared to standard cytotoxic chemotherapy. The study compared gefitinib with carboplatin and paclitaxel. In the EGFR mutated group, progression-free survival was significantly longer among those who received gefitinib than among those who received carboplatin and paclitaxel (hazard ratio for progression or death, 0.48; 95% CI, 0.36–0.64; $P < .001$) (16).

Even though patients with EGFR mutated NSCLC have good response to gefitinib or erlotinib, they eventually develop resistance and progress. One mechanism of this acquired resistance is due to a secondary mutation in exon 20, which leads to substitution of methionine for threonine at position 790 (T790M) in the kinase domain. A study by Pao et al. discovered this new mutation in patients who had developed resistance to gefitinib but did not detect this mutation in any untreated patients (17). The T790M mutation has however been reported in combination with the L858R mutation in untreated patients, and studies suggest that tumors with both mutations are very aggressive (18).

Another mechanism of resistance to gefitinib and erlotinib in EGFR mutated NSCLC is through MET amplification, and in vivo combination of EGFR and MET inhibition overcomes this resistance (19).

A recent study by Sequist et al., investigating the mechanism of acquired TKI resistance in EGFR mutated NSCLC, revealed that all drug-resistant tumors retained their original activating EGFR mutation and some acquired the T790M mutation or MET amplification. Some resistant cancers showed unexpected genetic changes including EGFR amplification and mutations in the PIK3CA gene, whereas others underwent a pronounced epithelial to mesenchymal transition. Also seen was that 14% of the resistant tumor had transformed from NSCLC into SCLC and were sensitive to standard SCLC treatments. In a few of these patients, serial biopsies revealed that genetic mechanisms of resistance were lost in the absence of the continued selective pressure of EGFR inhibitor treatment and such cancers were sensitive to a second round of treatment with EGFR inhibitors (20).

Other EGFR mutations such as insertion mutations in exon 20 of EGFR have been implicated in primary resistance to the TKI erlotinib and gefitinib. This mutation confers resistance by precluding the binding of TKIs to the EGFR TK domain (9,21).

■ KRAS

Guanine nucleotide triphosphatases (GTPase) KRAS, also known as V-Ki-ras2 Kirsten rat sarcoma viral oncogene homolog and KRAS, is a protein that is encoded by the KRAS gene. KRAS protein, like other RAS protein family members, belongs to a class of proteins called small GTPase and is involved in cellular signal transduction. KRAS is involved in the EGFR signaling pathway, which is important in the pathogenesis and progression of malignancy. KRAS is downstream of the EGFR receptor and regulates downstream proteins that control cell cycle progression.

Ninety percent of RAS mutations in lung cancer are found in KRAS. Approximately 97% of KRAS mutations in NSCLC involve codons 12 or 13. KRAS mutations are uncommon in lung squamous cell carcinomas (22). A landmark study in 1984 reported finding malignant activation of a KRAS oncogene in lung carcinoma tissue but not in normal tissue of the same patient. This mutation involved a single genetic alteration, a guanine to cytosine transversion, which was responsible for the acquisition of malignant properties by KRAS gene. Consequently, arginine instead of the normal glycine is incorporated into the KRAS coded p21 proteins at amino acid position 12 (23). With this mutation, KRAS is permanently turned on, without being triggered by EGFR-mediated signaling, leading to persistent activation of the EGFR signaling pathway and hence tumor survival, growth, proliferation metastasis, and angiogenesis.

KRAS mutations are found in higher incidence not only in heavy smokers but also in never/light smokers (22). So unlike EGFR mutations, which occurs more frequently in tumors from never smoker, KRAS tumor status cannot be predicted on the basis of smoking history alone.

Numerous studies have shown that patients with KRAS mutation do not respond to the EGFR TKIs, erlotinib, and gefitinib (24–26). Presently there are ongoing clinical trials aimed at overcoming this resistance.

■ ECHINODERM MICROTUBULE-ASSOCIATED PROTEIN-LIKE 4–ANAPLASTIC LYMPHOMA KINASE FUSION GENE

Anaplastic lymphoma kinase (ALK), also known as ALK tyrosine kinase receptor or CD246 (cluster of differentiation 246), is an enzyme that is encoded by the ALK gene and mutations in this gene, which has been implicated in the pathogenesis of NSCLC. This mutation is caused by fusion of the EML4 gene with the signaling portion of the ALK gene resulting in the formation of the fusion protein EML4–ALK, which has been implicated as a driver of oncogenesis. An inversion on the short arm of chromosome 2 (Inv(2)(p21p23)) that joins exons 1 to 13 of EML4 to exons 20 to 29 of ALK leads to the formation of this EML4–ALK fusion oncogene. The resulting chimeric protein contains an N-terminus derived from EML4 and a C-terminus containing the entire intracellular tyrosine kinase domain of ALK. A study utilizing transgenic mouse lines that expressed EML4–ALK specifically in lung alveolar epithelial cells revealed that these mice developed hundreds of adenocarcinoma nodules in both lungs within a few weeks after birth, and in vivo treatment of these EMK4–ALK transgenic mice with an oral small-molecule inhibitor of the kinase activity of ALK resulted in tumor regression, confirming the potent oncogenic activity of this fusion gene (27).

EML4–ALK translocation was initially described in Japanese patients with NSCLC in 2007 (28), and is found in approximately 7% of patients with NSCLC (29). Although multiple variants exist, all encode a fusion between the same cytoplasmic portions of the ALK but contain different truncations of EML4. Various isoforms of this fusion gene have been reported, with each different isoform comprising segments from either exon 6, 13, 20, or exon 18 of the 5′ EML4 fused to the same 3′ ALK kinase domain. Fusions of ALK with other partners have been described in lung cancer. Examples include KIF5B–ALK (30) and TFG–ALK (31).

Patients with the EML4–ALK fusion gene have similar clinical features as patients with mutated EGFR in that they are usually former to light smokers (often defined as ≤ 10 pack years and quit ≥ 1 year ago), relatively younger age at onset and of adenocarcinoma histology. Even though the EML4–ALK fusion gene is seen mostly in NSCLC with adenocarcinoma histology, new data suggest that it can be present in any histology. Apart from rare exceptions, EML4–ALK, EGFR, and K-ras mutations are mutually exclusive (28, 32).

Recently, the Food and Drug Administration (FDA) approved crizotinib, a potent, orally bioavailable, ATP competitive small molecule inhibitor of the catalytic activity of MET and ALK kinases, for the treatment of patients with NSCLC that harbor this EML4–ALK fusion gene. Clinical trial with crizotinib had shown dramatic response, with an early phase trial involving 82 patients with the EML4–ALK translocation showing tumor shrinkage in almost all the patients. The mean duration of treatment was 6.4 months, with the overall response rate being 57% (47 of 82 patients with

46 confirmed partial responses and one patient confirmed complete response); 27 patients (33%) had stable disease with the disease control rate at 8 weeks being 87%. Response duration varied from 1 to 15 months. Of 82 patients, 63 (77%) continued to receive crizotinib (after the time of data cutoff), and the estimated probability of 6 months progression free survival was 72% with no median for the study reached. Most of these patients had previously been treated (33).

The FDA approved test to detect the EML4–ALK translocation is the Vysis ALK Break Apart FISH Probe Kit. There are other methods to detect the ALK translocation, including immunohistochemistry and reverse transcription polymerase chain reaction. It will be important to standardize these tests.

■ ROS

ROS was first discovered as the oncogene product of the avian sarcoma RNA virus UR2 (34). The avian sarcoma RNA virus was observed to be a highly invasive fibrosarcoma-derived virus that was efficient at transforming chicken embryo fibroblasts and chicken embryo neuroretinal cells (35, 36). The amino acid sequence coded by the one portion of UR2 (a 68-kDa polypeptide named $p68^{v\text{-}ros}$) coded for a protein with TK activity.

Naturally occurring oncogenic versions of ROS have recently been reported. A recent global survey of phosphotyrosine signaling detected a fusion of ROS to the transmembrane solute carrier protein SLC34A2. The N-terminal region of SLC34A2, ending just after the first transmembrane region is fused N-terminal to the transmembrane region of ROS producing a truncated fusion protein with two transmembrane domains. (31). The NaPi-2B-ROS fusion protein expressed both the fused in glioblastoma (FIG) and ROS genes. Other forms of this fusion protein are also observed.

A recent study showed that cell lines expressing FIG/ROS were found to be inhibited by an ALK inhibitor (37). This is because ROS TKs share high sequence homology with ALK and hence could be a potential target for ALK inhibitors.

■ MET

MET gene is a proto-oncogene that has been implicated in the pathogenesis of lung cancer and encodes for a protein known as the hepatocyte growth factor receptor. MET is a tyrosine kinase receptor for hepatocyte growth factor (HGF) and is its only known high-affinity receptor. Studies suggest that the signal pathway between HGF and its receptor plays an important role in oncogenesis.

The MET gene is located on chromosome 7q21-q31, and is 120 kb in length with 21 exons and 20 introns. The MET receptor is part of a larger family of growth factor receptors with identical architecture that include the Ron and Sea receptors. It is comprised of a 50-kD extracellular alpha chain and a 140-kD transmembrane beta chain, which are linked by disulfide bonds. It contains the following domains: a large seven-blade propeller (semma domain), PSI (plexins, semaphorins, integrins), four IPT repeats (immunoglobulins, plexins, transcription Factors), TM (transmembrane), JM (juxtamembrane), and TK (38,39).

MET is selectively expressed in several normal epithelial tissues. High levels of MET RNA have been found in liver, gastrointestinal tract, thyroid, and kidney. The tissue distribution of the MET/HGF receptor indicates that it is involved in growth control of epithelial cells other than hepatocytes and suggests that its increased expression may confer a growth advantage to neoplastic cells (40).

Amplification, translocation, or mutation of MET are different mechanisms that lead to the uncontrolled activation of MET frequently seen in lung cancer, with majority of MET mutations being germline in nature.

Studies have suggested that MET mutations may differ based on ethnicity, as seen in a study by Krishnaswamy et al. that amplified the individual exons of semaphorin, juxtamembrane, and

TK domains of MET using tissue genomic DNA from 141 Asians, 76 Caucasians, and 66 African American lung cancer patients by polymerase chain reaction. Nine nucleotide substitutions leading to MET mutations were detected, with six of them involving nonsynonymous amino acid changes. Four of the nonsynonymous substitutions were also detected in the adjacent normal tissue consistent with a germline origin. All the nonsynonymous mutations were clustered in the semaphorin domain, except R988C in the juxtammembrane domain. N375S was the most frequently seen nonsynonmyous amino acid substitution and occurred at a higher frequency in East Asians compared with Caucasians, and was not seen in African Americans (41).

Activation of MET/HGF signaling leads to stimulation of cellular proliferation, promotion of cell movement, angiogenesis, invasion into extracellular matrix, epithelial morphogenesis, tumorigenesis, and tissue regeneration. NSCLC patients with MET overexpression typical have worse outcomes after complete resection (42).

Apart from NSCLC, c-Met overexpression has also been found in other malignancies like SCLC (43), hereditary papillary renal cell cancer (44), gastric cancer (45), childhood hepatocellular carcinoma (46), and metastatic head and neck cancer (47).

There are various studies investigating the therapeutic implication of the inhibition of MET (48–50).

The new FDA approved crizotinib also targets MET.

■ B-RAF

B-Raf is a member of the Raf kinase family of serine/threonine-specific protein kinases and plays a role in regulating the MAPK/extracellular signal-regulated kinase (ERK) signaling pathway, which is involved in cellular division and differentiation. The RAF family has three members: A-RAF, B-RAF, and C-RAF.

The Raf serine/threonine kinases are the principal effectors of Ras in the MAPK pathway, and lie downstream of Ras making it an attractive target. Raf is principally activated by Ras, but may also be activated by Ras-independent elements, and hence propagate signals through diverse effectors that mediate proliferation, angiogenesis, metastases, and survival (51).

The structure of Raf consists of an amino terminus that contains the regulatory domain, an activation loop, and a carboxyl terminus that contains the kinase domain. All Raf kinases are composed of three conserved regions, CR1 (adjacent to the amino terminus), CR2, and CR3 (adjacent to the carboxyl terminus). Raf is activated by the interaction of active GTP-bound Ras with the RBD (Ras-binding domain) of Raf and the adjacent zinc-binding cysteine-rich domain of CR1, facilitating recruitment of Raf to the cell membrane for activation.

While mutations in ARAF and CRAF are rare, BRAF mutations are seen in approximately 8% of all malignancies (52). The most common BRAF mutation (> 90%) is a valine-to-glutamine substitution at residue 600 (V600E), which exhibits 12.5-fold higher basal kinase activity than that of wild-type BRAF (51,52). This BRAF V600E mutation leads to constitutive ERK activation and tumor formation in nude mice (51).

A recent study by Hongbin et al. revealed that lung specific expression of the BRAF V600E mutation induces the activation of the ERK/MAPK pathway, which leads to the development of lung adenocarcinoma with bronchioloalveolar carcinoma features in vivo. Also seen was that in vivo pharmacologic inhibition of MAPK/ERK kinase (MEK;MAPKK) using CI-1040—a specific MEK inhibitor—induced tumor regression associated with inhibition of cell proliferation and induction of apoptosis in these de novo lung tumors (52).

Results of clinical trial using CI-1040 have however been disappointing (53). PD 0325901, a second generation MEK inhibitor that exhibits higher potency against MEK, improved bioavailability, and longer duration of target suppression is now under clinical trial.

CONCLUSION

As our understanding of the molecular mechanisms that underlies the pathogenesis and progression of cancer grows, there will be the emergence of more targeted therapies. We have already seen success with the development of the TKIs, erlotinib, and gefitinib that has shown improved benefit in patients with specific EGFR mutations, and more recently crizotinib that has shown very promising results in patients with the ALK translocation. Presently, research is underway to target the components of the MAPK pathway, specifically RAS and RAF. There is some promise with targeting downstream effectors as these are less redundant.

As different cancers have different molecular signatures, the emphasis today is on personalized medicine, with patient's therapy being tailored based on their distinct molecular markers. Ultimately, we will need to personalize our therapeutics, prognosis, predictive signature based not only on clinical and pathological criteria but also on molecular and biomarker criteria.

REFERENCES

1. Siegel R, et al. Cancer statistics, 2011: The impact of eliminating socioeconomic and racial disparities on premature cancer deaths. *CA Cancer J Clin.* 2011;61(4):212–236.
2. Hynes NE, Lane HA.ERBB receptors and cancer: the complexity of targeted inhibitors. *Nat Rev Cancer.* 2005;5(5):341–354.
3. Cohen S. Isolation of a mouse submaxillary gland protein accelerating incisor eruption and eyelid opening in the new-born animal. *J Biol Chem.* 1962;237:1555–1562.
4. Gschwind A, Fischer OM, Ullrich A. The discovery of receptor tyrosine kinases: targets for cancer therapy. *Nat Rev Cancer.* 2004;4(5):361–370.
5. Cohen S. The stimulation of epidermal proliferation by a specific protein (EGF). *Dev Biol.* 1965;12(3):394–407.
6. Mitsudomi T, Yatabe Y. Epidermal growth factor receptor in relation to tumor development: EGFR gene and cancer. *FEBS J.* 2010;277(2):301–308.
7. Burgess AW, et al. An open-and-shut case? Recent insights into the activation of EGF/ErbB receptors. *Mol Cell.* 2003;12(3):541–552.
8. Cohen S. Nobel lecture. Epidermal growth factor. *Biosci Rep.* 1986;6(12):1017–1028.
9. Zhang Z, et al. EGFR-mutated lung cancer: A paradigm of molecular oncology. *Oncotarget.* 2010;1(7):497–514.
10. Kosaka T, et al. Mutations of the epidermal growth factor receptor gene in lung cancer: Biological and clinical implications. *Cancer Res.* 2004;64(24):8919–8923.
11. Foster JM, et al. Novel and existing mutations in the tyrosine kinase domain of the epidermal growth factor receptor are predictors of optimal resectability in malignant peritoneal mesothelioma. *Ann Surg Oncol.* 2009;16(1): 152–158.
12. Lynch TJ, et al. Activating mutations in the epidermal growth factor receptor underlying responsiveness of non-small-cell lung cancer to gefitinib. *N Engl J Med.* 2004;350(21):2129–2139.
13. Paez JG, et al. EGFR mutations in lung cancer: Correlation with clinical response to gefitinib therapy. *Science.* 2004;304(5676):1497–1500.
14. Pao W, et al. EGF receptor gene mutations are common in lung cancers from "never smokers" and are associated with sensitivity of tumors to gefitinib and erlotinib. *Proc Natl Acad Sci U S A.* 2004;101(36):13306–13311.
15. Mitsudomi T, Yatabe Y. Mutations of the epidermal growth factor receptor gene and related genes as determinants of epidermal growth factor receptor tyrosine kinase inhibitors sensitivity in lung cancer. *Cancer Sci.* 2007;98(12): 1817–1824.
16. Mok TS, et al. Gefitinib or carboplatin-paclitaxel in pulmonary adenocarcinoma. *N Engl J Med.* 2009;361(10):947–957.
17. Pao W, et al. Acquired resistance of lung adenocarcinomas to gefitinib or erlotinib is associated with a second mutation in the EGFR kinase domain. *PLoS Med.* 2005;2(3):e73.
18. Toyooka S, Kiura K, Mitsudomi T. EGFR mutation and response of lung cancer to gefitinib. *N Engl J Med.* 2005;352(20):2136; author reply 2136.

19. Turke AB, et al. Preexistence and clonal selection of MET amplification in EGFR mutant NSCLC. *Cancer Cell.* 2010;17(1):77–88.
20. Sequist LV, et al. Genotypic and histological evolution of lung cancers acquiring resistance to EGFR inhibitors. *Sci Transl Med.* 2011;3(75): 75ra26.
21. Wang SE, et al. HER2 kinase domain mutation results in constitutive phosphorylation and activation of HER2 and EGFR and resistance to EGFR tyrosine kinase inhibitors. *Cancer Cell.* 2006;10(1):25–38.
22. Riely GJ, Marks J, Pao W. KRAS mutations in non-small cell lung cancer. *Proc Am Thorac Soc.* 2009;6(2):201–205.
23. Santos E, et al. Malignant activation of a K-ras oncogene in lung carcinoma but not in normal tissue of the same patient. *Science.* 1984;223(4637):661–664.
24. Massarelli E, et al. KRAS mutation is an important predictor of resistance to therapy with epidermal growth factor receptor tyrosine kinase inhibitors in non-small-cell lung cancer. *Clin Cancer Res.* 2007;13(10):2890–2896.
25. Pao W, et al. KRAS mutations and primary resistance of lung adenocarcinomas to gefitinib or erlotinib. *PLoS Med.* 2005;2(1):e17.
26. Eberhard DA, et al. Mutations in the epidermal growth factor receptor and in KRAS are predictive and prognostic indicators in patients with non-small-cell lung cancer treated with chemotherapy alone and in combination with erlotinib. *J Clin Oncol.* 2005;23(25):5900–5909.
27. Soda M, et al. A mouse model for EML4-ALK-positive lung cancer. *Proc Natl Acad Sci U S A.* 2008;105(50):19893–19897.
28. Soda M, et al. Identification of the transforming EML4-ALK fusion gene in non-small-cell lung cancer. *Nature.* 2007;448(7153):561–566.
29. Choi YL, et al. Identification of novel isoforms of the EML4-ALK transforming gene in non-small cell lung cancer. *Cancer Res.* 2008;68(13): 4971–4976.
30. Takeuchi K, et al. KIF5B-ALK, a novel fusion oncokinase identified by an immunohistochemistry-based diagnostic system for ALK-positive lung cancer. *Clin Cancer Res.* 2009;15(9):3143–3149.
31. Rikova K, et al. Global survey of phosphotyrosine signaling identifies oncogenic kinases in lung cancer. *Cell.* 2007;131(6):1190–1203.
32. Takahashi T, et al. Clinicopathologic features of non-small-cell lung cancer with EML4-ALK fusion gene. *Ann Surg Oncol.* 2010;17(3):889–897.
33. Kwak EL, et al. Anaplastic lymphoma kinase inhibition in non-small-cell lung cancer. *N Engl J Med.* 2010;363(18):1693–1703.
34. Balduzzi PC, et al. Some biological properties of two new avian sarcoma viruses. *J Virol.* 1981;40(1):268–275.
35. Notter MF, et al. Infection of neuroretinal cells in vitro by avian sarcoma viruses UR1 and UR2: Transformation, cell growth stimulation, and changes in transducin levels. *Virology.* 1987;160(2):489–493.
36. Notter MF, Balduzzi PC. Cytoskeletal changes induced by two avian sarcoma viruses: UR2 and Rous sarcoma virus. *Virology.* 1984;136(1): 56–68.
37. Gu TL, et al. Survey of tyrosine kinase signaling reveals ROS kinase fusions in human cholangiocarcinoma. *PLoS One.* 2011;6(1):e15640.
38. Cipriani NA, et al. MET as a target for treatment of chest tumors. *Lung Cancer.* 2009;63(2): 169–179.
39. Stamos J, et al. Crystal structure of the HGF beta-chain in complex with the Sema domain of the Met receptor. *EMBO J.* 2004;23(12):2325–2335.
40. Di Renzo MF, et al. Expression of the Met/HGF receptor in normal and neoplastic human tissues. *Oncogene.* 1991;6(11):1997–2003.
41. Krishnaswamy S, et al. Ethnic differences and functional analysis of MET mutations in lung cancer. *Clin Cancer Res.* 2009;15(18):5714–5723.
42. Okuda K, et al. Met gene copy number predicts the prognosis for completely resected non-small cell lung cancer. *Cancer Sci.* 2008;99(11): 2280–2285.
43. Maulik G, et al. Modulation of the c-Met/hepatocyte growth factor pathway in small cell lung cancer. *Clin Cancer Res.* 2002;8(2):620–627.
44. Schmidt L, et al. Germline and somatic mutations in the tyrosine kinase domain of the MET proto-oncogene in papillary renal carcinomas. *Nat Genet.* 1997;16(1):68–73.

45. Lee JH, et al. A novel germ line juxtamembrane Met mutation in human gastric cancer. *Oncogene.* 2000;19(43):4947–4953.
46. Park WS, et al. Somatic mutations in the kinase domain of the Met/hepatocyte growth factor receptor gene in childhood hepatocellular carcinomas. *Cancer Res.* 1999;59(2):307–310.
47. Di Renzo MF, et al. Somatic mutations of the MET oncogene are selected during metastatic spread of human HNSC carcinomas. *Oncogene.* 2000;19(12):1547–1555.
48. Sattler M, et al. A novel small molecule met inhibitor induces apoptosis in cells transformed by the oncogenic TPR-MET tyrosine kinase. *Cancer Res.* 2003;63(17):5462–5469.
49. Christensen JG, et al. A selective small molecule inhibitor of c-Met kinase inhibits c-Met-dependent phenotypes in vitro and exhibits cytoreductive antitumor activity in vivo. *Cancer Res.* 2003;63(21):7345–7355.
50. Puri N, et al. A selective small molecule inhibitor of c-Met, PHA665752, inhibits tumorigenicity and angiogenesis in mouse lung cancer xenografts. *Cancer Res.* 2007;67(8):3529–3534.
51. Beeram M, Patnaik A, Rowinsky EK. Raf: A strategic target for therapeutic development against cancer. *J Clin Oncol.* 2005;23(27):6771–6790.
52. Ji H, et al. Mutations in BRAF and KRAS converge on activation of the mitogen-activated protein kinase pathway in lung cancer mouse models. *Cancer Res.* 2007;67(10):4933–4939.
53. Rinehart J, et al. Multicenter phase II study of the oral MEK inhibitor, CI-1040, in patients with advanced non-small-cell lung, breast, colon, and pancreatic cancer. *J Clin Oncol.* 2004;22(22):4456–4462.

demos MEDICAL

ECAT Emerging Cancer Therapeutics

Chemotherapy Options for Advanced Non-Small Cell Lung Cancer

Athanasios G. Pallis, Vassilis Georgoulias*, and Sophia Agelaki

Department of Medical Oncology, University General Hospital of Heraklion, Crete, Greece

ABSTRACT

Chemotherapy remains the cornerstone of treatment in advanced/metastatic non-small cell lung cancer (NSCLC). Chemotherapy doublets are superior to single agent treatment in first-line treatment, and three-drug combinations do not offer any benefit in terms of overall survival compared to two-drug regimens. A combination of a platinum agent plus a third generation cytotoxic (vinorelbine, taxane, gemcitabine, pemetrexed) represents the current standard of care; however, no particular combination can be recommended as clearly superior to the others. The evidence suggests that cisplatin combinations have a higher response rate than carboplatin and may improve survival when combined with third-generation agents while cisplatin-based doublets are preferred over platinum-free regimens because they are associated with a marginal 1-year survival benefit. Recently, the addition of bevacizumab or cetuximab to chemotherapy doublets and the use of EGFR tyrosine inhibitors kinase gefitinib and erlotinib improved the outcome in selected patients with advanced NSCLC. For second-line treatment docetaxel, pemetrexed, and erlotinib represent the standard options.

Keywords: NSCLC, chemotherapy, targeted therapy

Approximately 40% of patients with non-small cell lung cancer (NSCLC) are diagnosed with metastatic disease, and furthermore, the vast majority of patients who are treated with curative intent will eventually develop metastatic disease (1). Patients with advanced NSCLC when treated with best supportive care (BSC) have a median survival of 4 to 5 months and a 1-year survival of approximately 10% (2). During 1980s, cisplatin-based chemotherapy regimens most frequently in combination with etoposide, ifosfamide, vindesine, or vinblastine resulted in objective responses rates of approximately 20% to 30%, but median survival was only 6 to 8 months and few patients survived longer than 1 year. Several randomized trials demonstrated a

*Corresponding author, Department of Medical Oncology, University General Hospital of Heraklion, Crete, Greece
E-mail address: georgsec@med.uoc.gr

Emerging Cancer Therapeutics 3:1 (2012) 11–26.

DOI: 10.5003/2151–4194.3.1.11

small but statistically significant survival benefit for patients receiving chemotherapy over BSC alone. The same observation was confirmed by meta-analyses that were performed to address the same question (3–5). The more recent of these meta-analyses with data from 2,714 patients from 16 randomized controlled trials (RCTs) demonstrated a significant benefit of chemotherapy (hazard ratio [HR], 0.77; 95% confidence interval [CI], 0.71–0.83; $P \leq .0001$), equivalent to a relative increase in survival of 23% or an absolute improvement in survival of 9% at 12 months, increasing survival from 20% to 29% (5). Conceivably, cisplatin-based chemotherapy was considered as the standard of care in most patients with advanced NSCLC (6).

■ FIRST-LINE CHEMOTHERAPY

Doublet Chemotherapy of Platinum Agent Plus a New Agent Versus Doublets Using Older Agents

During the 1980s and early 1990s, several randomized trials evaluated numerous first-generation cisplatin-based chemotherapy regimens (7–10). These trials yielded no significant differences between regimens or between studies.

Le Chevalier et al. were the first to compare the combination of cisplatin plus a newer generation agent with a first-generation cisplatin-based doublet (11). This trial demonstrated a significant overall survival (OS) prolongation for patients treated with cisplatin/vinorelbine compared to those treated with cisplatin/vindesine (median OS: 40 weeks vs. 32 weeks; $P = .04$). Moreover, this study proved that cisplatin was necessary because cisplatin/vinorelbine was superior to vinorelbine alone in terms of OS (40 weeks vs. 31 weeks; $P = .01$).

Further randomized trials addressing the same question verified that third-generation regimens, generally, are associated with improved efficacy, toxicity, quality of life, or a combination of these endpoints although statistically significant survival gain was not uniformly present (12–20) (Table 1).

A meta-analysis by Baggstrom et al. (21) further clarified this issue by demonstrating that third-generation platinum-based doublets were associated with a 6% reduction in the risk of death at 1 year when compared with older platinum-based doublets.

Platinum-New Agent Doublets Versus New Agent or Platinum Agent Alone

Chemotherapy is recommended for all NSCLC patients with good performance status. However, the question as to whether adding a second agent to a single-agent regimen offers a substantial benefit has been debated (22). A meta-analysis by Lilenbaum et al. demonstrated that although doublet chemotherapy increased the objective tumor response rate, it resulted in greater toxicity compared with single-agent therapy and the benefit in terms of OS was found to be even more controversial (23).

However, more recent RCTs have demonstrated that two-drug combinations are superior to a single-agent treatment in terms of overall response rate, progression-free survival (PFS) (24–28), and in some studies OS (25,27,28), no matter which newer agent is used (cisplatin, carboplatin, paclitaxel, docetaxel, gemcitabine, and vinorelbine).

A published data-based meta-analysis reported by Delbaldo et al. (29) (57 trials with 11,160 patients) demonstrated that the addition of a second drug to a single-agent regimen was associated with a statistically significant increase in the objective tumor response rate (odds ratio [OR], 0.42; 95% CI, 0.37–0.47; $P < .001$), a significant increase in 1-year survival (OR, 0.80; 95% CI, 0.70–0.91; $P < .001$; 5% absolute benefit with an increase of 1-year survival from 30%–35%), as well as in median survival (median ratio, 0.83; 95% CI, 0.79–0.89; $P < .001$). This benefit was smaller in the cases where a single-agent was used a third-generation drug (docetaxel, vinorelbine, gemcitabine, and irinotecan) for both 1-year survival rate ($P = .03$) and median survival ($P = .007$). Toxicity, as expected, was higher with doublet regimens.

TABLE 1 Randomized trials of cisplatin plus a new agent versus cisplatin plus an old agent

Trial	Therapy	Number of Patients	OR (%)	Median Survival (weeks)	*P* Value	1-Year Survival (%)
Le Chevalier (11)	V/P	206	30	40	.04	40
	Vi/P	200	19	32		32
Bonomi (12)	Pa (low)/P[a]	198	25.3	41.2	.048[b]	37.4
	Pa (high)/P	201	27.7	43.3		40.3
	E/P	200	12.4	32.9		32
Giaccone (13)	Pa/P	166	28	42.9	NS	41
	Ten/P	166	41	42.0		43
Gebbia (14)	V/P	122	39	7.0 mo	NS	15.2
	M/Vi/P	125	42	8.0 mo		14.7
Crino (15)	G/P	155	38	9.6 mo	NS	33
	M/I/P	152	26	8.6 mo		34
Cardenal (16)	G/P	68	41	37.7	NS	26
	E/P	67	22	30.3		32
Baldini (17)	Carbo/V	43	14.0	7.9 mo	NS	NR
	M/Vi/P	49	14.3	8.4 mo		
	P/I/V	48	16.7	8.8 mo		
Negoro (18)	CPT/P	129	44	50	NS[c]	46
	Vi/P	122	32	46		38
Kubota (19)	D/P	151	37	49.3	NS	48
	Vi/P	151	21	41.9		43
Belani (20)	Carbo/Pa	190	23	7.7 mo	NS	32
	P/E	179	15	9.0 mo		37

[a]Paclitaxel (low) = 135 mg/m^2 intravenously over 24 hours; Paclitaxel (high) = 175 mg/m^2 intravenously over 24 hours plus granulocyte colony-stimulating factor.
[b]Comparing the two paclitaxel groups combined with the etoposide/cisplatin group; other comparisons were not significant.
[c]Survival differences were significant in the Stage IV subset.
P = cisplatin; Vin = vindesine; E = etoposide; V = vinorelbine; Carbo = carboplatin; Pa = paclitaxel; Ten = teniposide; G = gemcitabine; D = docetaxel; Vi = vindesine; CPT = irinotecan; M = mitomycin; I = ifosfamide; NS = nonsignificant; NR = not reported; mo = months.

Triplets Versus Doublets

Given that doublets were associated with better clinical outcome compared to single-agent treatment, a logical question was if triplets could result to even better outcome. Several randomized trials evaluated the potential role of three drug combinations to improve survival outcomes in NSCLC (Table 2) (15,30–36). Although three-drug combinations led to significantly higher response rates, in general, they failed to demonstrate any benefit in terms of time to tumor progression and OS, while they were associated with significantly higher toxicity.

Two meta-analyses further evaluated this issue (29,37). Both analyses were consistent in demonstrating that adding a third drug improves response rate but does not significantly improve OS, while it is associated with higher toxicity. On the basis of these data, the American Society of Clinical Oncology (ASCO) recommends against the use of three cytotoxic drug combinations in the treatment of NSCLC (6).

TABLE 2 Randomized trials comparing triplets versus doublets for the treatment of advanced NSCLC

Author	Regimen	Number of Patients	ORR (%)	Median Survival (months)	*P* Value
Alberola (30)	P/G	370	42	9.3	NS
	P/G/V		41	8.2	
Laack (31)	G/V	287	13	8.3	NS
	G/V/P		28	7.5	
Crino (15)	P/G	307	38	8.6	NS
	M/I/P		26	9.6	
Comella (33)	P/V	180	25	8.1	0.04[a]
	P/G		30	9.7	NS[b]
	P/G/V		47	11.8	
Danson (32)	Ca/G	372	30	8.5	NS
	M/I/P		33	8.7	
	M/Vin/P				
Comella (36)	G/V	433	35	10.5	NS
	G/Pa		48	10.8	
	P/G/V				
	P/G/Pa				
Paccagnella (35)	P/Pa	324	20.2	8.3	0.032
	P/Pa/G		43.6	10.8	
Comella (34)	P/G	343	28	38 weeks	< .05 for both
	P/G/Pa		48	51 weeks	
	P/G/V		44	51 weeks	

P = cisplatin; G = gemcitabine; V = vinorelbine; M = mitomycin; I = ifosfamide; Ca = carboplatin; Vin = vinblastine; Pa = paclitaxel.

[a]versus triplet
[b]versus triplet

TABLE 3 Selected Phase III trials comparing third-generation platinum-based doublets

Trial	Number of Patients	Regimen	Median Survival (months)	*P* Value
ECOG 1594 (38)	1207	P/Pa vs. P/G vs. P/D vs. Carbo/Pa	7.8 vs. 8.1 vs. 7.4 vs. 8.1	NS
TAX 326 (90)	1218	P/V vs. P/D vs. Carbo/D	10.1 vs. 11.3 vs. 9.4	0.04[a] NS[b]
Scagliotti et al. (39)	1725	P/G vs. P/Pem	10.3 vs. 10.3	NS

P = cisplatin; V = vinorelbine; Carbo = carboplatin; Pa =paclitaxel; G = gemcitabine; D = docetaxel; Pem = pemetrexed; NS = nonsignificant; NR = not reported.
[a]P/V vs. P/T $p = .04$ in favor of P/T.
[b]P/V vs. Carbo/T p = NS.

Is There a More Effective Doublet of a Platinum Agent Plus a New Agent?

Numerous Phase III trials have directly compared several platinum/new agent doublets and failed to demonstrate a particular combination to be clearly superior for NSCLC. Most illustrative, appropriately sized trials comparing second-generation platinum-based doublets are presented in Table 3.

The Eastern Cooperative Oncology Group (ECOG) 1594 study was a large randomized trial that assigned 1207 patients with advanced NSCLC to a reference regimen of cisplatin and paclitaxel or to one of three experimental regimens: cisplatin and gemcitabine, cisplatin and docetaxel, or carboplatin and paclitaxel (38). ECOG performance status (0 or 1 vs. 2), weight loss in the previous 6 months (<5% vs. ≥5%), the stage of disease (IIIB vs. IV or recurrent disease), and the presence or absence of brain metastases were used as stratification factors. This trial failed to demonstrate any significant OS difference between the different chemotherapy regimens; median OS ranged from 7.4 to 8.1 months. The cisplatin/gemcitabine arm was associated with a significant time to tumor progression prolongation when compared with the reference arm (4.2 vs. 3.4 months, P = .001). Cisplatin/gemcitabine doublet was associated with more thrombocytopenia, cisplatin/docetaxel caused more neutropenia, and the carboplatin/paclitaxel arm caused the lowest rate of potentially life-threatening adverse events.

An interesting Phase III trial reported by Scagliotti et al. (39) was the first that demonstrated a significant interaction between treatment efficacy and tumor histology. This noninferiority, Phase III trial randomized 1,725 chemotherapy-naive patients with Stage IIIB/IV NSCLC to cisplatin/gemcitabine or cisplatin/pemetrexed. OS for cisplatin/pemetrexed was noninferior to cisplatin/gemcitabine (median survival, 10.3 vs. 10.3 months, respectively; HR = 0.94; 95% CI, 0.84–1.05) in the whole cohort of patients. However, OS was statistically superior for cisplatin/pemetrexed versus cisplatin/gemcitabine in patients with adenocarcinoma (n = 847; 12.6 vs. 10.9 months, respectively) and large-cell carcinoma histology (n = 153; 10.4 vs. 6.7 months, respectively), while in patients with squamous cell histology, there was a significant improvement in survival with cisplatin/gemcitabine versus cisplatin/pemetrexed (n = 473; 10.8 vs. 9.4 months, respectively).

A meta-analysis reported by Grossi et al. was designed to evaluate the relative impact of different third-generation agents by using both response and progressive disease rates as outcome measures (40). This analysis included 45 trials (n = 11867) comparing several third-generation agents (gemcitabine, paclitaxel, docetaxel, and vinorelbine) containing doublets with third-generation-agent-free doublets. Overall response rate was similar across different regimens, with no significant heterogeneity observed between studies. On the other hand, data about progressive disease were different with gemcitabine-containing chemotherapy resulting in a 14% lower risk for immediate progression (OR, 0.86, 95% CI, 0.77–0.95; P = .005). Treatment with docetaxel was associated with 9% lower risk for progressive disease, but this difference failed to reach statistical significance (OR, 0.91; 95% CI, 0.80–1.04; P = .16). Patients receiving paclitaxel showed a 22% higher risk for having progressive disease as the best response (OR, 1.22; 95% CI, 1.09–1.37; P = .0008), while no difference in the risk of progression was observed between vinorelbine-containing and vinorelbine-free regimens.

Platinum-Based Versus Platinum Free Doublets

Platinum-based chemotherapy is associated with considerable toxicity and for that reason a platinum-free approach was evaluated in Phase III trials (Table 4) as a less toxic alternative (30,31,36,41–51). These trials in general failed to demonstrate a significant difference in favor of the platinum in terms of OS, although platinum-based treatment was in general associated with higher response rates. In three trials, a trend toward better OS was observed in patients treated with platinum-based combinations (43–45). On the other hand, another study

TABLE 4 Platinum-based versus platinum-free regimens in first-line treatment of NSCLC

Author	Regimen	Number of Patients	Median PFS (months)	Median OS (months)	*P* Value	1-Year Survival (%)
Georgoulias (41)	D/P	441	9.5	10		NR
	D/G		8	9.5	NS	
Kosmidis (42)	Pa/C	502	6.3	10.4	.32	41.7
	Pa/G		6.1	9.8		41.4
Gridelli (43)	G/V	501	17 weeks	32 weeks	.08	NR
	G/P		22 weeks	38 weeks		
	P/V		22 weeks	38 weeks		
Smit (44)	G/P	490	5.6	8.9	NS	32.6
	Pa/P		4.4	8.1		35.5
	Pa/G		3.9	6.7		26.5
Alberola (30)	G/P	557	6.3	9.3		38
	G/P/V				NS	
	G/V-V/If		5.7	8.1		34
Laack (31)	GVP	287	19.3	32.4 weeks	NS	27.5
	GV		22.3	35.9 weeks		33.6
Georgoulias (45)	V/P	251	8.5	9.7	0.965	34.3
	D/G		8	9		40.8
Tan (46)	V/P	316	3.9	8.6	0.001	34.4
	V/G		4.4	11.5		48.9
Kubota (47)	C/Ta	401	5.8	14.1	NS	55.5
	VG→D		5.5	13.6		55.6
Treat (48)	G/C	1135	NR	7.9	NS	NR
	G/Pa			8.5		
	Pa/C			8.7		
Comella (36)	P/G (V)	433	6.1	10.7	NS	NR
	G/Pa		5.5	10.5		
Greco (49)	C/Pa/G	337	6	10.3	NS	38
	G/V		3.9	10.7		45
Pujol (50)	P/V	311	4.0	9.6	NS	46
	G/D		4.2	11.1		42
Stathopoulos (51)	C/Pa	360	NR	11.0	NS	42.7
	Pa/V			10.0		37.8

P = cisplatin; V = vinorelbine; G = gemcitabine; D = docetaxel; If = ifosfamide; Pa = paclitaxel; C = carboplatin; Epi = epirubicin; NR = not reported; NS = nonsignificant; ORR = overall response rate; TTP = time to tumor progression; OS = overall survival.

demonstrated that the combination of vinorelbine and gemcitabine was superior to vinorelbine plus carboplatin in terms of response rate, progression-free survival, OS, and clinical benefit (46).

Three meta-analyses have tried to further elucidate this issue. The first one by Pujol et al. (52) (11 Phase III studies with 4,602 patients) demonstrated a reduction of borderline significance in the risk of death at 1-year in favor of platinum-based doublets (OR, 0.88; 95% CI, 0.78–0.99; $P = .044$), corresponding to a 2.94% survival benefit at 1 year. The second one by D' Addario et al. (53) (37 trials with 7,633 patients) demonstrated an increase of 5% in 1-year survival rate with platinum-based regimens (34% vs. 29%; OR, 1.21; 95% CI, 1.09–1.35; $P < .0003$). However, no statistically significant increase in 1-year survival was found when platinum therapies were compared to third-generation-based combination regimens (OR, 1.11; 95% CI, 0.96–1.28; P = .17). Finally, in a third meta-analysis reported by Rajeswaran et al. (54) (17 trials with a total of 4,792 patients), the use of a platinum-based regimen resulted in a slightly higher 1-year survival (RR, 1.08; 95% CI, 1.01–1.16, P = .03). All three meta-analyses demonstrated higher response rate and higher toxicity for the platinum-based arm.

On the basis of these meta-analyses, the more recent ASCO guidelines for NSCLC support that platinum-based doublets should be preferred over nonplatinum ones because of their higher response rate and marginal superiority in OS (6).

Cisplatin Versus Carboplatin

In an attempt to circumvent cisplatin-induced toxicities, carboplatin—another platinum analog—was developed for clinical use (55). Several randomized Phase III trials have evaluated carboplatin-based regimens and found them to be feasible and active as first-line NSCLC treatment (56–58) but concerns still exist about whether carboplatin has equivalent efficacy to cisplatin or not (59).

Three meta-analyses have tried to answer this question. A meta-analysis based on abstracted data (eight trials, n = 2,948) comparing cisplatin versus carboplatin was reported by Hotta et al. (60). Cisplatin-based chemotherapy produced a higher response rate, but the survival advantage was not significant (HR, 1.050; 95% CI, 0.907–1.216; P = .515). Subgroup analysis revealed that combination chemotherapy consisting of cisplatin plus a new agent yields 11% longer survival than carboplatin plus the same new agent (HR, 1.106; 95% CI, 1.005–1.218; P = .039). A second meta-analysis was published by Ardizzoni et al. (61). This was an individual patient data meta-analysis (nine trials with 2,968 patients). Cisplatin-treated patients had a median survival of 9.1 months and a 1-year survival probability of 37%, while for carboplatin-treated patients, the median survival was 8.4 months and the 1-year survival probability of 34%. Carboplatin was associated with a higher risk of death although the difference was not statistically significant (HR, 1.07, 95% CI, 0.99–1.15, P = .100). However, this difference was significant in favor of cisplatin in patients treated with third-generation regimens (HR, 1.11; 95% CI, 1.01–1.21). Statistically, significant heterogeneity between trials was observed. Finally, a third meta-analysis was reported by Jiang et al. (62) (18 trials, n = 6,906 patients). This analysis demonstrated a comparable 1-year survival rate for cisplatin and carboplatin-based regimens (RR, 1.00, 95% CI, 0.94–1.07; P = .93). All three meta-analyses also demonstrated a higher response rate in favor of cisplatin containing regimens.

■ TARGETED AGENTS IN FIRST-LINE TREATMENT OF NSCLC

Bevacizumab

Angiogenesis is the formation of new blood vessels and is considered as a crucial process for the development of solid tumors and to the growth of secondary metastatic lesions (63). Vascular endothelial growth factor (VEGF) acts to promote normal and tumor angiogenesis (64). Bevacizumab is a recombinant, humanized, monoclonal antibody against VEGF (65). Bevacizumab when added to chemotherapy doublets in the context of first-line treatment offers a clinical benefit in terms of PFS (Avastin in Lung [AVAiL] study and ECOG 4599 study) (66,67) or OS (ECOG 4599) (67). AVAiL trial failed to demonstrate an OS benefit but it should be noted that its primary endpoint was PFS, and the study was not powered to demonstrate an OS difference. In these trials, bevacizumab was continued until disease progression. The optimal dose of bevacizumab was not determined because ECOG 4599 trial (67) used a dose of 15mg/kg while the European AVAiL trial (66) yielded positive results for both doses tested (7.5mg/kg and 15mg/kg). Exclusion criteria of both trials included squamous histology, history of hemoptysis (greater than one-half teaspoon of bright red blood per event), CNS metastases, history of thrombotic or hemorrhagic disorders, therapeutic anticoagulation, patients with tumors invading or abutting major blood vessels, clinically significant cardiovascular disease, or medically uncontrolled hypertension due to significant risk of hemorrhage. Thus, bevacizumab should be used only in selected patients with NSCLC.

Epidermal Growth Factor Receptor

Cetuximab

Epidermal growth factor receptor (EGFR) is a transmembrane receptor, which is highly expressed in NSCLC (68). EGFR is activated upon binding of ligands (epidermal growth factor, tumor growth factor-α, beta-cellulin, epiregulin, and amphiregulin) and then initiates an intracellular signal transduction cascade that affects cell proliferation, motility, and survival (68).

Cetuximab is a monoclonal antibody against the extracellular part of EGFR. Cetuximab in combination with chemotherapy has been evaluated in the context of Phase III trials as first-line treatment of NSCLC (69,70). A trial by Pirker et al. (69) (FLEX trial) evaluated cisplatin/vinorelbine doublet plus or minus cetuximab in 1,125 chemo-naive NSCLC patients with EGFR immunohistochemistry positive tumors. Cetuximab arm resulted in a statistically significant although moderate OS prolongation (11.3 vs. 10.1 months; $P = .044$) (69). A second smaller Phase III trial (BMS099 study) of taxane/carboplatin with cetuximab also failed to show any improvement in the study's primary endpoint, that is, PFS (70). On the basis of these results, cetuximab was not registered by EMEA for first-line treatment and further studies are needed to elucidate its role in the treatment of NSCLC.

EGFR Tyrosine Kinase Inhibitors

Erlotinib and gefitinib are orally administered, which are inhibitors of the tyrosine kinase domain of the intracellular part of EGFR (47). Mutations of the tyrosine kinase coding domain (exons 18–21) of the *EGFR* gene have been identified as the strongest predictive factor for clinical benefit for treatment with EGFR tyrosine kinase inhibitors (71).

The effects of single agent gefitinib versus chemotherapy as first-line treatment of NSCLC have been tested in the context of three Phase III studies (72–74). The trial by Mok et al. (72) (IPASS trial) enrolled clinically selected patients (Asian ethnicity only, with adenocarcinoma histology, and never or light ex-smokers [<100 cigarettes lifetime]), while the other two enrolled patients selected on the basis of the *EGFR* mutation status of their tumor (73,74). All these trials demonstrated a provocative PFS (primary endpoint in all three trials) benefit in favor of gefitinib over chemotherapy in patients bearing tumors with EGFR mutations. Furthermore, gefitinib was associated with a more favorable toxicity profile in all trials. Similarly, two Phase III trials evaluated erlotinib versus chemotherapy in the first-line treatment of NSCLC in patients with EGFR mutated tumors (75,76) and demonstrated a striking PFS difference in favor of erlotinib. These data support the use of EGFR tyrosine kinase inhibitors as first-line treatment for NSCLC patients with activating *EGFR* mutations.

■ PATIENT POPULATIONS WITH SPECIAL CONSIDERATIONS

Elderly Patients

Due to the aging of the Western world population, there is significant increase in the number of older patients diagnosed with NSCLC. Approximately 50% of NSCLC incidence occurs in patients older than 65 years, while 30% to 40% of cases are diagnosed in patients older than 70 years; therefore, the median age at diagnosis in NSCLC patients is 69 years (77). Despite this high part of disease burden in older patients, these patients are generally underrepresented in clinical trials due to considerations for increased toxicity (78) although the chemotherapy efficacy in the elderly is similar to that in younger patients and age has not been established as a negative prognostic factor for survival (79).

A number of prospective, randomized Phase III trials have evaluated the role of chemotherapy in the elderly NSCLC patients (80–84) (Table 5). Although published trials have clearly demonstrated that single-agent chemotherapy offers a survival benefit versus BSC in older NSCLC patients (80), the role of platinum-free chemotherapy doublets is controversial (81,83). The South Italian Cooperative Oncology Group (SICOG) reported a significant OS prolongation in favor of the vinorelbine/gemcitabine doublet compared to single-agent vinorelbine (81). However, a much bigger Phase III trial, the multicenter Italian lung cancer in the elderly Phase III trial (MILES) failed to yield any benefit in terms of OS or time to tumor progression in favor of vinorelbine/gemcitabine doublet compared with either single agent (83). The conflicting results between the SICOG (81) and MILES (83) trials could be due to differences regarding patient sample. However, it should be noted that the SICOG trial reported a very poor median survival of 18 weeks for patients treated with single-agent vinorelbine, unusually lower than the 28 weeks median survival reported for vinorelbine monotherapy in Phase III trials for elderly population (80,83) and is similar to that reported for BSC in the ELVIS trial (80).

Conflicting results also exist regarding the role of platinum-based doublets in the treatment of elderly NSCLC patients. A recently

TABLE 5 Elderly-specific, prospective randomized Phase III trials

Trial	Number of Patients	PFS (weeks)	*P* Value	OS (weeks)	*P* Value	1-Year OS
ELVIS (80)						
VNB	78			28		32%
BSC	76			21	.03	14%
SICOG (81)						
VNB	60			18		13%
VNB/GMB	60			29		30%
WJTOG 99004 (82)						
VNB	92	3.1 mo		9.9 mo		36.7%
D	90	5.5 mo	< .001	14.3 mo	.138	58.6%
MILES (83)						
VNB	233	18		36	.93[a]	38%
GMB	233	17		28	.65[a]	28%
VNB/GMB	232	19		30		30%
IFCT-0501 (84)						
Single agent (VNB or GMB)	226	3.0 mo		6.2 mo		
wPa/mCarbo	225	6.1 mo	$< 10^{-6}$	10.3 mo	.00004	
JCOG0803/WJOG4307 (85)						
D	137	4.4 mo	.37	14.8 mo	.824	58.2%
D/C	139	4.7 mo		13.3 mo		54.5%

BSC = best supportive care; VNB = vinorelbine; D = docetaxel; GMB = gemcitabine; mCarbo = monthly carboplatin; wPa = weekly paclitaxel; C = cisplatin; ELVIS = Elderly Lung Cancer Vinorelbine Italian Study; SICOG = Southern Italy Cooperative Oncology Group; WJTOG = West Japan Thoracic Oncology Group; MILES = Multicenter Italian Lung Cancer in the Elderly Study; IFCT = Intergroupe Francophone de Cancerologie Thoracique; JCOG = Japan Clinical Oncology Group.

[a]Versus combination treatment.

published Phase III trial reported by Quoix et al. (84) with 451 elderly patients compared a combination regimen of monthly carboplatin with weekly paclitaxel versus single-agent treatment with either vinorelbine or gemcitabine. This trial demonstrated a significant PFS and OS benefit in favor of the combination regimen (84). On the contrary, a Phase III trial reported by a Japanese group comparing a combination regimen of weekly docetaxel plus weekly cisplatin versus single-agent docetaxel (every 3 weeks) failed to demonstrate any benefit for the combination regimen (85).

■ SECOND-LINE TREATMENT

Docetaxel has received approval as second-line treatment on the basis of the results of a randomized Phase III trial that demonstrated a time to tumor progression and an OS prolongation over placebo (86). This study established single-agent docetaxel as the standard second-line treatment and as standard comparator arm for subsequent randomized trials. A more recent, noninferiority Phase III study compared docetaxel with pemetrexed as second-line therapy in NSCLC (87). No significant difference was observed in OS or 1-year survival, while pemetrexed was associated with a more favorable toxicity profile. This trial led to the approval of pemetrexed in the second-line treatment of NSCLC. Erlotinib has received approval by health authorities as second-line treatment of patients with locally advanced or metastatic NSCLC after failure of at least one prior chemotherapy regimen on the basis of the results of BR.21 trial, a Phase III trial by the National Cancer Institute of Canada (88). Patients treated with erlotinib experienced significantly longer PFS and OS over placebo. Gefitinib was compared to docetaxel in the context of a Phase III, noninferiority trial (89) (INTEREST trial). This trial met its primary endpoint of confirming noninferiority of gefitinib compared with docetaxel for OS. Thus, docetaxel, erlotinib, gefitinib, or pemetrexed could be considered as "standard" choices for second-line therapy.

■ REFERENCES

1. Carney DN, Hansen HH. Non-small-cell lung cancer—stalemate or progress? *New Engl J Med.* 2000;343:1261–1262.
2. Laskin JJ, Sandler AB. State of the art in therapy for non-small cell lung cancer. *Cancer Invest.* 2005;23:427–442.
3. Souquet PJ, Chauvin F, Boissel JP, et al. Meta-analysis of randomised trials of systemic chemotherapy versus supportive treatment in non-resectable non-small cell lung cancer. *Lung Canc.* 1995;12(Suppl. 1):S147-S154.
4. Chemotherapy in non-small cell lung cancer: A meta-analysis using updated data on individual patients from 52 randomised clinical trials. Non-small Cell Lung Cancer Collaborative Group. *BMJ.* 1995;311:899–909.
5. Chemotherapy in addition to supportive care improves survival in advanced non-small-cell lung cancer: A systematic review and meta-analysis of individual patient data from 16 randomized controlled trials. *J Clin Oncol.* 2008;26: 4617–4625.
6. Azzoli CG, Baker S, Jr., Temin S, et al. American Society of Clinical Oncology Clinical Practice Guideline update on chemotherapy for stage IV non-small-cell lung cancer. *J Clin Oncol.* 2009;27: 6251–6266.
7. Kris MG, Gralla RJ, Kalman LA, et al. Randomized trial comparing vindesine plus cisplatin with vinblastine plus cisplatin in patients with non-small cell lung cancer, with an analysis of methods of response assessment. *Canc Treat Rep.* 1985;69:387–395.
8. Ruckdeschel JC, Finkelstein DM, Ettinger DS, et al. A randomized trial of the four most active regimens for metastatic non-small-cell lung cancer. *J Clin Oncol.* 1986;4:14–22.
9. Bonomi PD, Finkelstein DM, Ruckdeschel JC, et al. Combination chemotherapy versus single agents followed by combination chemotherapy in stage IV non-small-cell lung cancer: A study of

the Eastern Cooperative Oncology Group. *J Clin Oncol.* 1989;7:1602–1613.

10. Weick JK, Crowley J, Natale RB, et al. A randomized trial of five cisplatin-containing treatments in patients with metastatic non-small-cell lung cancer: A Southwest Oncology Group study. *J Clin Oncol.* 1991;9:1157–1162.
11. Le Chevalier T, Brisgand D, Douillard JY, et al. Randomized study of vinorelbine and cisplatin versus vindesine and cisplatin versus vinorelbine alone in advanced non-small-cell lung cancer: Results of a European multicenter trial including 612 patients. *J Clin Oncol.* 1994;12:360–367.
12. Bonomi P, Kim K, Fairclough D, et al. Comparison of survival and quality of life in advanced non-small-cell lung cancer patients treated with two dose levels of paclitaxel combined with cisplatin versus etoposide with cisplatin: Results of an Eastern Cooperative Oncology Group trial. *J Clin Oncol.* 2000;18:623–631.
13. Giaccone G, Splinter TA, Debruyne C, et al. Randomized study of paclitaxel-cisplatin versus cisplatin-teniposide in patients with advanced non-small-cell lung cancer. The European Organization for Research and Treatment of Cancer Lung Cancer Cooperative Group. *J Clin Oncol.* 1998;16:2133–2141.
14. Gebbia V, Galetta D, Riccardi F, et al. Vinorelbine plus cisplatin versus cisplatin plus vindesine and mitomycin C in stage IIIB-IV non-small cell lung carcinoma: A prospective randomized study. *Lung Canc.* 2002;37:179–187.
15. Crino L, Scagliotti GV, Ricci S, et al. Gemcitabine and cisplatin versus mitomycin, ifosfamide, and cisplatin in advanced non-small-cell lung cancer: A randomized phase III study of the Italian lung cancer project. *J Clin Oncol.* 1999;17:3522–3530.
16. Cardenal F, Lopez-Cabrerizo MP, Anton A, et al. Randomized phase III study of gemcitabine-cisplatin versus etoposide-cisplatin in the treatment of locally advanced or metastatic non-small-cell lung cancer. *J Clin Oncol.* 1999;17:12–18.
17. Baldini E, Tibaldi C, Ardizzoni A, et al. Cisplatin-vindesine-mitomycin (MVP) vs cisplatin-ifosfamide-vinorelbine (PIN) vs carboplatin-vinorelbine (CaN) in patients with advanced non-small-cell lung cancer (NSCLC): A FONICAP randomized phase II study. Italian Lung Cancer Task Force (FONICAP). *Br J Canc.* 1998;77:2367–2370.
18. Negoro S, Masuda N, Takada Y, et al. Randomised phase III trial of irinotecan combined with cisplatin for advanced non-small-cell lung cancer. *Br.J Canc.* 2003;88:335–341.
19. Kubota K, Watanabe K, Kunitoh H, et al. Phase III randomized trial of docetaxel plus cisplatin versus vindesine plus cisplatin in patients with stage IV non-small-cell lung cancer: The Japanese Taxotere Lung Cancer Study Group. *J Clin Oncol.* 2004;22:254–261.
20. Belani CP, Lee JS, Socinski MA, et al. Randomized phase III trial comparing cisplatin-etoposide to carboplatin-paclitaxel in advanced or metastatic non-small cell lung cancer. *Ann Oncol.* 2005;16: 1069–1075.
21. Baggstrom MQ, Stinchcombe TE, Fried DB, et al. Third-generation chemotherapy agents in the treatment of advanced non-small cell lung cancer: A meta-analysis. *J Thorac Oncol.* 2007;2:845–853.
22. Bunn PA, Jr. Treatment of advanced non-small-cell lung cancer with two-drug combinations. *J Clin Oncol.* 2002;20:3565–3567.
23. Lilenbaum RC, Langenberg P, Dickersin K. Single agent versus combination chemotherapy in patients with advanced nonsmall cell lung carcinoma: A meta-analysis of response, toxicity, and survival. *Cancer.* 1998;82:116–126.
24. Lilenbaum RC, Herndon JE, List MA, et al. Single-agent versus combination chemotherapy in advanced non-small-cell lung cancer: The cancer and leukemia group B (study 9730). *J Clin Oncol.* 2005;23:190–196.
25. Sederholm C, Hillerdal G, Lamberg K, et al. Phase III trial of gemcitabine plus carboplatin versus single-agent gemcitabine in the treatment of locally advanced or metastatic non-small-cell lung cancer: The Swedish Lung Cancer Study Group. *J Clin Oncol.* 2005;23:8380–8388.
26. Georgoulias V, Ardavanis A, Agelidou A, et al. Docetaxel versus docetaxel plus cisplatin as front-line treatment of patients with advanced non-small-cell lung cancer: A randomized, multicenter phase III trial. *J Clin Oncol.* 2004;22:2602–2609.
27. Sandler AB, Nemunaitis J, Denham C, et al. Phase III trial of gemcitabine plus cisplatin versus

cisplatin alone in patients with locally advanced or metastatic non-small-cell lung cancer. *J Clin Oncol.* 2000;18:122–130.

28. Wozniak AJ, Crowley JJ, Balcerzak SP, et al. Randomized trial comparing cisplatin with cisplatin plus vinorelbine in the treatment of advanced non-small-cell lung cancer: A Southwest Oncology Group study. *J Clin Oncol.* 1998;16:2459–2465.
29. Delbaldo C, Michiels S, Syz N, et al. Benefits of adding a drug to a single-agent or a 2-agent chemotherapy regimen in advanced non-small-cell lung cancer: a meta-analysis. *JAMA.* 2004;292: 470–484.
30. Alberola V, Camps C, Provencio M, et al. Cisplatin plus gemcitabine versus a cisplatin-based triplet versus nonplatinum sequential doublets in advanced non-small-cell lung cancer: A Spanish Lung Cancer Group phase III randomized trial. *J Clin Oncol.* 2003;21:3207–3213.
31. Laack E, Dickgreber N, Muller T, et al. Randomized phase III study of gemcitabine and vinorelbine versus gemcitabine, vinorelbine, and cisplatin in the treatment of advanced non-small-cell lung cancer: From the German and Swiss Lung Cancer Study Group. *J Clin Oncol.* 2004;22:2348–2356.
32. Danson S, Middleton MR, O'Byrne KJ, et al. Phase III trial of gemcitabine and carboplatin versus mitomycin, ifosfamide, and cisplatin or mitomycin, vinblastine, and cisplatin in patients with advanced nonsmall cell lung carcinoma. *Cancer.* 2003;98:542–553.
33. Comella P, Frasci G, Panza N, et al. Randomized trial comparing cisplatin, gemcitabine, and vinorelbine with either cisplatin and gemcitabine or cisplatin and vinorelbine in advanced non-small-cell lung cancer: Interim analysis of a phase III trial of the Southern Italy Cooperative Oncology Group. *J Clin Oncol.* 2000;18:1451–1457.
34. Comella P. Phase III trial of cisplatin/gemcitabine with or without vinorelbine or paclitaxel in advanced non-small cell lung cancer. *Semin.Oncol.* 2001;28:7–10.
35. Paccagnella A, Oniga F, Bearz A, et al. Adding gemcitabine to paclitaxel/carboplatin combination increases survival in advanced non-small-cell lung cancer: Results of a phase II-III study. *J Clin Oncol.* 2006;24:681–687.
36. Comella P, Filippelli G, De CG, et al. Efficacy of the combination of cisplatin with either gemcitabine and vinorelbine or gemcitabine and paclitaxel in the treatment of locally advanced or metastatic non-small-cell lung cancer: A phase III randomised trial of the Southern Italy Cooperative Oncology Group (SICOG 0101). *Ann Oncol.* 2007;18:324–330.
37. Azim HA, Jr., Elattar I, Loberiza FR, Jr., et al. Third generation triplet cytotoxic chemotherapy in advanced non-small cell lung cancer: A systematic overview. *Lung Canc.* 2009;64:194–198.
38. Schiller JH, Harrington D, Belani CP, et al. Comparison of four chemotherapy regimens for advanced non-small-cell lung cancer. *N Engl J Med.* 2002;346:92–98.
39. Scagliotti GV, Parikh P, von PJ, et al. Phase III study comparing cisplatin plus gemcitabine with cisplatin plus pemetrexed in chemotherapy-naive patients with advanced-stage non-small-cell lung cancer. *J Clin Oncol.* 2008;26:3543–3551.
40. Grossi F, Aita M, Defferrari C, et al. Impact of third-generation drugs on the activity of first-line chemotherapy in advanced non-small cell lung cancer: A meta-analytical approach. *Oncologist.* 2009;14:497–510.
41. Georgoulias V, Papadakis E, Alexopoulos A, et al. Platinum-based and non-platinum-based chemotherapy in advanced non-small-cell lung cancer: A randomised multicentre trial. *Lancet.* 2001;357:1478–1484.
42. Kosmidis P, Mylonakis N, Nicolaides C, et al. Paclitaxel plus carboplatin versus gemcitabine plus paclitaxel in advanced non-small-cell lung cancer: A phase III randomized trial. *J Clin Oncol.* 2002;20:3578–3585.
43. Gridelli C, Gallo C, Shepherd FA, et al. Gemcitabine plus vinorelbine compared with cisplatin plus vinorelbine or cisplatin plus gemcitabine for advanced non-small-cell lung cancer: A phase III trial of the Italian GEMVIN Investigators and the National Cancer Institute of Canada Clinical Trials Group. *J Clin Oncol.* 2003;21:3025–3034.
44. Smit EF, van Meerbeeck JP, Lianes P, et al. Three-arm randomized study of two cisplatin-based regimens and paclitaxel plus gemcitabine in advanced non-small-cell lung cancer: A phase III trial of the

European Organization for Research and Treatment of Cancer Lung Cancer Group—EORTC 08975. *J Clin Oncol.* 2003;21:3909–3917.

45. Georgoulias V, Ardavanis A, Tsiafaki X, et al. Vinorelbine plus cisplatin versus docetaxel plus gemcitabine in advanced non-small-cell lung cancer: A phase III randomized trial. *J Clin Oncol.* 2005;23:2937–2945.
46. Tan EH, Szczesna A, Krzakowski M, et al. Randomized study of vinorelbine–gemcitabine versus vinorelbine–carboplatin in patients with advanced non-small cell lung cancer. *Lung Canc.* 2005;49:233–240.
47. Kubota K, Kawahara M, Ogawara M, et al. Vinorelbine plus gemcitabine followed by docetaxel versus carboplatin plus paclitaxel in patients with advanced non-small-cell lung cancer: A randomised, open-label, phase III study. *Lancet Oncol.* 2008;9:1135–1142.
48. Treat JA, Gonin R, Socinski MA, et al. A randomized, phase III multicenter trial of gemcitabine in combination with carboplatin or paclitaxel versus paclitaxel plus carboplatin in patients with advanced or metastatic non-small-cell lung cancer. *Ann Oncol.* 2010;21:540–547.
49. Greco FA, Spigel DR, Kuzur ME, et al. Paclitaxel/Carboplatin/gemcitabine versus gemcitabine/vinorelbine in advanced non-small-cell lung cancer: A phase II/III study of the Minnie Pearl Cancer Research Network. *Clin Lung Canc.* 2007;8:483–487.
50. Pujol JL, Breton JL, Gervais R, et al. Gemcitabine-docetaxel versus cisplatin-vinorelbine in advanced or metastatic non-small-cell lung cancer: A phase III study addressing the case for cisplatin. *Ann Oncol.* 2005;16:602–610.
51. Stathopoulos GP, Veslemes M, Georgatou N, et al. Front-line paclitaxel-vinorelbine versus paclitaxel-carboplatin in patients with advanced non-small-cell lung cancer: A randomized phase III trial. *Ann Oncol.* 2004;15:1048–1055.
52. Pujol JL, Carestia L, Daures JP. Is there a case for cisplatin in the treatment of small-cell lung cancer? A meta-analysis of randomized trials of a cisplatin-containing regimen versus a regimen without this alkylating agent. *Br J Cancer.* 2000;83:8–15.
53. D'Addario G, Pintilie M, Leighl NB, et al. Platinum-based versus non-platinum-based chemotherapy in advanced non-small-cell lung cancer: A meta-analysis of the published literature. *J Clin Oncol.* 2005;23:2926–2936.
54. Rajeswaran A, Trojan A, Burnand B, et al. Efficacy and side effects of cisplatin- and carboplatin-based doublet chemotherapeutic regimens versus non-platinum-based doublet chemotherapeutic regimens as first line treatment of metastatic non-small cell lung carcinoma: A systematic review of randomized controlled trials. *Lung Canc.* 2008;59:1–11.
55. Muggia FM. Overview of carboplatin: Replacing, complementing, and extending the therapeutic horizons of cisplatin. *Semin Oncol.* 1989;16:7–13.
56. Zatloukal P, Petruzelka L, Zemanova M, et al. Gemcitabine plus cisplatin vs. gemcitabine plus carboplatin in stage IIIb and IV non-small cell lung cancer: A phase III randomized trial. *Lung Canc.* 2003;41:321–331.
57. Jelic S, Mitrovic L, Radosavljevic D, et al. Survival advantage for carboplatin substituting cisplatin in combination with vindesine and mitomycin C for stage IIIB and IV squamous-cell bronchogenic carcinoma: A randomized phase III study. *Lung Canc.* 2001;34:1–13.
58. Kelly K, Crowley J, Bunn PA, Jr., et al. Randomized phase III trial of paclitaxel plus carboplatin versus vinorelbine plus cisplatin in the treatment of patients with advanced non-small-cell lung cancer: A Southwest Oncology Group trial. *J Clin Oncol.* 2001;19:3210–3218.
59. Rosell R, Gatzemeier U, Betticher DC, et al. Phase III randomised trial comparing paclitaxel/carboplatin with paclitaxel/cisplatin in patients with advanced non-small-cell lung cancer: A cooperative multinational trial. *Ann Oncol.* 2002;13:1539–1549.
60. Hotta K, Matsuo K, Ueoka H, et al. Meta-analysis of randomized clinical trials comparing cisplatin to carboplatin in patients with advanced non-small-cell lung cancer. *J Clin Oncol.* 2004;22:3852–3859.
61. Ardizzoni A, Boni L, Tiseo M, et al. Cisplatin-versus carboplatin-based chemotherapy in first-line treatment of advanced non-small-cell lung

cancer: An individual patient data meta-analysis. *JNCI Cancer Spectrum.* 2007;99:847–857.

62. Jiang J, Liang X, Zhou X, et al. A meta-analysis of randomized controlled trials comparing carboplatin-based to cisplatin-based chemotherapy in advanced non-small cell lung cancer. *Lung Canc.* 2007;57:348–358.
63. Folkman J. Role of angiogenesis in tumor growth and metastasis. *Semin Oncol.* 2002;29:15–18.
64. Poon RT, Fan ST, Wong J: Clinical implications of circulating angiogenic factors in cancer patients. *J Clin Oncol.* 2001;19:1207–1225.
65. Pallis AG, Serfass L, Dziadziusko R, et al. Targeted therapies in the treatment of advanced/metastatic NSCLC. *Eur J Cancer.* 2009;45:2473–2487.
66. Reck M, von PJ, Zatloukal P, et al. Phase III trial of cisplatin plus gemcitabine with either placebo or bevacizumab as first-line therapy for nonsquamous non-small-cell lung cancer: AVAil. *J Clin Oncol.* 2009;27:1227–1234.
67. Sandler A, Gray R, Perry MC, et al. Paclitaxel-carboplatin alone or with bevacizumab for non-small-cell lung cancer. *N Engl J Med.* 2006;355: 2542–2550.
68. Ciardiello F, Tortora G. EGFR antagonists in cancer treatment. *N Engl J Med.* 2008;358:1160–1174.
69. Pirker R, Pereira JR, Szczesna A, et al. Cetuximab plus chemotherapy in patients with advanced non-small-cell lung cancer (FLEX): An open-label randomised phase III trial. *Lancet.* 2009;373: 1525–1531.
70. Lynch TJ, Patel T, Dreisbach L, et al. Cetuximab and first-line taxane/carboplatin chemotherapy in advanced non-small-cell lung cancer: Results of the randomized multicenter phase III trial BMS099. *J Clin Oncol.* 2010;28:911–917.
71. Pallis AG, Fennell DA, Szutowicz E, et al. Biomarkers of clinical benefit for anti-epidermal growth factor receptor agents in patients with non-small-cell lung cancer. *Br J Canc.* 2011;105:1–8.
72. Mok TS, Wu YL, Thongprasert S, et al. Gefitinib or carboplatin-paclitaxel in pulmonary adenocarcinoma. *N Engl J Med.* 2009;361:947–957.
73. Maemondo M, Inoue A, Kobayashi K, et al. Gefitinib or chemotherapy for non-small-cell lung cancer with mutated EGFR. *N Engl J Med.* 2010;362:2380–2388.
74. Mitsudomi T, Morita S, Yatabe Y, et al. Gefitinib versus cisplatin plus docetaxel in patients with non-small-cell lung cancer harbouring mutations of the epidermal growth factor receptor (WJTOG3405): An open label, randomised phase 3 trial. *Lancet Oncol.* 2010;11:121–128.
75. Zhou C, Wu YL, Chen G, et al. Erlotinib versus chemotherapy as first-line treatment for patients with advanced EGFR mutation-positive non-small-cell lung cancer (OPTIMAL, CTONG-0802): A multicentre, open-label, randomised, phase 3 study. *Lancet Oncol.* 2011;12:735–742.
76. Rossel R, Gervais R, Vergnenegre A, et al. Erlotinib versus chemotherapy (CT) in advanced non-small cell lung cancer (NSCLC) patients (p) with epidermal growth factor receptor (EGFR) mutations: Interim results of the European Erlotinib Versus Chemotherapy (EURTAC) phase III randomized trial. *J Clin Oncol.* 2011;29:abstr A7503.
77. Pallis AG, Gridelli C. Is age a negative prognostic factor for the treatment of advanced/metastatic non-small-cell lung cancer? *Cancer Treat Rev.* 2010;36:436–441.
78. Hutchins LF, Unger JM, Crowley JJ, et al. Underrepresentation of patients 65 years of age or older in cancer-treatment trials. *N Engl J Med.* 1999;341:2061–2067.
79. Pallis AG, Karampeazis A, Vamvakas L, et al. Efficacy and treatment tolerance in older patients with NSCLC: A meta-analysis of five phase III randomized trials conducted by the Hellenic Oncology Research Group. *Ann Oncol.* 2011;22(11):2448–2455.
80. Effects of vinorelbine on quality of life and survival of elderly patients with advanced non-small-cell lung cancer. The Elderly Lung Cancer Vinorelbine Italian Study Group. *JNCI Cancer Spectrum.* 1999;91:66–72.
81. Frasci G, Lorusso V, Panza N, et al. Gemcitabine plus vinorelbine yields better survival outcome than vinorelbine alone in elderly patients with advanced non-small cell lung cancer. A Southern Italy Cooperative Oncology Group (SICOG) phase III trial. *Lung Canc.* 2001;34(Suppl. 4): S65–S69.
82. Kudoh S, Takeda K, Nakagawa K, et al. Phase III study of docetaxel compared with vinorelbine

in elderly patients with advanced non-small-cell lung cancer: Results of the West Japan Thoracic Oncology Group Trial (WJTOG 9904). *J Clin Oncol.* 2006;24:3657–3663.

83. Gridelli C, Perrone F, Gallo C, et al. Chemotherapy for elderly patients with advanced non-small-cell lung cancer: The multicenter Italian lung cancer in the elderly study (MILES) phase III randomized trial. *JNCI Cancer Spectrum.* 2003;95: 362–372.
84. Quoix E, Zalcman G, Oster JP, et al. Carboplatin and weekly paclitaxel doublet chemotherapy compared with monotherapy in elderly patients with advanced non-small-cell lung cancer: IFCT-0501 randomised, phase 3 trial. *Lancet.* 2011;378:1079–1088.
85. Abe T, Yokoyama A, Takeda K, et al. Randomized phase III trial comparing weekly docetaxel (D)-cisplatin (P) combination with triweekly D alone in elderly patients (pts) with advanced non-small cell lung cancer (NSCLC): An intergroup trial of JCOG0803/WJOG4307L. *J Clin Oncol.* 2011;29:abstr 7509.
86. Shepherd FA, Dancey J, Ramlau R, et al. Prospective randomized trial of docetaxel versus best supportive care in patients with non-small-cell lung cancer previously treated with platinum-based chemotherapy. *J Clin Oncol.* 2000;18:2095–2103.
87. Hanna N, Shepherd FA, Fossella FV, et al. Randomized phase III trial of pemetrexed versus docetaxel in patients with non-small-cell lung cancer previously treated with chemotherapy. *J Clin Oncol.* 2004;22:1589–1597.
88. Shepherd FA, Rodrigues PJ, Ciuleanu T, et al. Erlotinib in previously treated non-small-cell lung cancer. *N Engl J Med.* 2005;353:123–132.
89. Kim ES, Hirsh V, Mok T, et al. Gefitinib versus docetaxel in previously treated non-small-cell lung cancer (INTEREST): A randomised phase III trial. *Lancet.* 2008;372:1809–1818.
90. Fossella F, Pereira JR, von PJ, et al. Randomized, multinational, phase III study of docetaxel plus platinum combinations versus vinorelbine plus cisplatin for advanced non-small-cell lung cancer: The TAX 326 study group. *J Clin Oncol.* 2003;21:3016–3024.

demos MEDICAL

ECAT Emerging Cancer Therapeutics

Pros and Cons of Maintenance Therapy for Advanced Non-Small Cell Lung Cancer

A. Kotsakis, E. Kontopodis, and V. Georgoulias*

Department of Medical Oncology, University Hospital of Heraklion, Heraklion, Crete, Greece

■ ABSTRACT

Maintenance therapy has emerged as a promising approach for the management of patients with advanced non-small cell lung cancer (NSCLC). Although the extension of first-line platinum-based chemotherapy beyond four to six cycles is not associated with a survival advantage, the continuation of selected agents included in the induction regimen has produced encouraging results ("continuation maintenance"). Another promising strategy has been maintenance therapy with an active agent that was not a part of the first-line regimen ("switch maintenance"). The choice of agent and the overall duration of treatment for advanced NSCLC remain empiric. In this chapter, we review current clinical data on maintenance therapy and discuss their implications on treatment strategies for NSCLC.

Keywords: non-small cell lung cancer, maintenance therapy, continuation maintenance, switch maintenance

■ INTRODUCTION

Non-small cell lung cancer (NSCLC) accounts for approximately 85% of all lung cancer cases and is the leading cause of cancer death in both men and women in the United States and worldwide (1,2). Although significant advances have been made in the treatment of NSCLC over the last decade, the prognosis for advanced stage disease remains poor with reported median survival rates following the first-line treatment ranging between 10 and 13 months (3–5).

Platinum-based chemotherapy has been the cornerstone of treatment for NSCLC (6). The incorporation of third-generation chemotherapy agents (taxanes, vinorelbine, gemcitabine, pemetrexed) produced a superior response rate (RR) and

*Corresponding author, Department of Medical Oncology, University Hospital of Heraklion, PO Box 1352, 711 10 Heraklion, Crete, Greece

E-mail address: georgsec@med.uoc.gr

Emerging Cancer Therapeutics 3:1 (2012) 27–44.

DOI: 10.5003/2151–4194.3.1.27

an improved overall survival (OS) when compared with older, more toxic regimens (7). However, survival results remain poor (8), which has prompted investigators to examine several treatment strategies to improve patient outcomes. The role of maintenance therapy has been extensively investigated, and it recently emerged as a promising treatment strategy in advanced NSCLC. Maintenance therapy is prescribed with the intent of maintaining a successful clinical outcome after several cycles of first-line (or induction) chemotherapy (9). Three different strategies involving longer duration of the first-line therapy can be distinguished as follows: (a) continuing induction cytotoxic therapy until progression or a preplanned additional number of cycles over the standard, (b) continuing only part of the induction chemotherapeutic treatment or the molecular component ("continuation maintenance"), and (c) switching to another active agent that has not been given in the induction therapy ("switch maintenance").

■ CONTINUING INDUCTION THERAPY

Several trials have investigated the optimal duration of the first-line chemotherapy in patients with NSCLC (Table 1). In a phase III trial, 308 patients with stage IIIB or IV NSCLC were randomly assigned to three versus six cycles of mitomycin, vinblastine, and cisplatin. No differences in median time to progression (5 months for both arms; $P = .4$) or median OS (6 vs. 7 months) for three versus six cycles, respectively ($P = .2$) were observed. Although early in the treatment course (after 9 weeks), the quality of life (QoL) was not influenced by chemotherapy, after completion of six cycles of chemotherapy, fatigue was significantly ($P = .03$) increased as well as nausea and vomiting ($P = .06$) (10). Socinski et al. (11) conducted a phase III trial in patients with advanced or metastatic NSCLC, comparing four cycles of paclitaxel and carboplatin (arm A) with the same regimen until disease progression (PD; arm B). At progression, all patients received prespecified second-line treatment with weekly paclitaxel. Fifty-seven percent of the patients in arm A completed the planned four cycles of chemotherapy; in arm B, only 42% of the patients received five or more cycles. There were no differences in terms of objective response rate (ORR; $P = .80$) or OS between the two arms ($P = .63$). The toxicity profile was similar in both groups, with the exception of neuropathy, which was more frequent in arm B. No differences in QoL parameters were noted. Less than half of the patients (42% in arm A and 47% in arm B) were able to receive second-line treatment ($P = .42$) (11). von Plessen et al. (12) randomly assigned 297 patients with stage IIIB or IV NSCLC to three or six cycles of carboplatin and vinorelbine. Seventy-eight percent of patients in the three cycles arm (arm A) completed the planned therapy as opposed to 54% of those assigned to the six cycles arm (arm B). OS ($P = .75$) and progression-free survival (PFS; $P = .21$) were similar between the two arms. Second-line chemotherapy was administered to 12% and 10%, in arms A and B, respectively ($P = .4$). There were no significant differences in QoL between the two arms (12). In a phase III study, 314 patients with stage IIIB (with pleural effusion) or IV NSCLC who did not progress after two cycles of platinum-based chemotherapy (cisplatin plus either paclitaxel, docetaxel, or gemcitabine) were randomized to receive two or four additional cycles of the same regimen. Median time to tumor progression (TTP) was 6.2 months (95% CI, 5.7–6.7) for patients who underwent four additional cycles and 4.6 months for those who received two additional cycles of chemotherapy ($P = .001$); however, this difference did not translate into OS benefit (15.9 months [95% CI, 12.4–19.4] versus 14.9 months [95% CI, 13.0–16.8], respectively; $P = .461$). The frequencies of hematologic and nonhematologic toxicities were not significantly different between the two arms. However, QoL was significantly better for the patients treated with four cycles of chemotherapy compared with those treated with six cycles ($P < .05$) (13).

TABLE 1 Phase III studies of continuing the induction chemotherapy regimen

Treatment	N	Outcome	References
Three vs. six cycles of cisplatin/ mitomycin/vinblastine	308	TTP: 5 months for both arms (P = .4); OS: 6 vs. 7 months (P = .2)	Smith et al. (10)
Four cycles of paclitaxel/ carboplatin vs. paclitaxel/ carboplatin until PD	230	OS: 6.6 vs. 8.5 months (P = .63)	Socinski et al. (11)
Three vs. six cycles of carboplatin/vinorelbine	297	PFS: 16 vs. 21 weeks (P = .21); OS: 28 vs. 32 weeks (P = .75)	von Plessen et al. (12)
Four vs. six cycles of platinum-based doublet (if no progression after the first two cycles)[a]	314	TTP: 6.2 vs. 4.6 months (P = .001); OS: 15.9 vs. 14.9 months (P = .461)	Park et al. (13)

PD = disease progression; TTP = time to tumor progression; PFS = progression-free survival; OS = overall survival.
[a]Noninferiority trial.

■ CONTINUATION MAINTENANCE

Cytotoxic Agents (see Table 2)

Gemcitabine

Brodowicz et al. (14) conducted a randomized phase III trial to evaluate the effect of gemcitabine maintenance following four cycles of cisplatin and gemcitabine. Responding and stable disease (SD) patients (206 patients) were randomized 2:1 to gemcitabine or best supportive care (BSC). The primary endpoint was TTP. Almost half of the patients had a Karnofsky performance status (KPS) of ≤ 80. Patients on the gemcitabine arm had a significantly better TTP of 3.6 months (95% CI, 2.8–4.1), compared with 2 months (95% CI, 1.6–2.6) on the BSC arm (P < .001). Although median OS increased by 2 months in the maintenance arm (10.2 vs. 8.1 months), this difference was not statistically significant (P = .17). Remarkably, patients with KPS > 80 had significantly longer TTP and OS. Maintenance gemcitabine was well-tolerated and was not associated with deterioration of QoL. The most notable adverse events included neutropenia (14.9%), anemia (2.6%), and alopecia (4.3%). Approximately, 57% of patients in each arm received second-line treatment (14).

In a subsequent randomized phase III trial, patients responding to first-line treatment with carboplatin and gemcitabine were randomized to maintenance gemcitabine plus BSC versus BSC alone. The primary endpoint was OS. After randomization of 255 patients, the study was closed prematurely due to slow accrual. More than two-thirds of the patients had an Eastern Cooperative Oncology Group (ECOG) performance status (PS) of 2 and 28% had responded to the first-line treatment. Most common grade 3 and 4 adverse events on the gemcitabine arm were anemia (9%), neutropenia (13%), thrombocytopenia (9%), and fatigue (4%). A median number of four maintenance gemcitabine cycles were administered. The ORR was 28% with gemcitabine compared to 6% with BSC. Although both PFS (7.4 vs. 7.7 months) and OS (8.0 vs. 9.3 months) were numerically lower with gemcitabine compared with BSC, the differences were not statistically significant; notably, 16% of patients in the gemcitabine arm and 17% in the BSC arm received poststudy chemotherapy (15).

Pemetrexed

The PARAMOUNT trial evaluated the efficacy of maintenance pemetrexed compared with placebo in 539 patients with advanced nonsquamous NSCLC after four cycles of induction therapy with pemetrexed and cisplatin. In this phase III randomized trial of which the primary endpoint was PFS, patients were randomized (2:1) to pemetrexed versus placebo. All patients had an ECOG PS of 0 or 1 (PS 0: 91%), 87% had adenocarcinoma histology and 45% had responded to induction chemotherapy. Median number of administered cycles was four in both groups, whereas 23% of patients in the pemetrexed group and 14% in the placebo group were treated with more than six cycles of maintenance therapy. The most common grade 3/4 toxicities associated with pemetrexed included fatigue (4.2% vs. 0.6%), anemia (4.5% vs. 0.6%), and neutropenia (3.6% vs. 0%). Treatment discontinuation due to toxicity was required in 5% of the patients on the pemetrexed arm and 3% on the placebo arm. The independently reviewed ORR was 2.8% for pemetrexed compared with 0.6% for placebo ($P = .176$); however, disease control rate was significantly higher on the pemetrexed arm (72% vs. 60%; $P = .009$). Similarly, the independently reviewed median PFS was 3.9 months on the pemetrexed arm and 2.6 months on the placebo arm (hazard ratio [HR] = 0.64; 95% CI, 0.51–0.81; $P = .00025$). QoL was not different between two groups. Survival data have not been reported yet (16).

Pemetrexed plus Bevacizumab

The results of a randomized phase III trial (AVAPERL1) were recently presented. Patients with advanced, recurrent, or metastatic NSCLC who had not progressed after completion of four cycles of front-line treatment with cisplatin, pemetrexed, and bevacizumab (253 patients) were randomized 1:1 to continue their treatment with pemetrexed plus bevacizumab or bevacizumab alone. The primary endpoint was PFS from the initiation of first-line treatment (17). The occurrence of grade 3/4 adverse events was more common in the combination arm (33% vs. 18%) (18). PFS was improved with the combination regimen (median PFS 10.2 vs. 6.6 months; HR = 0.50; $P < .001$). However, a trend toward an improved QoL in favor of bevacizumab alone was observed (19). The median OS had not been reached for pemetrexed plus bevacizumab arm and was 15.7 months for bevacizumab arm (HR = 0.75; $P = .23$) (17).

Molecularly Targeted Agent (see Table 2)

Bevacizumab

Two phase III trials tested the role of the addition of bevacizumab to a standard platinum-based doublet therapy in stage IIIB (with pleural effusion) or IV nonsquamous NSCLC (4,20). In these trials, the control arm consisted of up to six cycles of chemotherapy (carboplatin and paclitaxel or cisplatin and gemcitabine), whereas the experimental arms included the same chemotherapy regimen and bevacizumab administered until PD or unacceptable toxicity. In E4599 ($n = 878$), the addition of bevacizumab to paclitaxel plus carboplatin conferred an improved ORR (35% vs. 15%; $P < .001$), PFS (6.2 vs. 4.5 months; HR = 0.66; 95% CI, 0.57–0.77; $P < .001$), and OS (12.3 vs. 10.3 months; HR = 0.79; 95% CI, 0.67–0.92; $P < .001$) (4). In the AVAiL trial, 1,043 patients were randomly assigned to cisplatin and gemcitabine plus either bevacizumab (7.5 mg/kg), bevacizumab (15 mg/kg), or placebo every 3 weeks. PFS was significantly improved with bevacizumab 7.5 mg and bevacizumab 15 mg (HR = 0.75; 95% CI, 0.62–0.91; $P = .003$ and HR = 0.82; 95% CI, 0.68–0.98; $P = .03$, respectively) compared with placebo; the median PFS was 6.7, 6.5, and 6.1 months for the 7.5 mg/kg, 15 mg/kg, and placebo groups, respectively (20); the difference in OS was not statistically significant (13.6, 13.4, and 13.1 months, respectively) (21). Notably, these trials were not designed to evaluate the efficacy of the maintenance approach. Thus, they did not address the incremental benefit of maintenance bevacizumab, since they did not include an arm without continuation of bevacizumab after front-line therapy.

TABLE 2 Completed phase III studies of continuation maintenance treatment in NSCLC

Maintenance Schedule	*N*	First-Line Treatment	Outcome	References
Gemcitabine plus BSC vs. BSC	206	Cisplatin/gemcitabine	TTP: 3.6 vs. 2 months ($P < .001$); OS: 10.2 vs. 8.1 months ($P = .172$)	Brodowicz et al. (14)
Gemcitabine plus BSC vs. BSC	255	Carboplatin/gemcitabine	PFS: 7.4 vs. 7.7 months (HR = 0.97; $P = .575$); OS: 8.0 vs. 9.3 months (HR = 1.09; $P = .838$)	Belani et al. (15)
Pemetrexed vs. placebo	539	Ciplatin/pemetrexed	PFS: 3.9 vs. 2.6 months (HR = 0.64; $P = .00025$); OS: not reported	Paz-Ares et al. (16)
Pemetrexed plus bevacizumab vs. bevacizumab	253	Ciplatin/pemetrexed/ bevacizumab	PFS[a]: 10.2 vs. 6.6 months (HR = 0.50; $P < .001$); OS[a]: NR vs. 15.7 months (HR = 0.75; $P = .23$)	Barlesi et al. (17)
Bevacizumab vs. observation	878	Paclitaxel/carboplatin/ bevacizumab vs. paclitaxel/carboplatin	PFS: 6.2 vs. 4.5 months ($P < .001$); OS: 12.3 vs. 10.3 months ($P < .001$)	Sandler et al. (4)
Bevacizumab (7.5 mg/kg) vs. bevacizumab (15 mg/kg) vs. placebo	1,043	Cisplatin/gemcitabine plus bevacizumab (7.5 mg/ kg)/bevacizumab (15 mg/kg)/placebo	PFS: 6.7 vs. 6.5 vs. 6.1 months ($P = .03$); OS: 13.6 vs. 13.4 vs. 13.1 ($P = .761$)	Reck et al. (20,21)
Cetuximab vs. observation	1,125	Cisplatin/vinorelbine/ cetuximab vs. cisplatin/ vinorelbine	PFS: 4.8 months in both groups; OS: 11.3 vs. 10.1 months ($P = .044$)	Pirker et al. (22)
Cetuximab vs. observation	676	Carboplatin/taxane/ cetuximab vs. carboplatin/taxane	PFS: 4.40 vs. 4.24 months ($P = .2358$); OS: 9.69 vs. 8.38 months ($P = .1685$)	Lynch et al. (23)

TTP = time to tumor progression; PFS = progression-free survival; OS = overall survival; BSC = best supportive care; NR = not reached.
[a]From start of first-line treatment.

Cetuximab

In the FLEX trial, 1,125 patients with stage IIIB (with pleural effusion) or IV NSCLC expressing epidermal growth factor receptor (EGFR) were randomized to receive vinorelbine and cisplatin for up to six cycles or the same chemotherapy regimen plus cetuximab administered until PD or unacceptable toxicity. The addition of cetuximab to chemotherapy significantly increased the ORR (36% vs. 29% with chemotherapy alone) and OS (11.3 vs. 10.1 months; HR = 0.87; 95% CI, 0.762–0.996; $P = .044$); PFS did not differ between the two groups (4.8 months in both groups; HR = 0.94; 95% CI, 0.83–1.08) (22). Similarly, the BMS-099 phase III trial compared carboplatin plus a taxane (paclitaxel or docetaxel) for up to six cycles with the same regimen plus cetuximab in 676 patients with stage IIIB (with pleural effusion) or IV NSCLC, not selected on the basis of EGFR expression. Cetuximab was offered until PD or unacceptable toxicity. The addition of cetuximab improved the ORR (26% vs. 17%; $P = .007$), but not the PFS (4.4 vs. 4.2 months; HR = 0.90; 95% CI, 0.76–1.07; $P = .24$) or the OS (9.69 vs. 8.38

months; HR = 0.89; 95% CI, 0.75–1.05; $P = .17$) (23). These two phase III trials with cetuximab did not examine the incremental benefit from maintenance cetuximab.

■ SWITCH CONTINUATION

Cytotoxic Agents (see Table 3)

Vinorelbine

Westeel et al. (24) examined the role of vinorelbine in the maintenance setting in a phase III randomized trial. Patients with stage IIIB and IV NSCLC were eligible for the study. Four cycles of induction treatment with mitomycin-C, ifosfamide, and cisplatin (MIC), or two cycles of MIC followed by radiation in patients with stage IIIB without pleural or pericardial effusion, or supraclavicular node involvement were offered. Responders to induction treatment were then randomized to weekly intravenous vinorelbine for up to 6 months or to observation alone. Forty-eight percent out of the 181 randomized patients had stage IV disease. The mean duration of therapy in the vinorelbine group was 13.8 weeks. Three quarters of the patients in the vinorelbine arm discontinued their therapy earlier, primarily due to PD (38%) or toxicity (21%). Most frequent grade 3/4 toxicities included leukopenia (46%) and infection (12.6%). Although more than half of the patients (53%) responded to the treatment, no significant difference in the OS (12.3 months in both arms) or PFS (5 vs. 3 months) was observed (24).

Docetaxel

Fidias et al. (25) investigated switch maintenance therapy with docetaxel in patients with NSCLC who had an objective response or SD after four cycles of gemcitabine and carboplatin. Three hundred nine patients were assigned to immediate (maintenance) docetaxel for up to six cycles or delayed administration of the same drug at PD (second-line treatment). Among them, more than 90% had an ECOG PS of 0 or 1 and 46% had responded to a first-line regimen. Of 153 patients in the immediate docetaxel arm, 95% received at least one cycle compared with only 63% of the 156 patients in the delayed docetaxel arm. The incidence of severe grade 3/4 toxicities was similar between the two arms. ORR was 12% and 11% in immediate and delayed docetaxel arms, respectively. Despite a statistically significant improvement in median PFS in favor of the immediate docetaxel (5.7 vs. 2.7 months; $P = .001$), a numerical improvement in median OS did not reach statistical significance (12.3 vs. 9.7 months; $P = .085$). QoL results were not statistically different between the two arms (25).

Pemetrexed

JMEN was a pivotal phase III randomized trial that tested the role of switch maintenance with pemetrexed in patients with advanced or metastatic NSCLC. After four cycles of a platinum-based doublet chemotherapy (not including pemetrexed), patients with no evidence of PD were randomly assigned 2:1 to pemetrexed versus placebo. A total of 663 patients with an ECOG PS of 0 or 1 were enrolled in the study and 49% had responded to first-line chemotherapy. The median number of maintenance cycles delivered was 5 in the pemetrexed group and 3.5 in the placebo group. Forty-eight percent of patients in the pemetrexed arm and 27% in the placebo arm received six or more cycles. Pemetrexed was generally well-tolerated with modest toxicity. Fatigue (5% vs. < 1% with placebo), neutropenia (3% vs. 0%), and anemia (3% vs. 0%) were the most common grade 3/4 adverse events. Treatment discontinuation due to drug-related toxic effects was rare (5% for pemetrexed and 1% for placebo). The ORR was higher in the pemetrexed group than in the placebo group, according to both investigator assessment (7% vs. 2%; $P = .005$) and independent review (3% vs. 0.5%; $P = .042$). Consistently, the disease control rate was significantly higher for pemetrexed, evaluated by investigators (52% vs. 33%; $P < .0001$) or by an independent review (49% vs.

TABLE 3 Completed phase III studies of switch maintenance therapy in NSCLC

Maintenance Schedule	*N*	First-Line Treatment	Outcome	References
Vinorelbine vs. observation	181	Mitomycin-C/ ifosfamide/cisplatin (MIC) or MIC + RT[a]	PFS: 5 vs. 3 months (HR = 0.77; *P* = .11); OS: 12.3 vs. 12.3 months (HR = 1.08; *P* = .65)	Westeel et al. (24)
Immediate docetaxel vs. docetaxel at PD	309	Carboplatin/ gemcitabine	PFS: 5.7 vs. 2.7 months (*P* = .001); OS: 12.3 vs. 9.7 months (*P* = .0853)	Fidias et al. (25)
Pemetrexed vs. placebo	663	Platinum-based doublet (not including pemetrexed)	PFS: 4.3 vs. 2.6 months (HR = 0.50; *P* < .0001); OS: 13.4 vs. 10.6 months (HR = 0.79; *P* = .012); For the nonsquamous NSCLC population: PFS: HR = 0.44; OS: HR = 0.70	Ciuleanu et al. (26)
Gefitinib until PD vs. three more cycles of first-line chemotherapy	604	Platinum-based doublet (three cycles)	PFS: 4.6 vs. 4.3 months (HR = 0.68; *P* < .001) OS: 13.7 vs. 12.9 months (HR = 0.86; *P* = .11)	Takeda et al. (28)
Gefitinib vs. placebo	173	Platinum-based doublet	PFS: 4.1 vs. 2.9 months (HR = 0.61; *P* = .0015) OS: 10.9 vs. 9.4 months (HR = 0.83; *P* = .2)	Gaafar et al. (29)
Erlotinib vs. placebo	889	Platinum-based doublet	PFS: 12.3 vs. 11.1 weeks (HR = 0.71; *P* < .0001) OS: 12.0 vs. 11.0 months (HR = 0.81; *P* = .0088)	Cappuzzo et al. (30)
Erlotinib plus bevacizumab vs. placebo plus bevacizumab	768	Platinum-based doublet plus bevacizumab	PFS: 4.8 vs. 3.7 months (HR = 0.722; *P* = .0012); OS: 15.9 vs. 13.9 months (HR = 0.90; *P* = .2686)	Miller et al. (32)
Gemcitabine or erlotinib vs. observation	464	Cisplatin/ gemcitabine	*Gemcitabine vs. observation:* PFS: 3.8 vs. 1.9 months (HR = 0.55; 95% CI, 0.43–0.70); OS: 12.1 vs. 10.7 months (HR = 0.86; 95% CI, 0.66–1.12); *Erlotinib vs. observation:* PFS: 2.9 vs. 1.9 months (HR = 0.82; 95% CI, 0.73–0.92); OS: 11.8 vs. 10.7 months (HR = 0.91; 95% CI, 0.8–1.04)	Perol et al. (34)

PFS = progression-free survival; OS = overall survival; PD = disease progression; BSC = best supportive care; RT = radiation therapy; 95% CI = 95% confidence interval.
[a]For patients with stage IIIB NSCLC without pleural effusion or supraclavicular lymph node involvement.

29%; *P* < .0001). PFS, the primary endpoint of the study (4.3 vs. 2.6 months; HR = 0.5; 95% CI, 0.42–0.61; *P* < .0001), and OS (13.4 vs. 10.6 months; HR = 0.79; 95% CI, 0.65–0.95; *P* = .012) were significantly improved with pemetrexed. Subgroup analysis revealed a significant benefit, in terms of PFS and OS, for patients with a nonsquamous histology who were treated with pemetrexed (PFS: HR = 0.44; 95% CI, 0.36–0.55 and OS: HR = 0.70; 95% CI, 0.56–0.88) compared with squamous histology (PFS: HR = 0.69; 95% CI, 0.49–0.98 and OS: HR = 1.07; 95% CI, 0.77–1.50). A significant treatment-by-histology interaction with both PFS (P = .036) and OS (P = .033) was noted. The prolonged treatment did not influence negatively the QoL of the patients. The rate of crossover to postdiscontinuation pemetrexed was only 18% (26,27).

Molecularly Targeted Agents (see Table 3)

Gefitinib

A randomized trial in advanced or metastatic NSCLC that enrolled 604 patients compared six cycles of platinum-doublet chemotherapy with three cycles of the same chemotherapy followed by gefitinib until PD. Approximately, 57% of patients in the latter arm received gefitinib after completion of three cycles of chemotherapy; one-third of patients developed early disease relapse and did not receive gefitinib. An additional 11% of patients refused to receive gefitinib because of a report about the risk for gefitinib-induced interstitial lung disease. The ORR was 29% for chemotherapy alone and 34% for chemotherapy followed by gefitinib (P = .20). The PFS was 4.3 months in the chemotherapy alone arm and 4.6 months in the gefitinib arm (HR = 0.68; 95% CI, 0.57–0.80; P < .001), while the median OS was 12.9 months for chemotherapy alone and 13.7 months for the gefitinib arm (HR = 0.86; 95% CI, 0.72–1.03; P = .11) (28). The European Organization for the Research and Treatment of Cancer (EORTC) conducted a randomized phase III trial (08021) that enrolled patients with stage IIIB (with pleural effusion) or IV NSCLC not progressing after standard first-line chemotherapy to gefitinib or placebo. After enrollment of 173 patients, the study closed prematurely due to low accrual. PFS was found to be significantly longer in the gefitinib arm (median PFS: 4.1 vs. 2.9 months; HR = 0.61; 95% CI, 0.45–0.83; P = .0015); there was no difference in OS between the two arms (median OS: 10.9 vs. 9.4 months; HR = 0.83; 95% CI, 0.60–1.15; P = .2) (29).

Erlotinib

The use of erlotinib as maintenance therapy was evaluated in a randomized, placebo-controlled trial comparing erlotinib with placebo (SATURN trial). In this trial, 889 patients with inoperable NSCLC not progressing after four cycles of platinum-based doublet chemotherapy were assigned. Approximately, 45% of patients had adenocarcinoma and 40% had squamous cell carcinoma histology in each arm. The primary endpoint was the PFS, and the patients were stratified by a number of clinical factors, including EGFR protein expression status assessed by immunohistochemistry (IHC) and EGFR gene copy number assessed by fluorescent in situ hybridization (FISH). All patients had an ECOG PS of 0 or 1, 44% had responded to first-line treatment and 5% had tumors with an EGFR-activating mutation. Grade 3/4 toxicities occurred in 12% of patients in the erlotinib arm compared with 1% in the placebo arm. Most common adverse events with erlotinib included rash (any grade: 60%) and diarrhea (any grade: 18%). Higher ORR was observed in maintenance erlotinib arm (12% vs. 5%; P = .0006). The study met its primary endpoint for PFS (HR = 0.71; P < .0001), although the improvement (12.3 vs. 11.1 weeks) was numerically small (1.2 week). The biomarkers' analysis revealed no significant interaction of EGFR protein expression or EGFR gene copy number. The benefit in PFS was observed in both patients with EGFR-activating mutations and those with wild-type EGFR, and was consistent across all patient subgroups (ECOG PS, smoking status, age, ethnic origin, sex, and histology). In the overall population, erlotinib conferred a statistically significant improvement in OS (12.0 vs. 11.0 months; HR = 0.81; 95% CI, 0.70–0.95; P = .0088). Similarly, patients with EGFR IHC-positive tumors had also a survival benefit (HR = 0.77; P = .0063).

The data for the erlotinib arm patients with EGFR-activating mutations in exon 19 or 21 showed a significantly improved PFS (HR = 0.10; $P < .0001$) compared to those with wild-type EGFR (HR = 0.78; $P = .018$). In contrast, a longer OS was not achieved presumably due to the extensive crossover to erlotinib at the time of progression. Interestingly, patients who had SD after first-line chemotherapy had a more pronounced OS benefit with maintenance erlotinib (11.9 vs. 9.6 months; HR = 0.72; $P = .002$) than those who had a previously complete or partial response (12.5 vs. 12.0 months; HR = 0.94; $P = .618$). The same proportion of patients in both groups (71%) received second-line treatment. QoL was not different between groups (30,31).

Erlotinib plus Bevacizumab

The combination of bevacizumab and erlotinib was compared with bevacizumab alone in the maintenance setting, following front-line chemotherapy plus bevacizumab, was evaluated in the ATLAS trial. This phase III randomized study enrolled 768 patients with advanced/metastatic disease. All patients had an ECOG PS of 0 or 1 and 82% had adenocarcinoma histology. The observed toxicity profile was characteristic and within the range expected based on a single-agent administration of both drugs. Rash (0.5% for bevacizumab plus placebo vs. 10% for bevacizumab plus erlotinib), diarrhea (0.8% vs. 9%), infection (5% vs. 4%), and hypertension (6% vs. 5%) were the most common grade 3/4 toxicities. Hemorrhagic grade 3/4 adverse events were rare. The trial stopped recruitment after the second planned interim efficacy analysis, because it met the primary endpoint. The median PFS in the intent-to-treat population was 4.76 months for the combination arm and 3.75 months for the bevacizumab/placebo arm (HR = 0.722; 95% CI, 0.59–0.88; $P = .0012$). Subsequent therapy was administered in 55% versus 50% (32). Although the median OS numerically favored the combination arm (15.9 vs. 13.9 months), this difference did not reach statistical significance (HR = 0.90; 95% CI, 0.74–1.09; $P = .2686$) (33).

Gemcitabine or Erlotinib

Perol et al. (34) designed a randomized clinical trial (Intergroupe Francophone de Cancérologie Thoracique [IFCT] trial) to evaluate the efficacy of maintenance gemcitabine or erlotinib versus observation in patients with NSCLC after four cycles of cisplatin and gemcitabine. The primary endpoint was PFS. The study was not powered to compare gemcitabine versus erlotinib. Second-line treatment with pemetrexed at PD was prespecified. Four hundred seventy-six patients with ECOG PS of 0 or 1 were randomized. Predominant grade 3/4 toxicities were neutropenia (20.8%) and thrombocytopenia (6.5%) with gemcitabine, and rash (9.0%) with erlotinib. Median PFS by independent review was 3.8 months with gemcitabine (HR = 0.55; 95% CI, 0.43–0.70 vs. observation), 2.9 months with erlotinib (HR = 0.82; 95% CI, 0.73–0.92 vs. observation), and 1.9 months with observation. OS data were not mature at the time of study analysis; in a preliminary analysis, OS was not significantly different with gemcitabine or erlotinib compared with observation (34).

■ WHICH PATIENTS MAY BENEFIT FROM MAINTENANCE?

It has been suggested that the patients with poor PS after first-line treatment, large tumors at the time of diagnosis, or modest response to the front-line therapy are less likely to receive second-line treatment (35). Although these factors are determinants of the likelihood of response to second-line treatment, it seems that they are also determinants for the outcome of maintenance therapy. Indeed, in the Central European Cooperative Oncology Group (CECOG) trial of maintenance gemcitabine, patients with good KPS (> 80) had significantly prolonged survival (22.9 vs. 8.3 months). In contrast, patients with KPS of 70 to 80 had almost identical survival regardless of receiving chemotherapy or not (14). Similarly, in a study presented by Socinski et al. (11), for patients who continued their front-line treatment beyond the standard four cycles, an improved survival of about 3 months in favor of the patients with better KPS was observed

(9.1 vs. 6.2 months) (11). The inclusion of patients with a PS ≥ 2 is one of the possible explanations for the negative results of the trial by Belani et al. (15) that evaluated gemcitabine maintenance. In their study, PS ≥ 2 was found as a prognostic factor for survival in the overall multivariate analysis (HR = 1.5; *P* = .009) (15). In contrast, all positive trials such as JMEN, SATURN, and the most recent PARAMOUNT and AVAPERL1 included patients with good PS (ECOG PS of 0–1) (16,17,26,30).

Response to front-line treatment has been suggested as a predictive marker for the outcome of maintenance therapy. In the SATURN study, patients who experienced disease stabilization derived greater survival benefit from the maintenance erlotinib than those who exhibited complete (CR) or partial response (PR). Patients with SD who received erlotinib had an OS of 11.9 months versus 9.6 months of those who were enrolled in the observational arm (HR = 0.72; *P* = .002). In contrast, for the patients whose disease responded to the first-line therapy, the survival was 12 and 12.5 months, respectively (HR = 0.92; *P* = .62) (30). Accordingly, in the JMEN study, patients with SD after completion of the front-line treatment achieved an OS of 16.6 months with pemetrexed maintenance versus 8.6 months for those treated with placebo (HR = 0.61; *P* = .0017). Among patients who achieved CR or PR, the median OS was 14.4 and 11.4 months for those treated with pemetrexed and placebo, respectively (HR = 0.81; *P* = .198) (36). However, the HR for PFS among the patients treated with gemcitabine in the IFCT trial was 0.44 for those who responded to the first-line treatment compared with 0.68 for those with SD (34).

The identification of biomarkers that are potentially predictive for the response to a particular treatment is under extensive investigation. So far, only the presence of activating EGFR mutations has been correlated with the clinical outcome of maintenance therapy. Indeed, in the SATURN trial patients with EGFR-sensitizing mutations treated with erlotinib had a profound PFS benefit with a reduced risk of PD by 90%. Furthermore, a highly significant interaction between treatment and EGFR mutations was observed (*P* < .001), confirming that EGFR mutation positivity can predict a favorable clinical outcome with erlotinib compared with EGFR wild type. Nevertheless, patients with EGFR-sensitizing mutations did not derive a significant improvement of OS from erlotinib versus placebo, which can be potentially explained by the small number of patients with EGFR mutations and the high level of crossover from the placebo group to erlotinib (67%) (37).

Histology has been proposed as another factor that plays a predictive role in the treatment of NSCLC (38,39). In the JMEN study, pemetrexed improved PFS and OS (HR = 0.51 and 0.73, respectively) among patients with adenocarcinoma The PFS for patients who received pemetrexed and placebo was 4.6 and 2.7 months, respectively and the OS was 15.5 and 10.3 months, respectively. On the other hand, the administration of pemetrexed to patients with squamous NSCLC was potentially detrimental (HR = 1.03 and 1.07, respectively) (26). A trend toward more pronounced benefit from erlotinib in patients with adenocarcinoma was observed in the SATURN trial; the HR for OS for the patients with squamous cell carcinoma treated with erlotinib was 0.76 compared with 0.60 for the patients with adenocarcinoma (30). Gefitinib maintenance also contributed to the reduction of the risk of death in adenocarcinoma patients only (HR = 0.79; *P* = .03), while the HR was 1.24 for those with nonadenocarcinoma (28).

UNANSWERED QUESTIONS ABOUT MAINTENANCE

The results of maintenance studies should be interpreted cautiously since their methodological design varies.

An important aspect is the variability among maintenance studies in the number of patients in the control arm who eventually received second-line treatment at the time of PD. About 40% to 50% of the NSCLC patients are unable to receive a second-line treatment due to PS deterioration

(40). In the maintenance trials that have been conducted so far, a large imbalance was shown among the patients in the observational arm who eventually received second-line treatment. Gerber et al. (41) have proposed that the insurance type, the number of administered cycles of chemotherapy in the first-line setting, and the prechemotherapy palliative radiation therapy negatively influence the patients' ability to receive second-line treatment (41).

The percentage of patients from the observational group who eventually receive second-line therapy ranges from 17% to 82%; furthermore, a similar discrepancy (3%–63%) appears regarding crossover in the second-line setting (15,25,26, 30,34,41).

In the JMEN study, as well as in others, second-line treatment was not prespecified but left to the discretion of treating physicians. Thus, it is not clear if the favorable results of the study can be attributed to the positive effect of the maintenance therapy or to the effectiveness of the selected second-line regimen. Moreover, given that only 19% of the patients in the placebo arm received pemetrexed at any time point, this study did not assess the potential impact of pemetrexed as second-line therapy in this group of patients. Similarly, in the SATURN trial, only 21% of patients in the placebo arm received erlotinib after progression. The Fidias' study was more appropriately designed from that perspective since patients in the observational group were to receive docetaxel at the time of PD. In this trial, the median OS of patients who did receive second-line treatment was almost identical to that of patients who proceeded to immediate treatment with docetaxel. However, an additional issue is the timing and type of imaging tests used for disease evaluation (42). In the Fidias' trial, the experimental group was being evaluated every 6 weeks as opposed to the 3 months of the control arm; it is obvious that a nonsymptomatic progression of the patients in the control arm could be detected with such delay, which likely influenced the study's results.

So far, the survival benefit observed with maintenance strategy has been primarily observed in studies using switch maintenance. The PARAMOUNT trial showed a superior PFS for the patients who continued receiving pemetrexed after completion of the prespecified number of cycles of cisplatin and pemetrexed. However, the OS analysis is still awaited (16). A phase II study testing maintenance pemetrexed in combination with bevacizumab in nonsquamous NSCLC following nonprogression after six cycles of pemetrexed, carboplatin, and bevacizumab showed promising results (43) and led to a phase III trial (AVAPERL1 study [MO22089]), which compared continued maintenance with bevacizumab versus the combination of bevacizumab and pemetrexed in nonsquamous patients with no progression after completion of four cycles of pemetrexed, cisplatin, and bevacizumab. Patients on the combination arm had a significantly longer PFS (10.2 vs. 6.6 months), which numerically far exceeded the outcome of other first-line trials, where PFS typically ranges between 5 and 7 months. However, no OS data have been presented from this study. A shortcoming of this study is that it did not answer whether bevacizumab maintenance is at all required in this setting. This question may be answered by the ongoing phase III trial conducted by ECOG (E5508), where patients with nonsquamous NSCLC who have no progression after front-line treatment with paclitaxel, carboplatin, and bevacizumab will be randomized to receive bevacizumab or pemetrexed or the combination (NCT01107626).

The best endpoint of the studies investigating the role of maintenance remains controversial. Most of the trials used PFS as primary endpoint (14,16,17,34). However, improvement in PFS does not necessarily translate into improvement in OS. In the trial by CECOG (14), as well as in the IFCT trial (34), although the PFS was significantly increased in the continuing arm, the OS was almost the same. Similarly, in most of the switch maintenance trials (25,32,34) that failed to demonstrate a prolongation of OS, eligibility criteria have varied between maintenance trials. Some trials included patients with a PS of 2 to 3, while other studies enrolled patients with a PS of 0 to 1 only. This factor is a known strong predictor of any survival benefit obtained from chemotherapy in NSCLC and poor PS has been associated with worse tolerability (44). The favorable results observed in JMEN (26), SATURN (30), and Fidias et al. (25) trials could also be attributed to the better PS of the patients who participated in those studies. These particular studies also revealed no difference in the QoL between the two arms, indicating that immediate therapy was better tolerated and was more effective in patients with good PS.

Several studies, as shown in Table 4, are currently ongoing and may shed light to many issues surrounding maintenance.

■ PATIENT SELECTION ISSUES

Histology has emerged as a major determinant of treatment selection in NSCLC (45,46). Accordingly, patient selection for maintenance therapy on the basis of histology has become essential. The SATURN trial demonstrated superiority of erlotinib in patients harboring EGFR mutations, although a modest survival benefit was observed in all patients regardless the EGFR status. Similarly, treatment with gefitinib showed survival benefit for adenocarcinomas only (28). Pemetrexed maintenance strikingly improved PFS and OS in the subset of patients with nonsquamous histology with a reported improvement in median OS of 5 months (26). Moreover, as stated above, other factors including SD as best response to first-line therapy and good PS should be also taken into consideration for the decision making given that maintenance therapy has been proven more efficacious in these subgroups of patients. The era of "one size fits all" seems old-fashioned, and the need of careful selection of the patients who are most likely to benefit from such approach has currently emerged as the primary goal of the modern oncology.

■ COST OF THERAPY AND QOL CONSIDERATIONS

In a U.S.-based cost-effectiveness analysis of switch maintenance therapy with pemetrexed, the incremental cost per life year gained was $122,371 for pemetrexed compared with observation and $150,260 for pemetrexed compared with erlotinib in the subset of NSCLC patients with nonsquamous histology (47). In an analysis performed for the United Kingdom's National Institute for Clinical Excellence, incremental cost-effectiveness ratio (ICER) for pemetrexed switch maintenance ranged between £33,732 and £51,192, per quality adjusted life year (QALY) gained, for patients with nonsquamous NSCLC (48). Similarly, the analysis for erlotinib, showed an ICERs of £44,812 and £68,120 per QALY gained for the SD in squamous and nonsquamous population; when erlotinib was compared with pemetrexed, the ICER was £84,029 per QALY gained (49).

So far, few studies have performed a cost-effectiveness analysis for the use of maintenance therapy in NSCLC. Most of the analyses have been done retrospectively, from data collected from the patients' charts (36). A prospective investigation of the cost-effectiveness of this approach is considered of great interest for the future maintenance trials and may help to the recognition of the patients who should proceed to the immediate administration of a potential active agent. Undoubtedly, the identification of patients who are likely to benefit more from the use of a specific maintenance agent, will increase benefits and lower the cost of the treatment. However, even the cost-effectiveness studies may not always reflect the real benefit of the maintenance therapy. A recently presented retrospective analysis by Bradbury et al. (50) surprisingly showed that the cost per year of life gained with maintenance erlotinib was not favorable for patients with EGFR-sensitizing mutations. This was because these patients stayed on treatment longer, thereby incurring considerably higher drug acquisition costs (50).

TABLE 4 Selected ongoing phase III studies of maintenance therapy in NSCLC

Regimen	First-Line Treatment	Sponsor	Primary Endpoint	Identification Number
Maintenance erlotinib vs. erlotinib at PD	Stage IIIB or IV, after four cycles of platinum-based chemotherapy without PD	Hoffmann–La Roche	OS	NCT01328951
Imetelstat plus standard of care (bevacizumab or observation) vs. standard of care (bevacizumab or observation)	Stage IV or recurrent locally advanced, after four to six cycles of platinum-based chemotherapy (with or without bevacizumab) without PD	Geron Corporation	PFS	NCT01137968
Pazopanib vs. pemetrexed	Stage IVA or IVB nonsquamous NSCLC, after four–six cycles of cisplatin or carboplatin plus pemetrexed without PD	GlaxoSmithKline	PFS	NCT01313663
Pemetrexed and carboplatin followed by maintenance pemetrexed vs. paclitaxel, carboplatin, and bevacizumab followed by maintenance bevacizumab	Stage IV nonsquamous NSCLC four cycles of initial treatment	Eli Lilly and Company	PFS without grade 4 toxicity	NCT00948675
Bevacizumab vs. pemetrexed plus bevacizumab	Stage IV or inoperable, locally advanced nonsquamous NSCLC, after four cycles of cisplatin, pemetrexed, and bevacizumab, with response	Hoffmann–La Roche	PFS	NCT00961415
Sunitinib vs. placebo	Stage IV or IIIB not candidate for chemoradiation NSCLC, after four cycles of platinum-based doublet chemotherapy with or without bevacizumab, without PD	Cancer and Leukemia Group B	PFS	NCT00693992
Gemcitabine vs. erlotinib vs. observation	Stage IV or IIIB with pleural effusion NSCLC, after four to six cycles of cisplatin and gemcitabine chemotherapy, without PD	Hospices Civils de Lyon, France	PFS	NCT00300586

(*Continued*)

TABLE 4 Selected ongoing phase III studies of maintenance therapy in NSCLC (*Continued*)

Regimen	First-Line Treatment	Sponsor	Primary Endpoint	Identification Number
Pemetrexed vs. bevacizumab	Stage IIIB or IV nonsquamous NSCLC, four cycles of paclitaxel, carboplatin, and bevacizumab, without progression	Eli Lilly and Company	OS	NCT00762034
Pemetrexed vs. bevacizumab vs. pemetrexed plus bevacizumab	Stage IV (M1a M1b) or IIIB not candidate for chemoradiation, after four cycles of paclitaxel, carboplatin, and bevacizumab, without PD	Eastern Cooperative Oncology Group	OS	NCT01107626
Pazopanib vs. placebo	Stage IIIB or IV, after four cycles of initial chemotherapy, without PD	European Organization for Research and Treatment of Cancer	OS	NCT01208064

OS = overall survival; PFS = progression-free survival.

It is likely that the extended use of chemotherapy has a deleterious effect on QoL (42). However, the results of some of the trials that prospectively investigated the effect of maintenance on QoL did not confirm these concerns (25,26,30). It is apparent that this issue needs to be addressed in the future trials' design.

■ CONCLUSIONS

Maintenance therapy is a proven strategy in the management of NSCLC. Erlotinib and pemetrexed are registered by regulatory agencies in the United States and Europe as maintenance therapy options in patients with NSCLC not progressing after four cycles of standard platinum-based doublet chemotherapy. The U.S. Food and Drug Administration (FDA) and the European Medicines Agency (EMEA) approved pemetrexed for maintenance therapy of patients with locally advanced or metastatic nonsquamous NSCLC whose disease has not progressed after four cycles of platinum-based doublet induction chemotherapy, whereas the FDA has approved erlotinib for the first-line maintenance therapy in unselected patients with locally advanced or metastatic NSCLC whose disease has not progressed after four cycles of platinum-based chemotherapy, while EMEA only for unselected patients who have SD after front-line therapy.

It is meaningful to discuss maintenance therapy with patients who are candidates for drug holiday after completion of the front-line therapy. Most of the studies in this setting have shown that the maintenance therapy prolongs tumor stability without deteriorating QoL. Patients with bulky and symptomatic disease should be considered for immediate treatment switch to take the advantage of receiving a potential active drug earlier in their disease course.

Clearly, maintenance therapy should not be offered to all patients. The identification of patients who are best suited to receive maintenance therapy will likely improve treatment outcomes. Furthermore, the identification of reliable, predictive biomarkers for agents used in maintenance therapy is of great interest.

REFERENCES

1. Jemal A, Siegel R, Ward E, Hao Y, Xu J, Thun MJ. Cancer statistics, 2009. *CA Cancer J Clin.* 2009; 59:225–249.
2. Owonikoko TK, Ragin CC, Belani CP, et al. Lung cancer in elderly patients: an analysis of the surveillance, epidemiology, and end results database. *J Clin Oncol.* 2007;25:5570–5577.
3. Longo-Sorbello GS, Chen B, Budak-Alpdogan T, Bertino JR. Role of pemetrexed in non-small cell lung cancer. *Cancer Invest.* 2007;25:59–66.
4. Sandler A, Gray R, Perry MC, et al. Paclitaxel–carboplatin alone or with bevacizumab for non-small-cell lung cancer. *N Engl J Med.* 2006;355: 2542–2550.
5. Scagliotti GV, Parikh P, von Pawel J, et al. Phase III study comparing cisplatin plus gemcitabine with cisplatin plus pemetrexed in chemotherapy-naive patients with advanced-stage non-small-cell lung cancer. *J Clin Oncol.* 2008;26:3543–3551.
6. Chemotherapy in non-small cell lung cancer: a meta-analysis using updated data on individual patients from 52 randomised clinical trials. Non-small Cell Lung Cancer Collaborative Group. *BMJ.* 1995;311:899–909.
7. Ramalingam S, Belani C. Systemic chemotherapy for advanced non-small cell lung cancer: recent advances and future directions. *Oncologist.* 2008;13(suppl 1):5–13.
8. Schiller JH, Harrington D, Belani CP, et al. Comparison of four chemotherapy regimens for advanced non-small-cell lung cancer. *N Engl J Med.* 2002;346:92–98.
9. Gridelli C, Maione P, Rossi A, et al. Potential treatment options after first-line chemotherapy for advanced NSCLC: maintenance treatment or early second-line? *Oncologist* 2009;14:137–147.
10. Smith IE, O'Brien ME, Talbot DC, et al. Duration of chemotherapy in advanced non-small-cell lung cancer: a randomized trial of three versus six courses of mitomycin, vinblastine, and cisplatin. *J Clin Oncol.* 2001;19:1336–1343.
11. Socinski MA, Schell MJ, Peterman A, et al. Phase III trial comparing a defined duration of therapy versus continuous therapy followed by second-line therapy in advanced-stage IIIB/IV non-small-cell lung cancer. *J Clin Oncol.* 2002;20:1335–1343.
12. von Plessen C, Bergman B, Andresen O, et al. Palliative chemotherapy beyond three courses conveys no survival or consistent quality-of-life benefits in advanced non-small-cell lung cancer. *Br J Cancer.* 2006;95:966–973.
13. Park JO, Kim SW, Ahn JS, et al. Phase III trial of two versus four additional cycles in patients who are nonprogressive after two cycles of platinum-based chemotherapy in non small-cell lung cancer. *J Clin Oncol.* 2007;25:5233–5239.
14. Brodowicz T, Krzakowski M, Zwitter M, et al. Cisplatin and gemcitabine first-line chemotherapy followed by maintenance gemcitabine or best supportive care in advanced non-small cell lung cancer: a phase III trial. *Lung Cancer.* 2006;52:155–163.
15. Belani CP, Waterhouse DM, Ghazal H, et al. Phase III study of maintenance gemcitabine (G) and best supportive care (BSC) versus BSC, following standard combination therapy with gemcitabine-carboplatin (G-Cb) for patients with advanced non-small cell lung cancer (NSCLC) [abstract 7506]. *J Clin Oncol.* 2010;28 (suppl 15).
16. Paz-Ares LG, De Marinis F, Dediu M, et al. PARAMOUNT: Phase III study of maintenance pemetrexed (pem) plus best supportive care (BSC) versus placebo plus BSC immediately following induction treatment with pem plus cisplatin for advanced nonsquamous non-small cell lung cancer (NSCLC) [suppl; abstract CRA7510]. *J Clin Oncol.* 2011;29.
17. Barlesi F, de Castro J, Dvornichenko V, et al. LATE BREAKING ABSTRACT: AVAPERL (MO22089): final efficacy outcomes for patients (pts) with advanced non-squamous non-small cell lung cancer (nsNSCLC) randomised to continuation maintenance (mtc) with bevacizumab (bev) or bev+pemetrexed (pem) after first-line (1L) bev-cisplatin (cis)-pem treatment (tx) [abstract 34]. *Eur J Cancer.* 2011;47 (suppl 2):16.

18. Ahn M, Gervais R, Mezger J, et al. AVAPERL1 (MO22089)—Interim safety of maintenance (mtc) bevacizumab (bev) + pemetrexed (pem) in patients (pts) with advanced non-squamous non-small cell lung cancer (nsnsclc) after first-line (1L) bev-cisplatin (cis)-pem treatment (tx) [abstract 9112]. *Eur J Cancer.* 2011;47(Suppl. 1):S626.
19. Rittmeyer A, Chouaid C, Kim JH, et al. An interim analysis of health-related quality of life (hrqol) in patients with non-squamous non-small-cell lung cancer (nsnsclc) receiving bevacizumab vs bevacizumab + pemetrexed for maintenance therapy in AVAPERL 1 [abstract 9076]. *Eur J Cancer.* 2011;47(suppl 1).
20. Reck M, von Pawel J, Zatloukal P, et al. Phase III trial of cisplatin plus gemcitabine with either placebo or bevacizumab as first-line therapy for nonsquamous non-small-cell lung cancer: AVAiL. *J Clin Oncol.* 2009;27:1227–1234.
21. Reck M, von Pawel J, Zatloukal P, et al. Overall survival with cisplatin-gemcitabine and bevacizumab or placebo as first-line therapy for non-squamous non-small-cell lung cancer: results from a randomised phase III trial (AVAiL). *Ann Oncol.* 2010;21:1804–1809.
22. Pirker R, Pereira JR, Szczesna A, et al. Cetuximab plus chemotherapy in patients with advanced non-small-cell lung cancer (FLEX): an open-label randomised phase III trial. *Lancet.* 2009;373:1525–1531.
23. Lynch TJ, Patel T, Dreisbach L, et al. Cetuximab and first-line taxane/carboplatin chemotherapy in advanced non-small-cell lung cancer: results of the randomized multicenter phase III trial BMS099. *J Clin Oncol.* 2010;28:911–917.
24. Westeel V, Quoix E, Moro-Sibilot D, et al. Randomized study of maintenance vinorelbine in responders with advanced non-small-cell lung cancer. *J Natl Cancer Inst.* 2005;97:499–506.
25. Fidias PM, Dakhil SR, Lyss AP, et al. Phase III study of immediate compared with delayed docetaxel after front-line therapy with gemcitabine plus carboplatin in advanced non-small-cell lung cancer. *J Clin Oncol.* 2009;27:591–598.
26. Ciuleanu T, Brodowicz T, Zielinski C, et al. Maintenance pemetrexed plus best supportive care versus placebo plus best supportive care for non-small-cell lung cancer: a randomised, double-blind, phase 3 study. *Lancet.* 2009;374:1432–1440.
27. Scagliotti G, Brodowicz T, Shepherd FA, et al. Treatment-by-histology interaction analyses in three phase III trials show superiority of pemetrexed in nonsquamous non-small cell lung cancer. *J Thorac Oncol.* 2011;6:64–70.
28. Takeda K, Hida T, Sato T, et al. Randomized phase III trial of platinum-doublet chemotherapy followed by gefitinib compared with continued platinum-doublet chemotherapy in Japanese patients with advanced non-small-cell lung cancer: results of a west Japan thoracic oncology group trial (WJTOG0203). *J Clin Oncol.* 2010;28:753–760.
29. Gaafar RM, Surmont VF, Scagliotti GV, et al. A double-blind, randomised, placebo-controlled phase III intergroup study of gefitinib in patients with advanced NSCLC, non-progressing after first line platinum-based chemotherapy (EORTC 08021/ILCP 01/03). *Eur J Cancer.* 2011;47: 2331–2340.
30. Cappuzzo F, Ciuleanu T, Stelmakh L, et al. Erlotinib as maintenance treatment in advanced non-small-cell lung cancer: a multicentre, randomised, placebo-controlled phase 3 study. *Lancet Oncol.* 2010;11:521–529.
31. Coudert B, Ciuleanu T, Park K, et al. Survival benefit with erlotinib maintenance therapy in patients with advanced non-small-cell lung cancer (NSCLC) according to response to first-line chemotherapy. *Ann Oncol.* 2012;23:388–394.
32. Miller VA, O'Connor P, Soh C, Kabbinavar F. A randomized, double-blind, placebo-controlled, phase IIIB trial (ATLAS) comparing bevacizumab (B) therapy with or without erlotinib (E) after completion of chemotherapy with B for first-line treatment of locally advanced, recurrent, or metastatic non-small cell lung cancer (NSCLC) [abstract LBA8002]. *J Clin Oncol.* 2009;27(suppl 18).
33. Kabbinavar FF, Miller VA, Johnson BE, O'Connor PG, Soh C. Overall survival (OS) in ATLAS, a phase IIIB trial comparing bevacizumab (B) therapy with or without erlotinib (E) after completion of chemotherapy (chemo) with B for first-line treatment of locally advanced, recurrent, or metastatic non-small cell lung cancer (NSCLC) [abstract 7526]. *J Clin Oncol.* 2010;28(suppl 15).

34. Perol M, Chouaid C, Milleron BJ, et al. Maintenance with either gemcitabine or erlotinib versus observation with predefined second-line treatment after cisplatin-gemcitabine induction chemotherapy in advanced NSCLC: IFCT-GFPC 0502 phase III study [abstract 7507]. *J Clin Oncol.* 2010;28(suppl 15).
35. Sun JM, Park JO, Won YW, et al. Who are less likely to receive subsequent chemotherapy beyond first-line therapy for advanced non-small cell lung cancer? Implications for selection of patients for maintenance therapy. *J Thorac Oncol.* 2010;5:540–545.
36. Coate LE, Shepherd FA. Maintenance therapy in advanced non-small cell lung cancer: evolution, tolerability and outcomes. *Ther Adv Med Oncol.* 2011;3:139–157.
37. Brugger W, Triller N, Blasinska-Morawiec M, et al. Prospective molecular marker analyses of EGFR and KRAS from a randomized, placebo-controlled study of erlotinib maintenance therapy in advanced non-small-cell lung cancer. *J Clin Oncol.* 2011;29: 4113–4120.
38. Kotsakis A, Yousem S, Gadgeel SM. Is histologic subtype significant in the management of NSCLC? *Open Lung Cancer J.* 2010;3:66–72.
39. Hirsch FR, Spreafico A, Novello S, Wood MD, Simms L, Papotti M. The prognostic and predictive role of histology in advanced non-small cell lung cancer: a literature review. *J Thorac Oncol.* 2008;3:1468–1481.
40. Eccles BK, Geldart TR, Laurence VM, Bradley KL, Lwin MT. Experience of first- and subsequent-line systemic therapy in the treatment of non-small cell lung cancer. *Ther Adv Med Oncol.* 2011;3:163–170.
41. Gerber DE, Rasco DW, Le P, Yan J, Dowell JE, Xie Y. Predictors and impact of second-line chemotherapy for advanced non-small cell lung cancer in the United States: real-world considerations for maintenance therapy. *J Thorac Oncol.* 2011;6: 365–371.
42. Owonikoko TK, Ramalingam SS, Belani CP. Maintenance therapy for advanced non-small cell lung cancer: current status, controversies, and emerging consensus. *Clin Cancer Res.* 2010;16: 2496–2504.
43. Patel JD, Hensing TA, Rademaker A, et al. Phase II study of pemetrexed and carboplatin plus bevacizumab with maintenance pemetrexed and bevacizumab as first-line therapy for nonsquamous non-small-cell lung cancer. *J Clin Oncol.* 2009;27: 3284–3289.
44. Blagden SP, Charman SC, Sharples LD, Magee LR, Gilligan D. Performance status score: do patients and their oncologists agree? *Br J Cancer* 2003;89:1022–1027.
45. Mok TS, Wu YL, Thongprasert S, et al. Gefitinib or carboplatin-paclitaxel in pulmonary adenocarcinoma. *N Engl J Med* 2009;361:947–957.
46. Mitsudomi T, Morita S, Yatabe Y, et al. Gefitinib versus cisplatin plus docetaxel in patients with non-small-cell lung cancer harbouring mutations of the epidermal growth factor receptor (WJTOG3405): an open label, randomised phase 3 trial. *Lancet Oncol.* 2010;11:121–128.
47. Klein R, Wielage R, Muehlenbein C, et al. Cost-effectiveness of pemetrexed as first-line maintenance therapy for advanced nonsquamous non-small cell lung cancer. *J Thorac Oncol.* 2010;5: 1263–1272.
48. Greenhalgh J, McLeod C, Bagust A, et al. Pemetrexed for the maintenance treatment of locally advanced or metastatic non-small cell lung cancer. *Health Technol Assess.* 2010;14:33–39.
49. Dickson R, Bagust A, Boland A, et al. Erlotinib monotherapy for the maintenance treatment of non-small cell lung cancer after previous platinum-containing chemotherapy: a NICE single technology appraisal. *Pharmacoeconomics.* 2011; 29:1051–1062.
50. Bradbury PA, Tu D, Seymour L, et al. Economic analysis: randomized placebo-controlled clinical trial of erlotinib in advanced non-small cell lung cancer. *J Natl Cancer Inst.* 2010;102:298–306.

demos MEDICAL

ECAT Emerging Cancer Therapeutics

Antiangiogenic Agents in Lung Cancer

Geetha Vallabhaneni[1] and Suresh S. Ramalingam[2*]

[1]*Department of Hematology and Medical Oncology, Winship Cancer Institute of Emory University, Atlanta, GA*

[2]*Department of Hematology and Medical Oncology, Winship Cancer Institute of Emory University, Atlanta, GA*

ABSTRACT

Vascular endothelial growth factor (VEGF) is one of the most important proangiogenic factors involved in tumorigenesis. Elevated VEGF expression is associated with poor prognosis in lung cancer. Extensive preclinical studies have proven that VEGF promotes neovascularization and metastatic foci in addition to facilitating growth of primary tumor itself in lung cancer. This chapter focuses on the role of antiangiogenic agents in the treatment of non-small cell lung cancer (NSCLC) and small cell lung cancer (SCLC). Bevacizumab, a recombinant humanized monoclonal antibody (rhuMAB) against VEGF, was approved by the United States FDA in 2006 for use in combination with carboplatin and paclitaxel in advanced diagnosed nonsquamous NSCLC. Several multitargeted tyrosine kinase inhibitors (TKIs) that bind to the internal domain of the VEGF receptor, including sunitinib, sorafenib, vandetanib, cediranib, and linifanib, have also been studied in lung cancer. So far, none of the VEGF TKIs have conferred survival benefit when used in combination with chemotherapy in NSCLC. Vascular disrupting agents that directly target existing tumor vasculature are also currently being studied in lung cancer. The lack of a predictive biomarker for patient selection has been the biggest hurdle in the development of antiangiogenic agents.

Keywords: lung cancer, angiogenesis, bevacizumab, VEGF, TKIs

*Corresponding author, Department of Hematology and Medical Oncology, Winship Cancer Institute, Emory University, 1365 Clifton Road NE, C-3090, Atlanta, GA 30322.

E-mail address: suresh.ramalingam@emory.edu

Emerging Cancer Therapeutics 3:1 (2012) 45–64.

DOI: 10.5003/2151–4194.3.1.45

INTRODUCTION

Lung cancer is the second most common cancer and the leading cause of cancer-related deaths in both men and women in the United States (1). There has been a gradual decrease in deaths from lung cancer in men over the past 50 years. Nearly 70% of patients have inoperable locally advanced tumors or metastatic disease at the time of diagnosis (2). Historically, the two most common histological types of lung cancer based on size and appearance of malignant cells seen under a conventional microscope are non-small cell lung cancer (NSCLC) and small cell lung cancer.

NSCLC accounts for nearly 85% of all cases of lung cancer (3,4). More than 50% of cases are seen in patients greater than 70 years of age (5,6). NSCLC can be further divided in to three major histologic subtypes: squamous-cell carcinoma, adenocarcinoma, and large cell lung cancer (4). Surgery is the preferred treatment for early-stage NSCLC with curative intent. Five-year survival rates for patients with Stage I and Stage II disease range from 54% to 73% and 38% to 48%, respectively (7). Platinum-based chemotherapy remains the standard treatment for advanced and metastatic NSCLC (8). Although treatment options for NSCLC have improved substantially in the past few years with newer generation chemotherapies and targeted agents, cure is still elusive. Hence, there is an urgent need to develop novel therapeutic options for systemic therapy of lung cancer. Approximately 40% of patients with advanced disease initially respond to cytotoxic chemotherapy, but they eventually will experience disease progression or recurrence (9). In the modern era, better understanding of the biology of cancer has led to exciting molecular targeted therapies. The vascular endothelial growth factor (VEGF) and epidermal growth factor receptor (EGFR) have been identified as key molecular targets in NSCLC.

ANGIOGENESIS AND LUNG CANCER

Angiogenesis

In 1971, Judah Folkman described the importance of tumor angiogenesis and laid the pathway for future antiangiogenic drugs. Angiogenesis is a fundamental event needed for growth of tumor cells and metastatic dissemination (10,11). It is a complex process where new blood vessels are formed from preexisting vasculature, and the process is implicated in a variety of disorders. Angiogenesis is crucial in normal physiologic processes, including fetal development, reproductive function, and wound healing. In normal physiologic processes, a balance is maintained between proangiogenic and antiangiogenic factors. However, during neoplastic growth, this well-controlled balance shifts toward proangiogenic activities, and this facilitates tumors to develop their own blood supply system. Proangiogenic factors include VEGF, fibroblast growth factor (FGF), tumor necrosis factor, platelet-derived growth factor (PDGF), integrins, nitric oxide, COX-2, interleukin-8, and others. Antiangiogenic factors include alpha, beta, and gamma interferons; angiostatin; endostatin; interleukin-12 (IL-12); platelet factor-4; and others (10,11). Thus, molecular basis of tumor angiogenesis has been of keen interest in the field of cancer research. Tumors can grow without neovascularization up to a certain size; however, angiogenesis is necessary for tumor growth beyond 1 to 2 mm and for metastasis (12). The critical role of angiogenesis is well established in lung cancers, and high microvessel density has been widely studied as a prognostic factor.

VASCULAR ENDOTHELIAL GROWTH FACTOR

VEGF is an important mediator of angiogenesis. VEGF expression is increased in a variety of tumors such as colorectal cancer, NSCLC, and

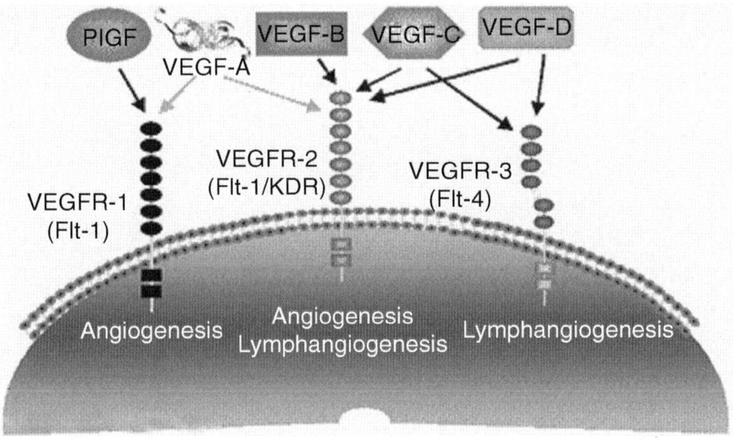

FIGURE 1
VEGF ligands and receptors. PIGF = placental growth factor.
Source: Image printed with permission from medscape.com, 2011.

breast and ovarian cancers (13). VEGF is one of the most important proangiogenic factors involved in tumor angiogenesis; hence, it has emerged as a key target for pharmacological inhibition of tumor angiogenesis. Hypoxia is the triggering event to VEGF production (13). When a cell becomes hypoxic, it produces hypoxia inducible factor, which stimulates the release of VEGF. Circulating VEGF then binds to VEGF receptors (VEGFRs) on endothelial cells, triggering the activation of tyrosine kinase pathway, which in turn leads to angiogenesis. VEGF family consists of five dimeric glycoproteins of approximately 40 kDa: VEGF-A, VEGF-B, VEGF-C, VEGF-D and placental growth factor (11,14). The major mediator in tumor angiogenesis is VEGF-A, which is commonly referred as VEGF (15). VEGF can facilitate tumor dissemination through increasing vascular permeability, hence increasing nutrient supply to tumor cells. This increased permeability can cause tumor dissemination through the blood circulation. VEGF ligands are secreted by tumor cells and macrophages. VEGF binds to three-cell surface distinct VEGFRs (Figure 1): VEGFR1 (fms-like tyrosine kinase 1 [Flt-1]), VEGFR2 (kinase domain region/fetal liver kinase 1 [kdr/flk-1]), and VEGFR3 (fms-like tyrosine kinase 4 [Flt-4]), which are located on the host vascular endothelial cells, monocytes, and hematopoietic precursors (10,11,16,17). The VEGFRs are made of an extracellular domain that binds specific VEGF ligand, a transmembrane domain and an intracellular region that contains a tyrosine kinase domain. When VEGF ligand–receptor interaction occurs, tyrosine kinase domain is activated; this in turn leads to the activation of intracellular signal transduction pathways. VEGFR2, which is commonly overexpressed by tumor vasculature, appears to play the most important role in tumor angiogenesis. Several strategies have been developed to target VEGF as blockade or as a therapeutic strategy for inhibiting angiogenesis, and hence tumor growth.

The proven approach to inhibit VEGF in lung cancer involves the use of an antibody directed against the endothelial receptor for VEGF. Other approaches to inhibit angiogenesis include, but are not limited to, VEGFR tyrosine kinase inhibitors (TKIs), matrix metalloproteinase inhibitors, and vascular disrupting agents (VDAs).

■ WHY IS VEGF IMPORTANT IN LUNG CANCER?

VEGF promotes neovascularization and in addition plays a key role in establishing new metastatic foci along with facilitating growth of primary tumor itself. Previous studies have shown that VEGF is overexpressed in 42% to 75% of NSCLC patients, and increased VEGF expression is associated with poor prognosis. VEGF expression and micro vessel density (MVD) are associated with a poor prognosis in NSCLC (18).

VEGF acts as a potent mitogen for endothelial cells and has minimal effects on other cell types. In addition, host vasculature is more stable compared with tumor vasculature and is therefore less susceptible to the effects of VEGF inhibition. In addition to promoting vascular growth, VEGF also causes inhibition of antitumor immune response, providing yet another mechanism by which VEGF inhibition could be effective for the treatment of cancer (11). Certain studies have also noted that VEGF inhibition improves delivery of chemotherapy to the tumor tissues, thereby allowing for enhanced efficacy of standard chemotherapeutic agents (17).

■ ANTI-VEGF AGENTS

Two classes of drugs have primarily gained importance in inhibition of VEGF function: Antibodies against VEGF or its receptor, and small-molecule TKIs (19) (Figure 2).

Anti-VEGF Monoclonal Antibodies

Bevacizumab (Avastin)

Bevacizumab is an anti-VEGF recombinant humanized monoclonal antibody (rhuMab VEGF). It comprises 93% human and 7% murine protein sequence (11,20). The human fraction and murine region constitutes the framework and complementary determining regions respectively. It inactivates all isoforms of VEGF and inhibits angiogenesis, tumor growth, and proliferation. It has a molecular weight of 149 kD and a half-life of 20 days. Bevacizumab has demonstrated clinical activity in variety of cancers including breast, colorectal, renal, and lung cancers (21). Bevacizumab was approved by Food and Drug Administration (FDA) in United States for metastatic NSCLC in October 2006, in combination with carboplatin and paclitaxel.

An initial three-arm Phase II study of newly diagnosed patients with advanced NSCLC showed that 15mg/kg of bevacizumab in combination with carboplatin and paclitaxel resulted in an improved time to progression (TTP), response rate and trend in overall survival (OS). Chemotherapy-naive patients were randomized to carboplatin and paclitaxel

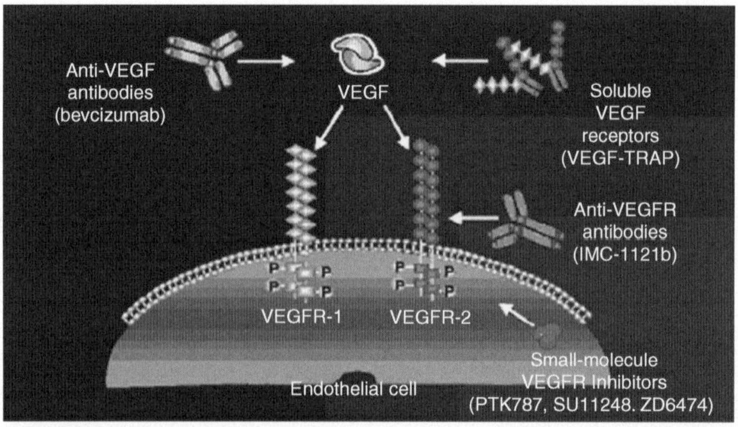

FIGURE 2
Agents targeting VEGF and the VEGF pathway.
Source: Image printed with permission from medscape.com, 2011.

with or without bevacizumab 7.5 or 15 mg/kg every 3 weeks. The median time to tumor progression was improved with the addition of bevacizumab to standard chemotherapy (7.4, 4.3, and 4.2 months for high–dose bevacizumab, low-dose bevacizumab, and chemotherapy-alone group, respectively) (22). Response rates were 32% for high-dose bevacizumab, 28% for low-dose bevacizumab, and 19% for chemotherapy-alone group. There were nine treatment-related deaths (four in each of the bevacizumab arms and one in the control arm). Six episodes of fatal hemoptysis occurred in bevacizumab-treated patients, out of which four episodes were in patients with squamous histology (22). This led to the exclusion of patients with squamous histology in subsequent confirmatory studies with bevacizumab in advanced NSCLC. The encouraging efficacy results with bevacizumab in the study laid the platform for the Phase III study by the Eastern Cooperative Oncology Group 4599 (ECOG 4599). The 15 mg/kg dose of bevacizumab was chosen for this study based on the favorable results over the lower dose in the Phase II study.

ECOG 4599 randomized 878 chemotherapy-naive patients with Stage IIIB and IV NSCLC to a combination of carboplatin (AUC = 6) and paclitaxel (200 mg/m^2) every 3 weeks for 6 cycles with or without bevacizumab at 15 mg/kg every 3 weeks until disease progression. The primary endpoint was the OS. Patients with squamous cell histology, brain metastasis, and history of gross hemoptysis and those on anticoagulation therapy were excluded. Patients receiving chemotherapy plus bevacizumab had a significantly increased objective response rate (35% vs. 15%, respectively), median OS (12.3 vs. 10.3 months, respectively), and progression-free survival (PFS) (6.2 vs. 4.5 months, respectively) compared with patients receiving chemotherapy alone. One-year and two-year survival rates in bevacizumab arm and chemotherapy-alone arm were 51% versus 44% and 23% versus 15%, respectively (23). There were 15 treatment-related deaths in the bevacizumab arm, of which 5 were related to fatal pulmonary hemorrhage. Other salient adverse events with the addition of bevacizumab included Grade 3 or 4 neutropenia, Grade 3 or 4 thromboembolism and Grade 3 hypertension. The favorable efficacy data resulted in the approval of bevacizumab for first line treatment in unresectable, recurrent, locally advanced, or metastatic NSCLC with non-squamous histology, in combination with carboplatin and paclitaxel (24).

Another Phase III trial AVAIL (Avastin in lung cancer) evaluated the combination of cisplatin and gemcitabine with bevacizumab in previously untreated Stage IIIB or IV or recurrent non-squamous NSCLC. PFS was the primary endpoint. In contrast to E4599, this trial was placebo-controlled. Patients were randomized to cisplatin plus gemcitabine with placebo or bevacizumab at 7.5 or 15 mg/kg. There was a statistically significant, but clinically modest, improvement in PFS with the addition of bevacizumab to chemotherapy (25). However, there was no improvement in OS. The efficacy results were similar between the two doses of bevacizumab.

Though these studies excluded patients with brain metastasis, recent evidence indicates the safety of using bevacizumab in this setting. Brain metastasis is a common in NSCLC and occurs in 25% to 30% of patients with NSCLC (26). A Phase II (PASSPORT) multi-center trial addressed the safety of bevacizumab in patients with non-squamous NSCLC and previously treated brain metastasis. This single-arm study enrolled 115 patients out of which majority received whole brain radiation with or without radiosurgery. The primary endpoint was to assess the incidence of symptomatic Grade ≥ 2 central nervous system (CNS) hemorrhage for bevacizumab treatment with first- or second-line systemic therapy. Patients received bevacizumab at 15 mg/kg every 3 weeks until disease progression or unacceptable toxicity, for a maximum of one year. When administered as first line, bevacizumab was given with platinum-based doublet chemotherapy for up to six cycles or erlotinib orally daily. Patients on second-line therapy received bevacizumab with single-agent erlotinib, pemetrexed, or docetaxel, or another chemotherapy regimen chosen at the investigator's discretion. There were no Grade 1 to Grade 5 CNS hemorrhages in patients treated with bevacizumab. The study demonstrated that bevacizumab could be safely administered in combination with a variety of chemotherapy regimens in first- and second-line settings, in patients with treated brain metastasis (26).

Table 1 summarizes the key Phase II and Phase III trials with bevacizumab in NSCLC.

■ DOSING AND ADMINISTRATION

The FDA-approved dose for bevacizumab in NSCLC is 15 mg/kg administered intravenously once every 3 weeks in combination with carboplatin and paclitaxel and then as maintenance monotherapy until disease progression. In patients who develop hypertensive crisis, gastrointestinal perforation, serious bleeding, or nephritic syndrome, permanent discontinuation of bevacizumab is recommended. Tracheoesophageal fistula (TEF) is a rare complication of lung cancer and its treatment, and it is often fatal. Spigel et al. described TEF as a new complication of bevacizumab in combination with chemotherapy and radiation based on two independent trials, one with limited-stage SCLC and other with locally advanced NSCLC (27).The study identified four confirmed and one suspected TEF. Bevacizumab's role in inhibition of angiogenesis and consequent delayed would heal likely accounts for this rare side effect (27,28). Therefore, the use of bevacizumab concurrently or immediately after thoracic radiation is not recommended.

■ VEGFR TYROSINE KINASE INHIBITORS

TKIs are small-molecule compounds that inhibit VEGFR activation (Table 2). Many of these agents target multiple other tyrosine kinases and hence have varying toxicity profiles. Table 3 summarizes the key Phase III trials with VEGF TKIs in NSCLC.

Sunitinib

Sunitinib (Sutent, Pfizer) is an oral small-molecule, multitargeted tyrosine kinase inhibitior, which prevents the growth of new tumor vessels and regression of existing tumor vasculature. It inhibits a wide range of protein kinases such as VEGFR1, VEGFR2, VEGFR3, PDGFR, c-kit, and Flt-3. Sunitinib has a higher affinity to PDGFR and Flt-3 than to VEGFR-2 and VEGFR-3, and hence it targets pathways that are not targeted by bevacizumab (29).

A Phase II trial evaluated the clinical activity of single-agent sunitinib in previously treated advanced NSCLC patients. Patients with Stage IIIB or IV received sunitinib 50 mg/day for 4 weeks followed by 2 weeks of treatment holiday. Of the 63 patients treated with sunitinib, 11.1% had partial responses and 28.6% had stable disease. The study showed that sunitinib had promising single-agent activity in patients with previously treated NSCLC, with an acceptable safety profile (30).

A Phase II trial SABRE-L treated patients with locally advanced, recurrent, or metastatic non-squamous NSCLC with a combination of carboplatin, paclitaxel, bevacizumab, and sunitinib (29). Preclinical model studies suggested that combining bevacizumab and sunitinib could have an additive effect. However, the study showed that addition of sunitinib to bevacizumab had an increased toxicity profile at 25-mg dose of sunitinib and could not be escalated to 37.5-mg dose secondary to frequent dose reductions and discontinuations (29). Unexpected high incidence of myelosuppression was a major concern in the study. Therefore, the combination of the four drugs was not tolerated well, and so it has not been developed further.

TABLE 1 Summary of bevacizumab trials in NSCLC patients

Trials	*N*	Setting	Schema	Type	Results
Johnson et al. (22)	99	First line; Stage IIIB, IV, or recurrent NSCLC	Carboplatin + Paclitaxel	Phase II, randomized	Median TTP: 4.2 months Median OS: 14.9 months RR: 18.8%
			Carboplatin + Paclitaxel + Bevacizumab 7.5 mg/kg		Median TTP: 4.3 months Median OS: 11.6 months RR: 28.1%
			Carboplatin + Paclitaxel + Bevacizumab 15 mg/kg		Median TTP: 7.4 months Median OS: 17.7 months RR: 31.5%
ECOG 4599 Sadler et al. (23)	878	First line; Stage IIIB, IV, or recurrent NSCLC	Carboplatin + Paclitaxel	Phase III, randomized	Median OS: 10.3 months Median PFS: 4.5 months RR: 35%
			Carboplatin + Paclitaxel + Bevacizumab 15 mg/kg		Median OS:12.3 months Median PFS: 6.2 months RR: 15%
AVAIL Manegold et al. (25)	1043	First line; Stage IIIB, IV, or recurrent non-squamous NSCLC	Gemcitabine + Cisplatin + placebo	Phase III, randomized	Median OS: 13.1 months Median PFS: 6.1 months
			Gemcitabine + Cisplatin + Bevacizumab 7.5 mg/kg		Median OS: 13.6 months Median PFS: 6.7 months
			Gemcitabine + Cisplatin + Bevacizumab 15 mg/kg		Median OS: 13.4 months Median PFS: 6.5 months
PASSPORT (AVF3752) Socinski et al. (26)	115	First or second line; advanced non-squamous NSCLC with treated brain metastasis	Carboplatin + Paclitaxel (at least 1 week after RT completion) + bevacizumab (at least 4 weeks after RT completion) until PD or up to 12 months	Single arm, Phase II	No grade ≥ CNS hemorrhage observed in study

(Continued)

TABLE 1 Summary of bevacizumab trials in NSCLC patients (*Continued*)

Trials	*N*	Setting	Schema	Type	Results
Herbst et al. (9)	120	Second line; Locally advanced or metastatic non-squamous NSCLC	Erlotinib 150 mg/kg + bevacizumab 15 mg/kg	Phase II, randomized	Median PFS: 4.4 months Median OS: 13.7 months
			Chemotherapy (Pemetrexed or Docetaxel) + Bevacizumab 15 mg/kg		Median PFS: 4.8 months Median OS: 12. 6 months
			Pemetrexed or Docetaxel alone		Median PFS: 3 months Median OS: 8.6 months
BeTa Hainsworth et al. (2)	636	Second line; Recurrent or refractory NSCLC	Erlotinib 150 mg/day + Placebo	Phase III, randomized	Median PFS:1.7 months Median OS: 9.2 months
			Erlotinib 150 mg/day + bevacizumab 15 mg/kg		Median PFS: 3.4 months Median OS: 9.3 months
ATLAS Miller et al. (50)	1160	First line; Stage IIIB or IV NSCLC	ERlotinib 150 mg/day + Placebo	Phase IIIb, randomized	Median PFS: 3.7 months
			Erlotinib 15 mg/day + bevacizumab 15 mg/kg		Median PFS: 4.8 months

N = Number of patients in study; TTP = time to progression; RR = response rate; CNS = central nervous system; PFS = progression-free survival; OS = overall survival.

A Phase III trial evaluated the combination of sunitinib and erlotinib versus erlotinib alone in previously treated advanced NSCLC patients. The study demonstrated a statistically significant improvement in PFS with sunitinib but no increase in OS (31).Based on these data, the optimal setting for use of sunitinib is not well defined. An ongoing study evaluates sunitinib as maintenance therapy in advanced NSCLC patients.

Sorafenib

Sorafenib (Nexavar, Bayer) inhibits VEGFR-2, VEGFR-3, PDGFR-B, Flt-3, and c-kit (32). Phase II studies of single-agent sorafenib in chemotherapy-naive or previously treated NSCLC patients have demonstrated modest benefits. A single-arm Phase II study enrolled 54 patients with relapsed or refractory NSCLC to sorafenib 400 mg oral twice daily until disease progression on acceptable toxicity. Primary objective of the study was to measure response rate. Fifty nine percent of the enrolled patients achieved stable disease, but there were no objective response (33). Most common adverse events in the study were diarrhea, hand-foot skin reaction, and fatigue. In ECOG 2501 Phase II trial, all patients received sorafenib 400 mg oral twice daily for 2 cycles, after progressing on at least 2 prior lines of chemotherapy (34). Patients with stable disease after 2 cycles were randomized to sorafenib or placebo. Results showed that sorafenib increased PFS (3.6 months versus 1.9 months) in heavily pretreated patients with slow growing disease and thus established evidence of biological effects with this agent.

A Phase III study ESCAPE (evaluation of sorafenib, carbopaltin, and paclitaxel efficacy) randomized 926 patients with unresectable Stage III or metastatic NSCLC to sorafenib at 400 mg oral twice daily or placebo on days 2 to 19, with carboplatin (AUC = 6) and paclitaxel (200 mg/m^2) therapy every 3 weeks for 6 cycles. The study was closed prematurely in 2008 as an interim analysis showed there was no benefit when sorafenib was added to carboplatin and paclitaxel in first-line setting (32). In patients with squamous histology, the combination of sorafenib with chemotherapy was inferior. These results were confirmed by a second Phase III study that showed no efficacy benefit with the combination of sorafenib with chemotherapy (35).

TABLE 2 Selected small-molecule inhibitors of VEGFRs

Inhibitors	VEGFR-1	VEGFR-2	VEGFR-3	PDGFR	c-KIT	EGFR
Sunitinib	+	+	+	+	+	–
Sorafenib	+	+	+	+	+	–
Vandetanib	–	+	+	+/–	–	+
Cediranib	+	++	+	+	–	–
Pazopanib	+	+	+			–
Linifanib	+	+	++			–

Source: Adapted from Ref. (75–77).
VEGFR = vascular endothelial growth factor receptor; PRGFR = platelet-derived growth factor receptor; EGFR = epithelial growth factor receptor.

TABLE 3 Phase III trials of TKIs in NSCLC (selected)

Drug	Trial	Setting/Type	Route of Administration	Treatment	Results
Cediranib	Goss et al. (43)	First line; Stage IIIB or IV NSCLC/Phase II/III	PO	Carboplatin + Paclitaxel + Cediranib	Median PFS: 5.6 months
				Carboplatin + Paclitaxel + Placebo	Median PFS: 5 months
	NCIC BR29 (44)	First line; Stage IIIB or IV NSCLC/Phase III		Carboplatin + Paclitaxel + Cediranib	Ongoing
				Carboplatin + Paclitaxel + Placebo	
Motesanib	Monet 1 Scagliotti et al. (78)	First line, Stage IIIB or IV or recurrent non-squamous NSCLC/Phase III	PO	Carboplatin + Paclitaxel + Motesanib	Median PFS: 5.6 months Median OS: 13 months
				Carboplatin + Paclitaxel + Placebo	Median PFS: 5.4 months Median OS: 11 months
Sunitinib	Govindan et al. (79)	Second or third line, recurrent Stage IIIB or IV NSCLC/Phase III	PO	Erlotinib + Sunitinib	Median OS: 9 months Median PFS: 3.6 months ORR: 10.6 months
				Erlotinib + Placebo	Median OS: 8.5 months Median PFS: 2.0 months ORR: 6.9 months
Sorafenib	Scagliotti et al. (32) Gatzmeier et al. (35)	First line, Stage IIIB or IV NSCLC/Phase III	PO	Carboplatin + Paclitaxel + Sorafenib	Median OS: 10.7 months
				Carboplatin + Paclitaxel + Placebo	Median OS: 10.6 months
		First line, Stage IIIB or IV non-squamous NSCLC/Phase III		Gemcitabine + Cisplatin + Sorafenib	Median PFS: 6.0 months Median OS: 12.4 months
				Gemcitabine + Cisplatin + Placebo	Median PFS: 5.5 months Median OS: 12.5 months

Vandetanib	Herbst et al. (38)	Second line, Stage IIIB or IV/Phase III	PO	Vandetanib + Docetaxel	Median PFS: 4.0 months Median OS: 10.3 months
				Docetaxel	Median PFS: 3.2 months Median OS: 9.9 months
	De Boer et al. (39)	Second line, Stage IIIB or IV/Phase III		Vandetanib + Pemetrexed	Median PFS: 4.4 months Median OS: 10.5 months
				Pemetrexed	Median PFS: 3.0 months Median OS: 9.2 months
	Natale et al. (40)	Second line, Stage IIIB or IV/Phase III		Vandetanib	Median PFS: 2.6 months Median OS: 6.8 months
				Erlotinib	Median PFS: 2.0 months Median OS: 7.7 months
	Lee et al. (41)	Second line, Stage IIIB or IV/Phase III		Vandetanib	Median OS: 8.5 months
				Placebo	Median OS: 7.8 months

TTP = time to progression; RR = response rate; ORR = objective response rate; OS = overall survival.

Vandetanib

Vandetanib (Caprelsa, Astrazeneca) is an oral antagonist of VEGFR-1, VEGFR-2, and VEGFR-3 and EGFR. It was approved by FDA in 2011 for treatment of patients with metastatic medullary thyroid cancer that are ineligible for surgery (36). A randomized Phase II study in 160 patients with advanced NSCLC compared the effects of 300 mg of vandetanib and 250 mg of gefitinib oral daily. Vandetanib showed a statistically significant improvement in TTP compared with gefitinib (11.9 and 8.1 weeks, respectively). Based on this study, further Phase III trials were designed (37).

Four Phase III trials, ZEST, ZEAL, ZEPHYR, and ZODIAC, evaluated the use of vandetanib in various settings of NSCLC. ZODIAC and ZEAL were second-line trials that combined docetaxel and pemetrexed, respectively, with vandetinib. ZODIAC study (docetaxel with or without vandetanib) showed a statistically significant PFS and a statistically nonsignificant OS improvement with vandetinib (38). No statistically significant PFS and OS were seen with addition of vandatenib with pemetrexed in the ZEAL study (39). The ZEST trial showed similar PFS and OS when vandetanib was compared with erlotinib (40). ZEPHYR trial compared vandetanib plus best supportive care and best supportive care in patients with locally advanced or metastatic NSCLC after prior therapy with an EGFR inhibitor (41). The trial did not meet its primary endpoint of prolonging OS in these patients. The common side effects of vandetanib include rash, diarrhea, neutropenia, hypertension, and QTc prolongation (42). Because of the disappointing results of these studies, vandetanib is not being developed further for lung cancer treatment.

Cediranib (AZD 2171)

Cediranib inhibits VEGFR-1, VEGFR-2, VEGFR-3, PDGFR-beta, and c-kit. A randomized Phase II/III study (NCIC BR24) compared carboplatin (AUC = 6) and paclitaxel (200 mg/m^2) with or without cediranib as initial chemotherapy for advanced NSCLC (43). Response rates were higher with cediranib (38% versus 16%), but there was significant toxicity even with a reduction in dose of cediranib to 30 mg/day. A follow-up study, NCIC BR29, evaluated a lower dose of cediranib (20 mg QD) in combination with chemotherapy for advanced NSCLC (44).

Pazopanib

Pazopanib, another oral angiogenesis inhibitor that targets VEGFR, PDGFR, and c-Kit, has demonstrated clinical activity as monotherapy in renal cell carcinoma, ovarian cancer, and sarcoma (45,46). A Phase II study evaluated the efficacy of pazopanib monotherapy in patients with operable Stage I/II NSCLC. Patients received pazopanib 800 mg oral daily preoperatively for 2 to 6 weeks. Approximately 86% of patients achieved tumor volume reduction after pazopanib treatment (47). Grade 2 hypertension, diarrhea, and fatigue are the most common side effects associated with pazopanib. This is the first study to demonstrate efficacy and safety of a targeted agent in preoperative setting in early-stage NSCLC.

Linifanib (ABT-869)

Linifanib is a novel, orally active dual inhibitor of VEGF and PDGFR tyrosine kinases and is being investigated in several different cancers. A Phase II trial assessed the activity and safety of linifanib in patients with locally advanced or metastatic NSCLC. Patients who received one or two prior systemic therapy were randomized to linifanib 0.10 mg/kg or 0.25 mg/kg once daily. Primary endpoint was progression free rate at 16 weeks. Secondary endpoints included objective response rate, TTP, PFS, and OS. Results showed that linifanib had an objective response rate of 5.0% (3.1% and 6.8% for low dose and high dose, respectively), progression-free rate at 16 weeks was 33.1% (32.3% and 33.8%), median TTP was 3.6 months (3.6 and

3.7 months), median PFS was 3.6 months (3.5 and 3.6 months), and median OS was 9 months (10.0 and 8.3 months) (48). The most common adverse events with linifanib were diarrhea, hypertension, and fatigue. Hence, linifanib has single-agent activity in advanced NSCLC patients in second- or third-line setting with an acceptable safety profile. It is presently being studied in a randomized study in combination with chemotherapy for first-line therapy of advanced non-squamous NSCLC.

Combined VEGF and EGFR Blockade

Preclinical studies suggest that multiple signaling pathways are dysregulated in tumorigenesis. Hence, combining drugs to target multiple critical molecular pathways is an attractive option. EGFR- and VEGF-dependent angiogenesis pathways play a crucial role in lung cancer, including disease progression. Erlotinib (Tarceva, Genentech) is a selective, reversible EGFR tyrosine kinase inhibitor (49). Preclinical studies demonstrated a favorable interaction when both EGFR and VEGF pathways were blocked simultaneously, compared with either blockade alone. The greater growth inhibition with the combination of these targeted drugs is attributed to the common downstream signaling of the VEGF and EGFR pathways (49). Several preclinical studies in xenograft models demonstrated that the combined inhibition of anti-VEGF and anti-EGFR produced a favorable outcome (49). Hence, a number of trials were designed focusing on the effects of erlotinib in combination with bevacizumab in a wide range of tumors including NSCLC.

A multicenter, Phase II trial randomized patients with refractory and relapsed non-squamous NSCLC to a combination of bevacizumab with erlotinib or bevacizumab with chemotherapy and compared it with chemotherapy alone (9). The trial showed a favorable OS with the combination of bevacizumab and erlotinib. To further assess the combination of bevacizumab with erlotinib, a Phase III trial BeTA randomized 636 patients with advanced NSCLC after failure of standard first-line chemotherapy to a combination of erlotinib at 150 mg oral daily with bevacizumab at 15 mg/kg every 3 weeks or erlotinib plus placebo (2). The study excluded patients with prior bevacizumab therapy. The primary endpoint was the OS. Median PFS was 3.4 months in the bevacizumab arm versus 1.7 months in placebo arm. The trial however failed to meet its primary end point, with similar OS between the two arms (9.3 months for bevacizumabarm versus 9.2 months in placebo arm) (2). The toxicitis of bevacizumab and erlotinib in the study were similar to the known toxicities of individual drugs.

The ATLAS trial (n = 1160) randomized patients with locally advanced, recurrent or metastatic NSCLC to upfront platinum-based chemotherapy with bevacizumab for four cycles. If patients had stable disease, they were randomized to bevacizumab or placebo or a combination of bevacizumb with erlotinib. The study included patients with treated brain metastasis and patients on low–molecular weight heparin. Though the median PFS was 4.8 months in bevacizumab plus erlotinib arm versus 3.7 months for bevacizumab plus placebo arm, there was no improvement in the OS (50). Based on these results, the combined blockade of EGFR and angiogenesis does not appear to be a promising approach for the treatment of lung cancer in an unselected group of patients.

VEGF Trap

Aflibercept is a fusion protein containing VEGFR-1 and VEGFR-2 domains. The advantage of aflibercept over other VEGF inhibitors is that it has a high VEGF-A binding affinity, nearly 1000 times more than bevacizumab, and the ability to bind VEGF-B, and longer half-life (51). Leigh et al. showed that aflibercept had single agent activity in heavily pretreated patients with adenocarcinoma histology, resistant to platinum and erlotinib. It is well tolerated, and the most common adverse effects seen with this drug were hypertension, proteinuria, fatigue, arthralgia, and myalgia. A Phase III trial randomized patients with advanced or metastatic non-squamous NSCLC to aflibercept or placebo in combination with docetaxel in second-line setting. The study failed to meet its primary endpoint of OS. Median OS was 10.4 months in placebo arm and 10 months in aflibercept arm (52).

■ VASCULAR DISRUPTING AGENTS

VDAs cause disruption of existing tumor vasculature, leading to tumor necrosis. VDAs differ in mechanism of action from vascular targeting agents (VTAs) such as angiogenesis inhibitors; VDAs cause collapse of existing solid tumor vasculature, whereas VTAs prevent the formation of new blood vessels and do not target existing vasculature (53). Preclinical models have led to the development of two main classes of VDAs: tubulin polymerization inhibitors such as combretastatin A4 phosphate and the flavonoid class such as flavone acetic acid (FAA) and ASA404 (vadimezan) (54). One of the more promising VDAs in clinical trials in recent years is ASA404.

A Phase II study evaluated the feasibility of adding ASA404 to carboplatin (AUC 6) or paclitaxel 175 mg/m^2 in patients with untreated, advanced NSCLC. Patients were randomized to carboplatin plus paclitaxel or carboplatin plus paclitaxel plus ASA404 1200 mg/m^2. Tumor response rate (31% vs. 22%), median time to tumor progression (5.4 vs. 4.4 months) and median survival (14 vs. 8.8 months) were improved in the ASA404 combination group compared with standard chemotherapy group (55).These outcomes were confirmed in a single-arm evaluation of ASO404 1800 mg/m^2 with same chemotherapy. Median survival was 8.8 months in chemotherapy arm, 14 months in chemotherapy plus ASO 404 1200 mg/m^2 and 14.9 months in chemotherapy plus ASO 404 1800 mg/m^2 (55,56). These encouraging results have led to two Phase III trials: ATTRACT-1 (Antivascular Targeted Therapy: Researching ASA404 in Cancer Treatment) and ATTRACT-2.

ATTRACT-1 trial randomized patients with newly diagnosed advanced NSCLC to carboplatin, paclitaxel, and placebo, or carboplatin, paclitaxel, and ASA404 1800 mg/m^2. There was no difference in OS between the two arms; median OS was 13.4 months for ASO404 and 12.7 months for placebo arm; hence ASAO404 failed to improve outcomes in advanced NSCLC (57). ATTRACT-2 trial randomized patients with newly diagnosed advanced NSCLC to docetaxel with or without ASA404 1800 mg/m^2. The study was terminated after interim analysis showed that the study would not meet its primary endpoint of OS.

ABT-751 is an oral VDA that binds to the colchicine-binding site on B-tubulin, inhibiting polymerization of microtubules. A Phase I/II study of pemetrexed with and without ABT-751 was conducted on patients with recurrent advanced or metastatic NSCLC. Patients received pemetrexed 500 mg/m^2 on day 1 and ABT-751 or placebo on days 1 to 14 of 21-day cycles. PFS was primary endpoint. Median PFS in ABT-751 arm was 2.3 months versus 1.9 months in placebo arm, hence addition of ABT-751 to pemetrexed does not improve outcome in an unselected patient population (58).

■ BIOMARKERS

There is an important need to pursue biomarkers that can reflect the effect of drug and predict response to therapy in clinical practice. The classical endpoints used in clinical trials routinely may not be sufficient to evaluate the biological effects of antiangiogenic drugs (59). Identification of such markers may lead to better planning and interpretation of future studies.

An et al. sought to find blood-based biomarkers that can be used to predict efficacy in advanced and recurrent NSCLC treated with bevacizumab and chemotherapy. Based on the mechanisms of action of bevacizumab, it was hypothesized that plasma VEGF levels can be affected by addition of bevacizumab and predict clinical outcomes (60).

The study showed that VEGF levels decreased with marginal significance at 6 weeks or later, compared with the baseline. OS was improved in the low posttreatment VEGF levels group compared with the high group using the median posttreatment plasma VEGF level as the cutoff point (60). Disorganized expression of adhesion molecules has been observed in a variety of cancers including lung, gastric, breast, head-and-neck, and colorectal cancers. Major adhesion molecules involved in lung cancer include E-cadherin, intercellular adhesion molecule (ICAM)-1 and E-selectin. Gogali et al. showed that ICAM-1 serum levels were significantly elevated in both SCLC and NSCLC (61). Dowlati et al. evaluated VEGF, basic FGF (bFGF), ICAM, and E-selectin within the E4599 randomized trial to determine the prognostic and predictive value of these markers. Pretreatment VEGF, and pretreatment and week 7 bFGF, ICAM, and E-selectin were measured. The study showed that patients with a low baseline ICAM had a higher response rate and better OS than those with high baseline ICAM, irrespective of treatment arm (62). Patients with high VEGF levels were more likely to respond to carboplatin plus paclitaxel plus bevacizumab than to carboplatin and paclitaxel alone. The authors concluded that baseline ICAM levels were prognostic for survival and predictive of response to chemotherapy with or without bevacizumab, and VEGF levels were predictive of response to bevacizumab but not survival.

Circulating endothelial cell (CEC) is a surrogate of angiogenesis, so CEC number may reflect the extent of tumor angiogenesis. Previous studies have shown that CECs increase in lung cancer and decrease following antiangiogenic therapy (63,64). Heymach et al. showed that pazopanib therapy was associated with significant changes of eight cytokine and angiogenic factors in patients with early-stage NSCLC (65). Another study demonstrated that low baseline circulating VEGF may be predictive of PFS in advanced NSCLC receiving vandetanib versus gefitinib or vandetanib plus docetaxel versus docetaxel (66). Polymorphisms in VEGF gene have been identified that may have functional activity. Heist et al. showed that VEGF polymorphisms may affect survival in early-stage lung cancer (67). However, large, independent studies are needed to further investigate polymorphisms in VEGF for their predictive potential.

A number of invasive and noninvasive methods such as tissue biopsy, MVD, and imaging have been studied to accurately monitor the effects of antiangiogenic treatment, but no method so far has been universally validated. In particular, MVD has been indicated as a marker for disease progression and OS (68). However, its utility in evaluating response to antiangiogenic treatment has been disappointing. Future clinical trials of antiangiogenic agents should focus on discovery of new biomarkers and validate the markers already studied.

■ ANTIANGIOGENIC AGENTS IN SMALL CELL LUNG CANCER

Elevated VEGF expression is associated with poor prognosis in small cell lung cancer. Based on this idea, a Phase II trial ECOG 3501 was initiated, which investigated the safety and efficacy of bevacizumab in combination with cisplatin and etoposide in patients with extensive stage small cell lung cancer (ES-SCLC). Patients received cisplatin 60 mg/m^2 and etoposide 120 mg/m^2 with bevacizumab 15 mg/kg (69). Primary endpoint was PFS at 6 months. The study showed that addition of bevacizumab to chemotherapy results in improved favorable PFS and OS. The 6-month PFS was 30.2%, median PFS was 4.7 months, and 1 year OS was 38.1% with combination of bevacizumab to chemotherapy.

A Phase II study CALGB 30306 studied the combination of cisplatin 30 mg/m^2 and irinotecan 65 mg/m^2 on days 1 and 8 plus bevacizumab 15 mg/kg every 3 weeks for four cycles, in untreated ES-NSCLC (70). A higher response rate of 75%, PFS of 7.1 months, and OS of 11.7 months were reported (69,70). These results were followed by a randomized Phase II study to assess the efficacy of bevacizumab with first-line standard chemotherapy in patients with untreated ES-SCLC. Patients were randomized to bevacizumab or placebo with cisplatin or carboplatin plus etoposide for four cycles followed by single-agent bevacizumab or placebo until disease progression or unacceptable toxicity. Primary endpoint was PFS. The study showed a superior PFS in bevacizumab arm compared with that in placebo arm (5.5 months versus 4.4 months, respectively) (71).However, no improvement in OS was observed with bevacizumab.

BR20, a Phase II study, examined whether vandetanib could prolong PFS in SCLC after complete or partial response to induction chemotherapy. The study showed that median PFS for vandetanib and placebo was 2.7 and 2.8 months, respectively (72).OS for vandetanib was 10.6 months versus 11.9 months for placebo. Vandetanib was associated with higher degree of toxicity requiring dose adjustments, primarily gastrointestinal toxicity and rash. Hence, Vandetanib failed to demonstrate efficacy in maintenance setting for SCLC.

A Phase I trial, CALGB 30504, was planned to evaluate the dose of sunitinib that can be safely combined with cisplatin and etoposide in ES-SCLC patients. The study showed that sunitinib 25 mg/day on days 1 to 14 in combination with standard cisplatin and etoposide caused high treatment-related mortality, and hence it is not recommended (73).A Phase II trial analyzed the safety and efficacy of cediranib in previously treated SCLC with platinum-based regimen. Patients received cediranib 45 mg oral daily; however, the dose was reduced to 30 mg subsequently secondary to side effects. Cediranib failed to demonstrate any objective responses in refractory or recurrent SCLC at 30-mg or 45-mg dose (74). Taken together, the efficacy of antiangiogenic agents is unproven in patients with SCLC.

■ CONCLUSIONS

Antiangiogenic therapy has demonstrated modest benefits in patients with NSCLC. Bevacizumab is the only agent to gain approval by the FDA among the class of these drugs. While bevacizumab does not cause objective responses when used as monotherapy, several VEGF TKIs have demonstrated response rates of 7% to 10%. However, they have not been easy to combine with chemotherapy or have not led to improved survival when used in combination with chemotherapy. The inability to develop predictive biomarkers has been a stumbling block for continued evaluation of antiangiogenic agents in NSCLC patients. Given that the target is the host, responses in the host occur regardless of antitumor effects in patients treated with antiangiogenic therapy. This has been the major impediment to biomarker discovery.

A number of novel agents with distinct mechanisms of action are still under development for NSCLC. This includes the humanized monoclonal antibodies IMC-1121B (Ramucirumab), which targets VEGFR-2, and IMC-18F1, which targets VEGFR-1 (75). It remains to be seen if these agents will exert greater biological and clinical efficacy. An ongoing study will determine the addition of antiangiogenic therapy to patients with surgically resected early-stage NSCLC (ECOG 1505). Another area of investigation that might prove useful involves the combination of antiangiogenic therapy with other molecularly targeted agents. In addition, a greater understanding of the escape pathways that are activated in response to VEGF inhibition could lead to novel combination regimens.

■ REFERENCES

1. Jemal A, Siegel R, Xu J, Ward E. Cancer statistics 2010. *CA Cancer J Clin*. 2010;60(5):277–300.
2. Herbst RS, Ansari R, Bustin F, et al. Efficacy of bevacizumab plus erlotinib versus erlotinib alone in advanced non-small-cell lung cancer after failure of standard first-line chemotherapy (BeTa): A double-blind, placebo-controlled, phase 3 trial. *Lancet*. 2011;377(9780):1846–1854.
3. Quoix E, Westeel V, Zalcman G, Milleron B. Chemotherapy in elderly patients with advanced

non-small cell lung cancer. *Lung Cancer*, 2011;74(3):364–368.
4. Herbst RS, Heymach JV, Lippman SM. Lung cancer. *N Engl J Med*. 2008;359(13):1367–1380.
5. Davidoff AJ, Tang M, Seal B. Chemotherapy and survival benefit in elderly patients with advanced non-small-cell lung cancer. *J Clin Oncol*. 2010;28(13):2191–2197.
6. Owonikoko TK and Ramalingam S. The role of targeted agents in the treatment of elderly patients with non-small cell lung cancer (NSCLC). *Curr Treat Options Oncol*. 2008;9(4–6):313–325.
7. Rami-Porta R, Ball D, Crowley J, et al. The IASLC Lung Cancer Staging Project: Proposals for the revision of the T descriptors in the forthcoming (seventh) edition of the TNM classification for lung cancer. *J Thorac Oncol*. 2007;2(7):593–602.
8. Ramalingam SS and Belani CP. Antiangiogenic agents in the treatment of nonsmall cell lung cancer: Reality and hope. *Curr Opin Oncol*. 2010; 22(2):79–85.
9. Herbst RS, O'Neill VJ, Fehrenbacher L, et al. Phase II study of efficacy and safety of bevacizumab in combination with chemotherapy or erlotinib compared with chemotherapy alone for treatment of recurrent or refractory non small-cell lung cancer. *J Clin Oncol*. 2007; 25(30):4743–4750.
10. Rossi A, Maione P, Sacco P, et al. Vascular endothelial growth factor receptor as target for advanced non-small cell lung cancer therapy. *Curr Drug Targets*. 2010; 11(7):865–8784.
11. Moreira IS, Fernandes PA, and Ramos MJ. Vascular endothelial growth factor (VEGF) inhibition—A critical review. *Anticancer Agents Med Chem*. 2007;7(2):223–245.
12. Folkman J. What is the evidence that tumors are angiogenesis dependent? *J Natl Cancer Inst*. 1990;82(1):4–6.
13. Midgley R, Kerr D. Bevacizumab—current status and future directions. *Ann Oncol*. 2005;16(7): 999–1004.
14. Ellis LM and Hicklin DJ. VEGF-targeted therapy: Mechanisms of anti-tumour activity. *Nat Rev Cancer*. 2008;8(8):579–591.
15. Gressett SM, Shah SR. Intricacies of bevacizumab-induced toxicities and their management. *Ann Pharmacother*. 2009;43(3):490–501.
16. Ferrara N, Gerber HP, and LeCouter J. The biology of VEGF and its receptors. *Nat Med*. 2003; 9(6):669–676.
17. Gerber HP and Ferrara N. Pharmacology and pharmacodynamics of bevacizumab as monotherapy or in combination with cytotoxic therapy in preclinical studies. *Cancer Res*. 2005;65(3):671–680.
18. Guo X, Chen Y, Xu Z, et al. Prognostic significance of VEGF-C expression in correlation with COX-2, lymphatic microvessel density, and clinicopathologic characteristics in human non-small cell lung cancer. *Acta Biochim Biophys Sin*. 2009;41(3):217–222.
19. Sandler AB, Johnson DH, and Herbst RS. Anti-vascular endothelial growth factor monoclonals in non-small cell lung cancer. *Clin Cancer Res*. 2004;10(12 Pt 2):4258s–4262s.
20. Presta LG, Chen H, O'Connor SJ, et al. Humanization of an anti-vascular endothelial growth factor monoclonal antibody for the therapy of solid tumors and other disorders. *Cancer Res*. 1997;57(20):4593–4599.
21. Shih T, Lindley C. Bevacizumab: An angiogenesis inhibitor for the treatment of solid malignancies. *Clin Ther*. 2006;28(11):1779–1802.
22. Johnson DH, Fehrenbacher L, Novotny WF, et al. Randomized phase II trial comparing bevacizumab plus carboplatin and paclitaxel with carboplatin and paclitaxel alone in previously untreated locally advanced or metastatic non-small-cell lung cancer. *J Clin Oncol*. 2004;22(11):2184–2191.
23. Sandler A, Gray R, Perry MC, et al. Paclitaxel-carboplatin alone or with bevacizumab for non-small-cell lung cancer. *N Engl J Med*. 2006;355(24):2542–2550.
24. Cohen MH, Gootenberg J, Keegan P. FDA drug approval summary: Bevacizumab (Avastin) plus Carboplatin and Paclitaxel as first-line treatment of advanced/metastatic recurrent non-squamous non-small cell lung cancer. *Oncologist*, 2007;12(6):713–718.
25. Reck M, von Pawel J, Zatloukal P, et al. Phase III trial of cisplatin plus gemcitabine with either placebo or bevacizumab as first-line therapy for nonsquamous non-small-cell lung cancer: AVAIL. *J Clin Oncol*. 2009;27(8): 1227–1234.

26. Socinski MA, Langer CJ, Huang JE, et al. Safety of bevacizumab in patients with non-small-cell lung cancer and brain metastases. *J Clin Oncol.* 2009;27(31):5255–5261.
27. Spigel DR, Hainsworth JD, Yardley DA, et al. Tracheoesophageal fistula formation in patients with lung cancer treated with chemoradiation and bevacizumab. *J Clin Oncol.* 2010;28(1): 43–48.
28. Goodgame B, Veeramachaneni N, Patterson A, et al. Tracheo-esophageal fistula with bevacizumab after mediastinal radiation. *J Thorac Oncol.* 2008;3(9):1080–1081.
29. Socinski MA, Scappaticci FA, Samant M, et al. Safety and efficacy of combining sunitinib with bevacizumab + paclitaxel/carboplatin in non-small cell lung cancer. *J Thorac Oncol.* 2010;5(3): 354–360.
30. Socinski MA, Novello S, Brahmer JR, et al. Multicenter, phase II trial of sunitinib in previously treated, advanced non-small-cell lung cancer. *J Clin Oncol.* 2008;26(4):650–656.
31. Scagliotti G, Krakowski M, Szczesna A, et al. Sunitinib (SU) in combination with erlotinib (E) for the treatment of advanced/metastatic non-small cell lung cancer (NSCLC) a phase III study. *ESMO (European Society for Medical Oncology).* 2010.
32. Scagliotti G, Novello S, von Pawel J, et al. Phase III study of carboplatin and paclitaxel alone or with sorafenib in advanced non-small-cell lung cancer. *J Clin Oncol.* 2010;28(11):1835–1842.
33. Blumenschein GR, Jr., Gatzemeier U, Fossella F, et al. Phase II, multicenter, uncontrolled trial of single-agent sorafenib in patients with relapsed or refractory, advanced non-small-cell lung cancer. *J Clin Oncol.* 2009;27(26):4274–4280.
34. Schiller JH, Lee JW, Hanna NH, Traynor AM, Carbone DP. A randomized discontinuation phase II study of sorafenib versus placebo in patients with non-small cell lung cancer who have failed at least two prior chemotherapy regimens: E2501. *J Clin Oncol.* 2008;26(May 20 suppl): abstr 8014.
35. Gatzmeier U, Eisen T, Santoro A, et al. Sorafenib + Gemcitabine/cisplatin (GC) vs GC alone in the first-line treatment of advanced non-small cell lung cancer: Phase III NSCLC research experience utilizing sorafenib. Nexus trial. *Ann Oncol.* 2010;21:viii7, LBA no. 15, 2010.
36. Commander H, Whiteside G, Perry C. Vandetanib: First global approval. *Drugs.* 2011; 71(10):1355–1365.
37. Natale RB, Bodkin D, Govindan R, et al. Vandetanib versus gefitinib in patients with advanced non-small-cell lung cancer: Results from a two-part, double-blind, randomized phase ii study. *J Clin Oncol.* 2009;27(15):2523–2529.
38. Herbst RS, Sun Y., Korfee S, et al. Vandetanib plus docetaxel versus docetaxel as second-line treatment for patients with advanced non-small cell lung cancer (NSCLC): A randomized, double-blind phase III trial (ZODIAC). *J Clin Oncol.* 2009;27(suppl; abstr CRA8003):18s.
39. De Boer R, Arrieta Ó, Gottfried M, et al. Vandetanib plus pemetrexed versus pemetrexed as second-line therapy in patients with advanced non-small cell lung cancer (NSCLC): A randomized, double-blind phase III trial (ZEAL). *J Clin Oncol.* 2009;27(15s):suppl, abstr 8010.
40. Natale RB, Thongprasert S, Greco FA, et al. Vandetanib versus erlotinib in patients with advanced non-small cell lung cancer (NSCLC) after failure of at least one prior cytotoxic chemotherapy: A randomized, double-blind phase III trial (ZEST). *J Clin Oncol.* 2009;27(15s):suppl, abstr 8009.
41. Lee J, Hirsh V, Park K, et al. Vandetanib versus placebo in patients with advanced non-small cell lung cancer (NSCLC) after prior therapy with an EGFR tyrosine kinase inhibitor (TKI): A randomized, double-blind phase III trial (ZEPHYR). *J Clin Oncol.* 2010;28(15s):suppl, abstr 7525.
42. Herbst RS., Toxicities of antiangiogenic therapy in non-small-cell lung cancer. *Clin Lung Cancer.* 2006;8(1):S23–S30.
43. Goss GD, Arnold A, Shepherd FA, et al. Randomized, double-blind trial of carboplatin and paclitaxel with either daily oral cediranib or placebo in advanced non-small-cell lung cancer: NCIC clinical trials group BR24 study. *J Clin Oncol.* 2010;28(1):49–55.
44. Laurie et al. A Double Blind Randomized Trial of Cediranib Versus Placebo in Patients Receiving

Paclitaxel/Carboplatin Chemotherapy for the Treatment of Advanced or Metastatic Non-Small Cell Lung Cancer (NCIC BR29).

45. Melichar B, Studentova H, Zezulova M. Pazopanib: A new multiple tyrosine kinase inhibitor in the therapy of metastatic renal cell carcinoma and other solid tumors. *J Buon*. 2011; 16(2):203–209.
46. Burger RA. Overview of anti-angiogenic agents in development for ovarian cancer. *Gynecol Oncol*. 2011; 121(1):230–238.
47. Altorki N, Lane ME, Bauer T, et al. Phase II proof-of-concept study of pazopanib monotherapy in treatment-naive patients with stage I/II resectable non-small-celllungcancer. *JClinOncol*. 2010;28(19): 3131–3137.
48. Tan EH, Goss GD, Salgia R, et al. Phase 2 trial of Linifanib (ABT-869) in patients with advanced non-small cell lung cancer. *J Thorac Oncol*. 2011;6(8):1418–1425.
49. Sandler A, Herbst R. Combining targeted agents: Blocking the epidermal growth factor and vascular endothelial growth factor pathways. *Clin Cancer Res*. 2006;12(14 Pt 2):4421s–4425s.
50. Miller VA, O'Connor P, Soh C, Kabbinavar F. A randomized, double-blind, placebo-controlled, phase IIIb trial (ATLAS) comparing bevacizumab (B) therapy with or without erlotinib (E) after completion of chemotherapy with B for first-line treatment of locally advanced, recurrent, or metastatic non-small cell lung cancer (NSCLC). *J Clin Oncol*. 2009;27(18s):suppl, abstr LBA8002.
51. Leighl NB, Raez LE, Besse B, et al. A multicenter, phase 2 study of vascular endothelial growth factor trap (Aflibercept) in platinum- and erlotinib-resistant adenocarcinoma of the lung. *J Thorac Oncol*. 2010;5(7):1054–1059.
52. Novello S, Ramlau R, Gorbunova VA, et al. Aflibercept in combination with docetaxel for second-line treatment of locally advanced or metastatic non small cell lung cancer (NSCLC): Final results of a multinational placebo-controlled phase III trial (EFC10261-VITAL). Abstract associated with oral presentation at: *The 14th Biennial World Conference on Lung Cancer*, July 3-7, 2011; Amsterdam, The Netherlands.
53. Thorpe PE. Vascular targeting agents as cancer therapeutics. *Clin Cancer Res*. 2004;10(2):415–427.
54. Baguley BC. Preclinical efficacy of vascular disrupting agents in non-small-cell lung cancer. *Clin Lung Cancer*. 2011. 12(2):81–86.
55. McKeage MJ, Von Pawel J, Reck M, et al. Randomised phase II study of ASA404 combined with carboplatin and paclitaxel in previously untreated advanced non-small cell lung cancer. *Br J Cancer*. 2008; 99(12):2006–2012.
56. McKeage MJ, Reck M, Jameson MB, et al. Phase II study of ASA404 (vadimezan, 5,6-dimethylxanthenone-4-acetic acid/DMXAA) 1800mg/m(2) combined with carboplatin and paclitaxel in previously untreated advanced non-small cell lung cancer. *Lung Cancer*. 2009; 65(2):192–197.
57. Lara PN, Jr., Douillard JY, Nakagawa K, et al. Randomized phase III placebo-controlled trial of carboplatin and paclitaxel with or without the vascular disrupting agent vadimezan (ASA404) in advanced non-small-cell lung cancer. *J Clin Oncol*. 2011; 29(22):2965–2971.
58. Rudin CM, Mauer A, Smakal M, et al. Phase I/II study of pemetrexed with or without ABT-751 in advanced or metastatic non-small-cell lung cancer. *J Clin Oncol*. 2011; 29(8):1075–1082.
59. Ruegg C, Meuwly JY, Driscoll R, et al. The quest for surrogate markers of angiogenesis: A paradigm for translational research in tumor angiogenesis and anti-angiogenesis trials. *Curr Mol Med*. 2003; 3(8):673–691.
60. An SJ, Huang YS, Chen ZH, et al. Posttreatment plasma VEGF levels may be associated with the overall survival of patients with advanced non-small cell lung cancer treated with bevacizumab plus chemotherapy. *Med Oncol*. 2011.[Epub ahead of print]
61. Gogali A, Charalabopoulos K, Zampira I, et al. Soluble adhesion molecules E-cadherin, intercellular adhesion molecule-1, and E-selectin as lung cancer biomarkers. *Chest*. 2010; 138(5): 1173–1179.
62. Dowlati A, Gray R, Sandler AB, et al. Cell adhesion molecules, vascular endothelial growth factor, and basic fibroblast growth factor in patients with non-smallcelllungcancertreatedwithchemotherapywith or without bevacizumab—an Eastern Cooperative Oncology Group Study. *Clin Cancer Res*. 2008; 14(5):1407–1412.

63. Kawaishi M, Fujiwara Y, Fukui T, et al. Circulating endothelial cells in non-small cell lung cancer patients treated with carboplatin and paclitaxel. *J Thorac Oncol.* 2009;4(2):208–213.
64. Morita R, Sato K, Nakano M, et al. Endothelial progenitor cells are associated with response to chemotherapy in human non-small-cell lung cancer. *J Cancer Res Clin Oncol.* 2011; 17:17.
65. Nikolinakos PG, Altorki N, Yankelevitz D, et al. Plasma cytokine and angiogenic factor profiling identifies markers associated with tumor shrinkage in early-stage non-small cell lung cancer patients treated with pazopanib. *Cancer Res.* 2010;70(6):2171–2179.
66. Hanrahan EO, Ryan AJ, Mann H, et al. Baseline vascular endothelial growth factor concentration as a potential predictive marker of benefit from vandetanib in non-small cell lung cancer. *Clin Cancer Res.* 2009;15(10):3600–3609.
67. Heist RS, Zhai R, Liu G, et al. VEGF polymorphisms and survival in early-stage non-small-cell lung cancer. *J Clin Oncol.* 2008;26(6):856–862.
68. Brown AP, Citrin DE, Camphausen KA, Clinical biomarkers of angiogenesis inhibition. *Cancer Metastasis Rev.* 2008; 27(3):415–434.
69. Horn L, Dahlberg SE, Sandler AB, et al. Phase II study of cisplatin plus etoposide and bevacizumab for previously untreated, extensive-stage small-cell lung cancer: Eastern Cooperative Oncology Group Study E3501. *J Clin Oncol.* 2009;27(35):6006–6011.
70. Ready N, Dudek AZ, Wang XF, Graziano S, Green MR, Vokes EE, CALGB 30306: A phase II study of cisplatin (C), irinotecan (I) and bevacizumab (B) for untreated extensive stage small cell lung cancer (ES-SCLC). *J Clin Oncol.* 2007;25(18S): 7563.
71. Spigel DR, Townley PM, Waterhouse DM, et al. Randomized phase II study of bevacizumab in combination with chemotherapy in previously untreated extensive-stage small-cell lung cancer: Results from the SALUTE trial. *J Clin Oncol.* 2011;29(16):2215–2222.
72. Arnold AM, Seymour L, Smylie M, et al. Phase II study of vandetanib or placebo in small-cell lung cancer patients after complete or partial response to induction chemotherapy with or without radiation therapy: National Cancer Institute of Canada Clinical Trials Group Study BR.20. *J Clin Oncol.* 2007;25(27):4278–4284.
73. Ready N, Dunphy F, Pang H, Heinze R, Crawford R, Vokes EE. Combination chemotherapy with sunitinib (IND 74019; NSC 736511) for untreated extensive-stage small cell lung cancer (SCLC): CALGB 30504 phase IB safety results. 2010 ASCO Annual Meeting, 2010. *J Clin Oncol.* 2010;28(5s):suppl, abstr 7056.
74. Ramalingam SS, Belani CP, Mack PC, et al. Phase II study of Cediranib (AZD 2171), an inhibitor of the vascular endothelial growth factor receptor, for second-line therapy of small cell lung cancer (National Cancer Institute #7097). *J Thorac Oncol.* 2010;5(8):1279–1284.
75. Clement-Duchene C, Wakelee H. Antiangiogenic agents and vascular disrupting agents for the treatment of lung cancer: A review. *J Thorac Oncol.* 2010;5(1):129–139.
76. Pallis AG, Serfass L, Dziadziusko R, et al. Targeted therapies in the treatment of advanced/metastatic NSCLC. *Eur J Cancer.* 2009;45(14):2473–2487.
77. Reinmuth N, Thomas M, Meister M, et al. Current data on predictive markers for anti-angiogenic therapy in thoracic tumours. *Eur Respir J.* 2010;36(4):915–924.
78. Scagliotti G, Vynnychenko I,, Ichinose Y, et al. An international, randomized, placebo-controlled, double-blind phase III study (MONET1) of motesanib plus carboplatin/paclitaxel (C/P) in patients with advanced nonsquamous non-small cell lung cancer (NSCLC). *J Clin Oncol.* 2011;29:suppl, abstr LBA7512.
79. Govindan R, Krzakowski M, Szczesna A, et al. Sunitinib in Combination with Erlotinib for the Treatment of Advanced/Metastatic Non-Small cell Lung Cancer (NSCLC): A Phase III Study. *Eur Soc Med Oncol.* (ESMO), 2010.

Emerging Novel Targeted Agents for Lung Cancer

Rathi N. Pillai and Taofeek K. Owonikoko*

Department of Hematology and Medical Oncology, Emory University, Atlanta, GA

ABSTRACT

Lung cancer has evolved from an incurable, uniformly fatal disease to a disease where competing therapeutic options offer clinical benefit for an increasing proportion of the patients. While recent observations showed that tumor histology may assist in optimizing patient care, the use of cytotoxic agents in unselected patients is no longer a winning strategy for the future. Exciting findings from basic research of lung cancer have now led to the emergence of aberrant genetic and molecular changes that present valid target that can be exploited for clinical benefit in patients. This chapter focuses on the emergence of echinoderm microtubule-associated protein-like 4-translocated lung cancer and anaplastic lymphoma kinase-translocated lung cancer and the promise of new generation of HSP90 inhibitors as examples of the recent advances in lung cancer therapeutics and a model for the future evolution of novel therapies in this disease.

Keywords: lung cancer, EML4–ALK, heat shock protein, crizotinib, ganetespib

INTRODUCTION

Lung cancer remains the most common and highly fatal cancer encountered in the United States. (1). The lack of a validated and effective screening strategy until very recently meant that the majority of cases present with advanced disease at diagnosis. Platinum-based doublet regimen was established in the last decade as the bedrock of systemic therapy. This regimen provided the foundation to incorporate newer agents such as bevacizumab and cetuximab as a means of improving efficacy outcomes (2). Improved understanding of the biology and pathogenesis of lung cancer has led to the identification of an increasing number of signaling pathways whose alteration serves as key driver events and, therefore, presents potential targets for novel therapeutic agents. This review provides an overview of emerging and newly established treatment strategies in lung cancer with particular emphasis on patients harboring the anaplastic lymphoma

*Corresponding author, Department of Hematology and Medical Oncology, Emory University, 1365 Clifton Road NE, Rm C-3080, Atlanta, GA 30322

E-mail address: towonik@emory.edu

Emerging Cancer Therapeutics 3:1 (2012) 65–72.

DOI: 10.5003/2151–4194.3.1.65

kinase (ALK) and the echinoderm microtubule-associated protein-like 4 (EML4) translocation.

■ ALK-REARRANGEMENT AS A THERAPEUTIC TARGET IN NON-SMALL CELL LUNG CANCER

The chromosomal translocation involving the ALK and the EML4 genes was first described in 2007 as a driver molecular aberration in lung adenocarcinoma (3). This translocation results in an inversion of the short arm of chromosome 2, fusing the N-terminal domain of EML4 to the intracellular kinase domain of ALK, resulting in a constitutively active kinase. EML4–ALK activity modulates many downstream pathways, which mediate cell proliferation and cell survival, including the PI3K/Akt and Ras/Mek/Erk pathways (Figure 1) (4). The transforming activity of this fusion protein was demonstrated using both tumor xenograft and transgenic mouse models (3,5). Furthermore, ALK mutation has been shown to be mutually exclusive of both epidermal growth factor receptor (EGFR) and KRAS mutations (6–8).

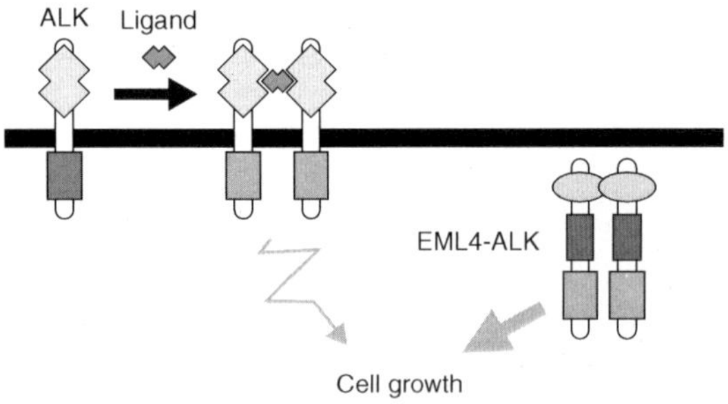

FIGURE 1
Activation mechanisms for EML4–ALK.
Wild-type ALK undergoes transient homodimerization in response to specific ligand receptor binding, which results in activation and downstream mitogenic signal transduction. Constitutively oligomerized EML4–ALK via the coiled coil domain of EML4 results in persistent mitogenic signaling and malignant transformation.
Source: Adapted from Ref. (28).

The EML4–ALK translocation has been described in up to 7% of non-small cell lung cancer (NSCLC) patients. ALK-rearranged NSCLC occurs more frequently in patients with history of never having used tobacco or light smokers defined as less than 10 pack years (9). This is similar to patients with EGFR mutations. However, unlike the female predominance seen in EGFR-mutated lung cancer, patients with EML4–ALK translocation tend to be male (58%) versus only 26% in EGFR patients. Also, patients with EML4–ALK fusion protein tend to be younger than the general population of lung cancer patients, with a median age of 52 years compared with 66 years in EGFR-mutated lung cancer and 64 years in wild-type group (6). Similar to other driver genetic and molecular aberrations described in NSCLC, EML4–ALK translocations occur more commonly in adenocarcinomas (10,11). Depending on the population studied, such tumors tend to have unique histology. For instance, a review of patients with EML4–ALK-translocated tumors in a U.S. lung cancer population found that 60% of tumors have sheet-like pattern, and 82% have signet-ring cell appearance (6,8). In contrast, ALK-positive tumors in Asian patients tend to have acinar pattern of growth (65%) with mucin production (7).

Shortly after the initial characterization of the EML4–ALK translocation, a small molecule inhibitor PF-02341066, which acts as a competitive inhibitor at the adenosine triphosphate (ATP) binding site of tyrosine kinases, was found to be active against the ALK fusion protein in cell lines (12). This compound, later named crizotinib, was subsequently tested in a multicenter Phase I study enriched for ALK-translocated tumors (13). The dose escalation phase employed broad solid tumor patient population with treatment-refractory disease to define toxicities and maximum tolerated dose of the compound. Subsequently, an expansion cohort exclusively made up of patients with ALK-rearranged lung cancer identified by fluorescence in situ hybridization (FISH) testing was treated at the recommended Phase 2 dose of 250 mg BID. The demographics of the 82-patient expansion cohort were similar to other ALK-positive cohorts: 96% adenocarcinomas, younger age patients with median age 51 years, and 94% never or light smokers. Although it was a heavily pretreated group as 79 patients (94%) had received prior therapy, the overall response rate was 57% (47 of 82 patients) with mean duration of therapy of 6.4 months, and estimated progression-free survival (PFS) at 6 months was 72%. The treatment was well tolerated with notable adverse events being Grade 1 or 2 nausea and diarrhea as well as transient visual disturbances such as flashing or trailing lights following moving objects, floaters, or blurry vision with light adaptation. The visual disturbance started at a median of 2 weeks into treatment and usually resolved with continued therapy. This Phase I study demonstrated the safety of crizotinib and confirmed that interrupting aberrant ALK signaling with a small molecule inhibitor could result in clinical benefit. An updated report from a total of 119 patients enrolled on the study was presented at the 2011 American Society of Clinical Oncology annual meeting (14). Out of 116 patients evaluable for response, the overall response was 61% (71 of 116 patients) including 2 patients with complete response after a median follow-up period of 11 months. The median time to response and median duration of response were 8 and 48 weeks, respectively, while the median PFS was 10 months (95% confidence interval [CI]: 8.2–14.7).

Based on the promising results seen in Phase I setting, a number of confirmatory Phase II and Phase III studies were initiated to better define the efficacy of crizotinib. PROFILE 1005 is a Phase II study of crizotinib in patients with advanced NSCLC with disease progression after prior chemotherapy (15). The study enrolled a total of 136 patients to receive crizotinib 250 mg BID continuously until disease progression. During interim analysis, 88% of patients remained on therapy with median treatment duration of 9 weeks, and objective tumor shrinkage was reported in 83% of patients. The adverse event profile mirrored the experience in Phase I setting with the most frequently reported events being nausea (46%), vomiting (39%), and diarrhea (29%) and visual (45%) disturbances. There were nine deaths including two that were deemed treatment-related. The impressive clinical benefit observed in these early phase trials led to an expedited approval by the U.S. Food and Drug Administration (FDA) for crizotinib for the treatment of patients with locally advanced or metastatic NSCLC, whose tumor harbors the ALK rearrangement as determined by break-apart FISH probe.

It is noteworthy that despite the impressive objective response with crizotinib and the expedited FDA approval, definitive evidence for an overall survival benefit remains to be proven in a prospective fashion. A recent retrospective analysis reported on the survival of patients with ALK-translocated tumors treated with crizotinib compared with ALK-positive control patients that did not receive crizotinib as well as ALK-negative and EGRR mutation-positive patients treated with EGFR tyrosine kinase inhibitors (16). Among 82 ALK-positive patients treated with crizotinib, median overall survival from the time of initiation of crizotinib had not been reached at the time of reporting (95% CI: 17 months to not reached) with 1-year and 2-year overall survival rates of 74% (95% CI: 63–82) and 54% (95% CI: 40–66). This survival outcome was not impacted by age, gender, or ethnicity. ALK-positive patients treated with crizotinib had a superior survival outcome compared with those treated with other agents: 1-year and 2-year overall survival of 70% (95% CI: 50–83) versus 44% (CI: 23–64), and 55% (CI: 33–72) versus 12% (CI: 2–30); hazard ratio, 0.36; 95% CI: 0.17 to 0.75; $P = .004$. The survival in ALK-positive patients who did not receive crizotinib was similar to that in 253 patients without ALK translocation (median overall survival 20 months [95% CI: 13–26] vs. 15 months [CI: 13–17]; $P = 0.244$) suggesting that ALK translocation did not confer any prognostic benefit. Although this analysis suggests that crizotinib therapy is associated with a survival benefit in patients with ALK-rearranged NSCLC, definitive evidence is awaited from ongoing prospective studies of crizotinib.

Development of resistance is a well-recognized setback when biologically targeted agents are introduced into the clinic as witnessed with erlotinib and gefitinib in NSCLC as well as imatinib in chronic myelogenous leukemia. Not surprising therefore, resistance to crizotinib has been described both under experimental laboratory condition as well as in the clinic in patients receiving crizotinib. Two gatekeeper mutations, C1156Y and L1196M, similar to the T315 mutation in BCR-ABL and the T790M gatekeeper mutation in EGFR, were described in a patient who developed resistance to therapy approximately 6 months into his treatment with crizotinib (17). Protein crystal structure analysis showed that both of these mutations are located close to the ATP-binding pocket of the kinase domain of the ALK enzyme, thereby interfering with the binding of the inhibitor to the tyrosine kinase. Similarly, an in vitro model of acquired resistance to crizotinib using continuous exposure of a highly sensitive EML4–ALK-positive NSCLC cell line to crizotinib until the emergence of resistance revealed two mechanisms of resistance. There was gene amplification involving the EML4–ALK gene in cells exposed to intermediate concentrations of crizotinib, and the L1196M gatekeeper mutation was detected in cells resistant to higher drug concentration (18). Intriguingly, two structurally different ALK inhibitors, NVP-TAE684 and AP26113, retained activity against the resistant cells in vitro and in vivo, thus indicating potential use of these agents in patients who are resistant to crizotinib. Furthermore, the fortuitous observation that 17-AAG, a geldanamycin Hsp90 inhibitor, was also active against the crizotinib-resistant cell lines provided further preclinical support for the clinical efficacy of the new generation, non-geldanamycin heat shock protein (HSP) inhibitors against ALK-translocated NSCLC (18).

Other small molecule inhibitors are currently in various stages of preclinical and clinical evaluation including CH5424802, which is unaffected by the L1196M gatekeeper mutation since its kinase-binding mechanism is dissimilar to that of crizotinib (19). X-376 and X-396 are potent ALK inhibitors from Xcovery pharmaceuticals with a 10-fold greater specific binding to the ALK kinase domain compared with crizotinib (20). These agents also displayed greater in vitro and in vivo potency than crizotinib against parental and resistant cell lines. While crizotinib is the established therapy for the ALK-positive subset of lung cancer, treatment strategies continue to evolve due to the emergence of acquired resistance to this agent and the need to further improve the clinical outcome of these patients in the future.

■ HEAT SHOCK PROTEIN (HSP) INHIBITORS IN LUNG CANCER

HSPs are chaperone proteins that play a central role in the regulation of protein folding to ensure accurate conformation and intracellular trafficking while preventing protein aggregation. Excessive accumulation of HSPs is known to accompany malignant transformation leading to a reduced efficiency of the cells to degrade oncogenic proteins. Many tumors show increased levels of HSPs, which promote cell survival, growth, and metastasis (21,22). Inhibition of different components of the HSP machinery as an anticancer treatment strategy is predicated on the expected degradation of these oncogenic proteins such as signal transducers, receptors, and growth factors.

Hsp90 is one of the important members of this family of chaperone proteins that act to stabilize a wide variety of intracellular client proteins. HSP90 is a constitutively expressed protein with five different isoforms. It binds to client proteins in cooperation with another chaperone, HSP70 and its cofactor HSP40. An adapter protein known as HSP organizing protein (HOP) binds through its small helical tetratricopeptide repeat (TPR) domains to link HSP90 and HSP70. The ATPase activity of HPS90 is stimulated by a cofactor, Aha1 leading to a conformational change that dissociates ADP from the HSP70/HSP40/HOP complex, thereby allowing ATP-dependent interaction with other members of the multiprotein complex such as CDC37 and p23 in order to form a mature complex (Figure 2). The mature complex prevents client protein degradation, thereby ensuring their maturation and activation under various states of cellular stresses. HSP90 inhibitors prevent mature complex formation by inhibiting ATP-binding, thereby causing a shortened half-life of the multichaperone protein complex and consequently rapid degradation of the oncogenic proteins by the proteasome machinery (23).

The initial attempt to exploit this dependence of cancer cells on HSP function met with little success due to poor pharmacological properties of the lead compounds derived from geldanamycin (24). More recently, encouraging clinical results are beginning to emerge through the use of improved drug formulation and the development of non-geldanamycin class of HSP90 inhibitors.

IPI-504 (or retaspimycin) is a water-soluble hydrochloride salt of 17-AAG. This agent was evaluated in a Phase II study that enrolled 76 patients with advanced NSCLC previously treated with EGFR TKI therapy (25). While the overall response rate was not impressive at 7% with a median PFS of 2.86 months, there was a very interesting observation in three patients with ALK-rearranged cancer. Two of these three patients achieved partial response and all three remained on study for approximately 7 months.

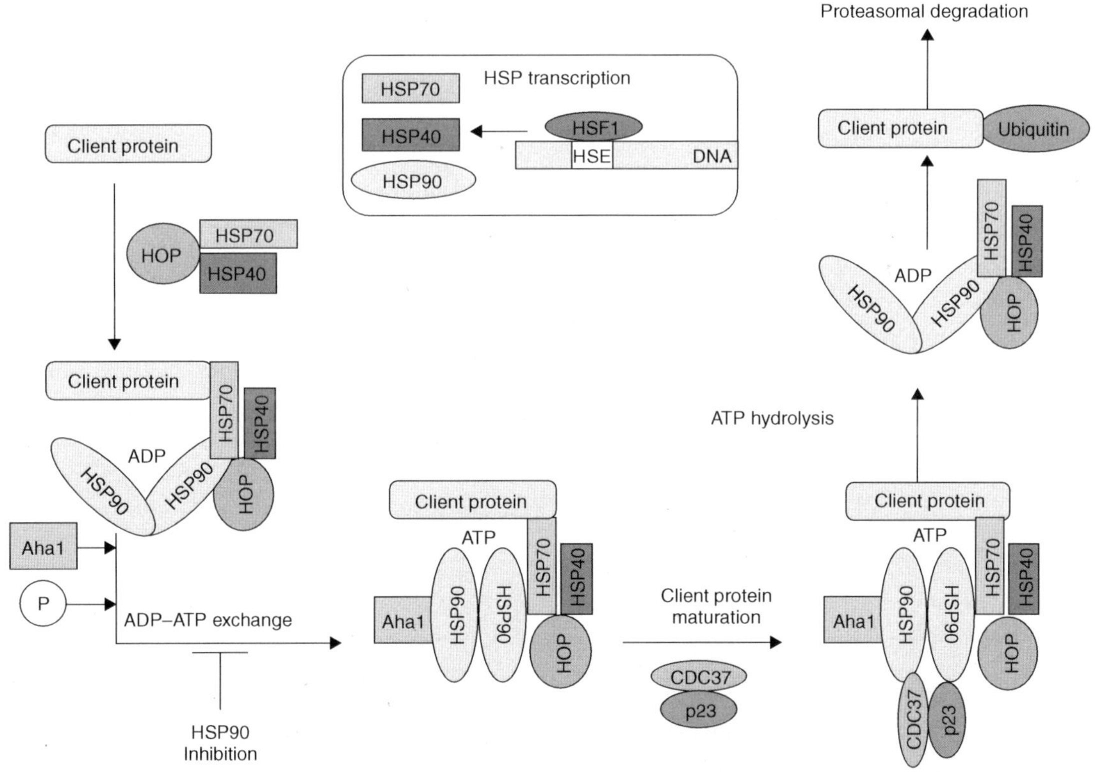

FIGURE 2
Schematic diagram of HSP chaperone function in intracellular trafficking and degradation of client proteins.
Source: Adapted from Ref. (23).

The molecular basis for this interesting observation remains to be fully elucidated. However, the fusion product of the EML4–ALK is an important client protein and undergoes degradation within 3 hours of HSP90 inhibition unlike EGFR protein whose degradation can take as much as 24 hours. IPI-504 was shown to induce a dose-dependent growth inhibition both in H3122 native cells and in crizotinib-resistant derivatives (26). This preclinical and clinical observation informed the design of an ongoing Phase II trial that is investigating the efficacy of IPI-504 in patients with ALK-positive NSCLC [NCT01228435].

Another agent called STA 9090 (or ganetespib) is a potent HSP90 inhibitor that is structurally unrelated to the first-generation ansamycin Hsp90 inhibitors. Ganetespib was evaluated in a biomarker-enriched NSCLC patient population who had failed prior treatments. A total of 76 evaluable patients were enrolled into cohorts of mutant EGFR, mutant KRAS, wild-type EGFR/KRAS, and adenocarcinoma histology of unknown mutational status at the time of enrolment. Consistent with preclinical model prediction, patients with mutant K-Ras demonstrated clinical benefit in terms of disease control. The eight patients with ALK-translocated tumors displayed the most provocative clinical efficacy with 88% achieving disease control lasting at least 16 weeks, 75% showing objective tumor shrinkage, and 50% achieving a confirmed partial response (27). This result will inform future developmental strategies for this compound in lung cancer. Potential population of interest will include KRAS mutant and ALK-translocated tumors.

The improved tolerability observed with IPI-504 and ganetespib along with the promising activity of these agents, especially in patients with ALK-rearranged NSCLC, has solidified HSP90 as a therapeutic target in NSCLC. These agents may offer important therapeutic options in the future for ALK-positive as well as other molecularly defined patient categories, such as K-Ras mutant tumors.

CONCLUSIONS

The era of personalized medicine has firmly taken root in oncology. The field of thoracic oncology has no doubt adopted this paradigm shift to drive the management of lung cancer. The success of tyrosine kinase inhibitors, gefitinib and erlotinib, against mutant EGFR has fueled the discovery of an increasing number of targets. EML4–ALK translocation is the most recently defined subset of patients with NSCLC, but other molecular subsets have been characterized including PIK3CA, Raf, and HER2 driven tumors. Several specific inhibitors of the constitutively active tyrosine kinase activity of this fusion protein are already in clinical testing with crizotinib, the most advanced of these agents, already approved for routine clinical use by the FDA. The development of resistance to ALK-targeted therapy has evolved quite rapidly from a laboratory curiosity to become an important clinical reality. Inhibitor of the protein chaperones, HSP90, offers potential treatment option for such patients. More importantly, this class of agents may also find use in other subsets of lung cancer including K-Ras mutant lung cancer and other oncogene-driven pathways.

REFERENCES

1. Lung Cancer Home Page. 2011. http://www.cancer.gov/cancertopics/types/lung
2. Schiller JH, Harrington D, Belani CP, et al. Comparison of four chemotherapy regimens for advanced non-small-cell lung cancer. *N Engl J Med*. 2002;346(2):92–98.
3. Soda M, Choi YL, Enomoto M, et al. Identification of the transforming EML4-ALK fusion gene in non-small-cell lung cancer. *Nature*. 2007; 448(7153):561–566.
4. Shaw AT, Solomon B. Targeting anaplastic lymphoma kinase in lung cancer. *Clin Cancer Res*. 2011;17(8):2081–2086.
5. Soda M, Takada S, Takeuchi K, et al. A mouse model for EML4-ALK-positive lung cancer. *Proc Natl Acad Sci U S A*. 2008;105(50):19893–19897.

6. Shaw AT, Yeap BY, Mino-Kenudson M, et al. Clinical features and outcome of patients with non-small-cell lung cancer who harbor EML4-ALK. *J Clin Oncol.* 2009;27(26):4247–4253.
7. Inamura K, Takeuchi K, Togashi Y, et al. EML4-ALK lung cancers are characterized by rare other mutations, a TTF-1 cell lineage, an acinar histology, and young onset. *Mod Pathol.* 2009;22(4):508–515.
8. Rodig SJ, Mino-Kenudson M, Dacic S, et al. Unique clinicopathologic features characterize ALK-rearranged lung adenocarcinoma in the western population. *Clin Cancer Res.* 2009;15(16): 5216–5223.
9. Sasaki T, Rodig SJ, Chirieac LR, Jänne PA. The biology and treatment of EML4-ALK non-small cell lung cancer. *Eur J Cancer.* 2010;46(10):1773–1780.
10. Takahashi T, Sonobe M, Kobayashi M, et al. Clinicopathologic features of non-small-cell lung cancer with EML4-ALK fusion gene. *Ann Surg Oncol.* 2010;17(3):889–897.
11. Inamura K, Takeuchi K, Togashi Y, et al. EML4-ALK fusion is linked to histological characteristics in a subset of lung cancers. *J Thorac Oncol.* 2008;3(1):13–17.
12. Koivunen JP, Mermel C, Zejnullahu K, et al. EML4-ALK fusion gene and efficacy of an ALK kinase inhibitor in lung cancer. *Clin Cancer Res.* 2008;14(13):4275–4283.
13. Kwak EL, Bang YJ, Camidge DR, et al. Anaplastic lymphoma kinase inhibition in non-small-cell lung cancer. *N Engl J Med.* 2010;363(18):1693–1703.
14. Camidge DR, Bang Y, Kwak EL, et al. Progression-free survival (PFS) from a Phase 1 study of crizotinib (PF-02341066) in patients with ALK-positive non-small cell lung cancer (NSCLC). Paper presented at: 2011 ASCO Annual Meeting; June 3–7, 2011; Chicago, IL.
15. Crino L, Kim D, Riely J, et al. Initial phase II results with crizotinib in advanced ALK-positive non-small cell lung cancer (NSCLC): PROFILE 1005. Paper presented at: 2011 ASCO Annual Meeting; June 3–7, 2011; Chicago, IL.
16. Shaw AT, Yeap BY, Solomon BJ, et al. Effect of crizotinib on overall survival in patients with advanced non-small-cell lung cancer harbouring ALK gene rearrangement: a retrospective analysis. *Lancet Oncol.* 2011;12(11):1004–1012.
17. Choi YL, et al. EML4-ALK mutations in lung cancer that confer resistance to ALK inhibitors. *N Engl J Med.* 2010;363(18):1734–1739.
18. Katayama R, Khan TM, Benes C, et al. Therapeutic strategies to overcome crizotinib resistance in non-small cell lung cancers harboring the fusion oncogene EML4-ALK. *Proc Natl Acad Sci U S A.* 2011;108(18):7535–7540.
19. Sakamoto H, Tsukaguchi T, Hiroshima S, et al. CH5424802, a selective ALK inhibitor capable of blocking the resistant gatekeeper mutant. *Cancer Cell.* 2011;19(5):679–690.
20. Lovly CM, Heuckmann JM, de Stanchina E, et al. Insights into ALK-driven cancers revealed through development of novel ALK tyrosine kinase inhibitors. *Cancer Res.* 2011;71(14):4920–4931.
21. Bagatell R, Whitesell L. Altered Hsp90 function in cancer: a unique therapeutic opportunity. *Mol Cancer Ther.* 2004;3(8):1021–1030.
22. Whitesell L, Lindquist SL. HSP90 and the chaperoning of cancer. *Nat Rev Cancer.* 2005; 5(10):761–772.
23. Mahalingam D, Swords R, Carew JS, Nawrocki ST, Bhalla K, Giles FJ. Targeting HSP90 for cancer therapy. *Br J Cancer.* 2009;100(10):1523–1529.
24. Solit DB, Chiosis G. Development and application of Hsp90 inhibitors. *Drug Discov Today.* 2008;13(1–2):38–43.
25. Sequist LV, Gettinger S, Senzer NN, et al. Activity of IPI-504, a novel heat-shock protein 90 inhibitor, in patients with molecularly defined non-small-cell lung cancer. *J Clin Oncol.* 2010;28(33):4953–4960.
26. Normant E, Paez G, West KA, et al. The Hsp90 inhibitor IPI-504 rapidly lowers EML4-ALK levels and induces tumor regression in ALK-driven NSCLC models. *Oncogene.* 2011;30(22): 2581–2586.
27. Wong K, Koczywas M, Goldman JW, et al. An open-label phase II study of the Hsp90 inhibitor ganetespib (STA-9090) as monotherapy in patients with advanced non-small cell lung cancer (NSCLC). Paper presented at: 2011 ASCO Annual Meeting; June 3–7, 2011; Chicago, IL.
28. Mano H. Non-solid oncogenes in solid tumors: EML4-ALK fusion genes in lung cancer. *Cancer Sci.* 2008;99(12):2349–2355.

demos MEDICAL

ECAT Emerging Cancer Therapeutics

State-of-the-Art Treatment of Lung Cancer in the Elderly

Antonio Rossi*

Division of Medical Oncology, "S.G. Moscati" Hospital, Avellino, Italy

■ ABSTRACT

Lung cancer, the leading cause of cancer-related deaths worldwide, with a median incidence age of 71 years, is a disease that is closely linked with the elderly. The limited representation of the elderly in most clinical trials, the presence of comorbidities, and the progressive reduction of organ functional reserve are the most important aspects influencing treatment decision. This means that heterogeneity represents the main characteristic of older patients. Thus, the comprehensive geriatric assessment, a useful but very complex tool in evaluating all of these aspects, could help in elderly patients' selection and in the best treatment choice. Non-small cell lung cancer (NSCLC) accounts for about 85% of all new lung cancer diagnoses, while small cell lung cancer (SCLC) makes up the remaining 15%. Most data address metastatic NSCLC, implying that recommendations can be drawn specifically for this subgroup. In early-stage and locally advanced NSCLC, the lack of adequate trials leaves the choice of the therapeutic approach dependent on the general condition of every single patient. Unfortunately, studies specifically addressing the treatment of elderly with SCLC have enrolled too few patients to produce any useful guideline. Thus, the treatment of elderly patients is still a challenge.

Keywords: NSCLC, SCLC, chemotherapy, targeted therapy, radiotherapy, surgery

■ INTRODUCTION

Cancer is an age-associated disease, and the number of people aged ≥65 years will double by the year 2040 (1). The increased risk for cancer associated with older age can be expected to increase the number of cancer patients by 60% in the next 30 years (2). Lung cancer is the most common cancer and the leading cause of cancer-related deaths worldwide, both in men and women (3). According to an analysis by the Surveillance Epidemiology End Results (SEER) database, on 373,489 lung cancer diagnoses, more than 50% were diagnosed in people aged ≥70 years, and about 15% of cases

*Corresponding author, Division of Medical Oncology, "S.G. Moscati" Hospital, Contrada Amoretta, 8, 83100 Avellino, Italy

E-mail address: arossi_it@yahoo.it

Emerging Cancer Therapeutics 3:1 (2012) 73–94.

DOI: 10.5003/2151–4194.3.1.73

in patients ≥80 years (4,5). These data suggest that with a median incidence age of 71 years, lung cancer is a disease that is closely linked with the elderly. The incidence and the mortality from lung cancer have decreased among individuals aged ≤50 years, but has increased among those aged ≥70 years (6). In particular, the 5-year survival rate was lower in the octogenarians compared with patients aged 70 to 79 or younger than 70 years (7.4% vs. 12.3% vs. 15.5%; $P < .0001$) across sex, histologic subtypes, stages, and racial categories (5).

There is no clear cut-off age to define an elderly. This is because aging is a highly individualized process in which all the changes involved cannot be predicted solely on the basis of chronological age. Thus, it is important to evaluate a patient's "functional age" rather than chronological age especially in oncology, where chemotherapy and radiotherapy have substantial side effects. Unfortunately, to establish the biologic age is still difficult nowadays due to the lack of adequate laboratory tests and tools. Consequently, the chronological age is the only indicator in defining the elderly, and 70 years may be the most appropriate threshold because the incidence of age-related changes starts to increase after this cut-off age (7).

Undoubtedly, lung cancer in elderly patients is an increasingly common problem which the practitioner of oncology must face.

■ FACTORS AFFECTING ELDERLY LUNG CANCER TREATMENT

Several factors influence the reluctance to use chemotherapy in the elderly. Among these, the most important are the general lack of studies in this age group and the limited representation of the elderly population in most clinical trials for cancer. A retrospective analysis of patients enrolled onto Southwest Oncology Group trials between 1993 and 1996 reported that the proportion of cancer patients aged ≥65 years was significantly smaller than the percentage of older patients in the U.S. population (25% vs. 63%, respectively; $P < .001$). When the age cut-off was set at 70 years, the proportions were 13% and 47%, respectively ($P < .001$) (8). The underrepresentation of the elderly in clinical trials might be due to trial protocol (restrictions on comorbidities or organ function requirements), physicians skepticism (the patient would not be able to tolerate treatment due to comorbidities and advanced age), and patient-related barriers (hospitals accessing difficulties, lack of adequate information) (9,10).

Comorbidities are serious medical conditions that are not directly related to the cancer itself but involve mainly metabolism or the cardiovascular, respiratory, renal, and hepatic systems, adversely affecting the patient's functional status. It has been reported that among individuals aged 65 to 74, the mean number of chronic diseases is 6. The most important coexisting pathologies in lung cancer patients are cardiovascular and pulmonary diseases, common among heavy smokers (11).

The physiological progressive reduction of functional reserve that occurs in several organs with aging might cause an increase in the susceptibility of elderly patients to adverse effects with a potential impairment of the quality of life (QoL) (12). A pooled analysis evaluated outcomes for elderly patients who participated in elderly specific (required age ≥65 years) or age-unspecified trials (required age ≥18 years), demonstrating that those who were treated on elderly specific trials experienced fewer severe adverse events with similar survival outcomes (13). Hence, the enrollment of elderly patients in specific trials improves the understanding of physiological and pharmacodynamic changes related to aging, with a substantial effect on outcomes and toxicities.

Elderly patients represent a very heterogeneous group. The comprehensive geriatric assessment (CGA) is a useful but very complex tool which includes several self-assessed questionnaires assessing the patient's functional status, presence of comorbidities, mental status and emotional conditions, social support, nutritional status, polypharmacy, and geriatric syndromes. This allows the classification of elderly patients into three categories: fit patients with no serious comorbidity and dependence; frail patients with significant dependency and comorbidities; and vulnerable patients with some instrumental activity of daily living (IADL) dependency with or without severe comorbidities (14,15). On the basis of the CGA results, fit patients, who have similar prognosis, treatment tolerance, and outcome compared with their younger counterparts, may receive the standard therapeutic approaches, while a less aggressive treatment or only the best supportive care (BSC) should be considered for the other categories. However, the CGA is too lengthy to be applied in the daily clinical practice (Table 1); therefore, other faster and easier tools such as the Cardiovascular Health Study (CHS), which includes only five items (16), and the Vulnerable Elderly Survey 13 (VES-13), which includes 13 simple questions (17), are being investigated in this setting.

All these considerations underline the need to perform an adequate baseline evaluation of the elderly patient to better choose the most appropriate therapy.

TABLE 1 Main parameters and methods of the assessment included in a CGA

Parameters	Methods of the Assessment
Functional status	Performance status
	Activities of daily living
	Instrumental activities of daily living
Comorbidities	Number of comorbid conditions
	Severity of comorbid conditions (comorbidity index)
Socioeconomic conditions	Living conditions
	Presence and adequacy of a caregiver
Cognitive conditions	Folstein mini-mental state evaluation
Emotional conditions	Geriatric depression scale
Pharmacy	Number of medications
	Appropriateness of medications
	Risk of drug interactions
Nutritional status	Mini-nutritional assessment
	Body mass index
Geriatric syndromes	Dementia
	Delirium
	Depression
	Falls
	Neglect and abuse
	Spontaneous bone fractures

■ NON-SMALL CELL LUNG CANCER

Non-small cell lung cancer (NSCLC), including squamous carcinoma, adenocarcinoma, and large cell carcinoma, accounts for about 85% of all new lung cancer diagnoses. Unfortunately, roughly one-third of these receive curatively intended treatment, leaving the majority of candidates to palliative chemotherapy (18).

Early Stages

About 35% of all patients affected by NSCLC were diagnosed having Stages I, II, and IIIA (19) with a 5-year survival rate of 60% to 70% for pathologic Stage I, 35% to 45% and 25% for pathologic Stages II and IIIA, respectively (20). The therapeutic strategy includes surgery for a complete resection of the tumor, whenever surgery is not feasible, curative radiotherapy could be a valid option. The postsurgical approach includes adjuvant chemotherapy and/or radiotherapy when indicated.

Surgery

NSCLC surgery still remains the treatment of choice offering the greatest likelihood of a cure for patients diagnosed with early-stage disease. Age used to be considered a relative contraindication to thoracic surgical procedures due to a limited life expectancy. However, the improvements in thoracic surgical techniques, anesthesia, and postoperative care allowed the inclusion of an increasing number of elderly patients in surgical trials. Retrospective analyses support that all the thoracic surgical procedures are feasible regardless of patient age (21). But since these data are retrospective, they could be susceptible to selection bias.

Comorbidities and the potential morbidity and mortality related to surgery are important key points in evaluating elderly patients for surgery. A careful patient selection with preoperative evaluation based on cardiac and respiratory assessment is crucial for the accurate prediction of operative risk, postoperative performance, and QoL leading to an improvement of the results (21). A marked difference was found in postoperative outcome between elective and emergency operations, pneumonectomy and lobectomy or wedge resection, regardless of age (22). In fact, analyzing patients aged ≥70 years, postoperative complications occurred in 78.5% of 42 patients who had undergone pneumonectomy and in 58% of 48 patients who had received lobectomy or wedge resections, and all postoperative deaths occurred in the patients undergoing pneumonectomy (23). In an attempt to reduce operative morbidity and mortality, video-assisted thoracic surgery (VATS) has been proposed, resulting particularly interesting in elderly patients, with encouraging results also in octogenarians (24,25). Hence, in experienced hands and after a careful selection of candidates, VATS may be a safe and acceptable procedure.

A very important point is the outcome of elderly patients. Age is not a negative prognostic factor for long-term postoperative overall survival (OS), with 5-year survival rates ranging between 21% and 58% depending on the stage of patients included in the study (21). Moreover, studies comparing outcomes between elderly and younger patients have not demonstrated significant differences in OS (26–30) or change in functional status (31,32). Yet, considering cancer-specific survival in the elderly, the importance of taking into account the cancer-unrelated deaths should be clearly underlined.

All in all, surgery should not be denied to early-stage NSCLC elderly only on the basis of chronological age. But, a careful selection of the patient is mandatory to optimize surgical results.

Radiotherapy With Curative Intent

Radiotherapy administered with curative intent could be a valid option for elderly patients not amenable for surgery due to medical concerns or who do not want to undergo surgery, thus resulting in a feasible and tolerable option also in the elderly population (33). Nevertheless, despite no significant differences were reported in terms of recurrence-free survival or OS, a greater number of elderly patients experienced weight loss compared with their younger counterparts (34–36).

More effective and better tolerated newer radiation techniques have been explored also in the elderly (37). Stereotactic body radiation is a safe and effective method of treating lung cancer in medically inoperable or elderly patients, with OS potentially comparable with those of surgery (38). In fact, when administered to 193 patients aged ≥75 years (73 octogenarians) with Stage I NSCLC, reported 1- and 3-year survival of 86% and 45%, respectively and minimal toxicity (39). Radio-surgery is a novel and promising concept which enables the selective delivery of an intense dose of high-energy radiation to destroy a tumor with precise targeting, without significant complications for inoperable patients (40).

Overall, radiotherapy and, in particular, stereotactic radio-surgery, which avoids the morbidity, recovery, and potential mortality connected with surgery, would be useful for a vulnerable population, including octogenarians.

Adjuvant Chemotherapy

Cisplatin-based adjuvant chemotherapy, improving OS after radical resection, is recommended in general patient population with Stages II to IIIA NSCLC (41,42). Unfortunately, to date, there are no prospective, elderly specific results but only retrospective analyses which show that the benefit of adjuvant chemotherapy is independent of age (43,44). In the JBR.10 trial, patients radically resected for Stages IB to II were randomized to four cycles of adjuvant cisplatin plus vinorelbine or control. OS by age revealed a trend favoring the young (age ≤65 years) in both univariate (hazard ratio [HR] for death 0.77, P = .084) and multivariate analyses (HR for death 0.75, P = .059). OS for patients aged >65 years was significantly better with chemotherapy versus observation, with a 5-year survival rate of 68% versus 48%, respectively (HR for death 0.61, P = .04). However, patients aged >75 years had significantly shorter OS than those aged 66 to 74 (HR for death 1.95, P = .02). The elderly received significantly fewer doses of both cisplatin and vinorelbine. Fewer elderly patients completed treatment and more refused treatment compared with the young (P = .03). There were no significant differences in hospitalization, toxicities, or granulocyte-colony stimulating factor (G-CSF) use (43). A pooled analysis evaluated the efficacy and toxicity of adjuvant cisplatin-based chemotherapy by three age groups: 3,269 young (<65 years), 901 midcategory (65–69 years) and 414 elderly (≥70 years). No difference in the severe toxicity rate was observed among the age groups. Elderly patients received significantly lower first and total cisplatin doses, and fewer chemotherapy cycles (P < .0001). In the young patients, the HR for death was 0.86 (95% confidence interval [CI] 0.78–0.94), 1.01 (95% CI 0.85–1.21) for the midcategory, and 0.90 (95% CI 0.70–1.16) for the elderly patients (P = .29). The HR for event-free survival was 0.82 (95% CI 0.75–0.90) for the young, 0.90 (95% 0.76–1.06) for the midcategory, and 0.87 (95% CI 0.68–1.11) for the elderly patients (P = .42). More elderly patients died from nonlung cancer-related causes (12% young, 19% midcategory, 22% elderly; P < .0001) (44).

A retrospective analysis, using the SEER database from 1992 to 2005, included 3,324 patients aged ≥65 years with resected Stages II to IIIA NSCLC. Platinum-based chemotherapy administered in 684 (21%) patients was associated with improved OS (HR 0.80, 95% CI 0.72–0.89) but also with increased serious adverse events (odds ratio [OR] 2.0, 95% CI 1.5–2.6). Moreover, chemotherapy was not beneficial for patients aged ≥80 years (HR 1.33, 95% CI 0.86–2.06) (45).

Thus, also the adjuvant cisplatin-based chemotherapy should not be withheld from elderly patients purely on the basis of age. However, the OS benefit comes from retrospective analyses based on highly selected patients and may be due to lack of potency; so their extrapolation to the general elderly population should be made with caution. To date, no data support the use of adjuvant chemotherapy in patients older than 75 years, implying individual decisions should be made on a case-by-case basis after a discussion of the risks, potential benefits, life expectancy, comorbidities, and available results.

Adjuvant Radiotherapy

There is no role for adjuvant radiotherapy in Stages I and II NSCLC, while its role in Stage IIIA/N2 remains controversial (46,47). A retrospective analysis of a Phase III randomized trial comparing cisplatin plus vinorelbine versus control in radically resected Stage IB to IIIA NSCLC patients showed a higher OS for the N2-positive subgroup receiving postoperative radiotherapy (48). A prospective randomized trial, addressing this question in the general population, is ongoing in Europe (49).

To sum up, due to an almost total lack of data regarding the role of adjuvant radiotherapy, especially for elderly NSCLC populations, and given the lack of demonstrated benefit for its use in the general population, it is not advisable to use this therapy in clinical practice for elderly NSCLC patients.

Neoadjuvant Therapy

The role of neoadjuvant chemotherapy for the treatment of early-stage NSCLC is still controversial in the general population. A systematic review suggests a 12% relative OS benefit with the addition of neoadjuvant chemotherapy (1,507 patients, HR 0.88, 95% CI 0.76–1.01, P = .07) (50). No data are available specifically for the elderly population. However, this topic is particularly interesting because preoperative chemotherapy is generally more tolerable than postoperative chemotherapy and, as a consequence, potentially more suitable for elderly patients than standard adjuvant chemotherapy.

Locally Advanced Disease

Patients affected by locally advanced unresectable NSCLC account for about 27% (19) with a 5-year survival rate of 10% (20). Concurrent chemo-radiotherapy is the standard approach reporting an OS improvement (HR 0.84, 95% CI 0.74–0.95; P = .004) a better locoregional control (HR 0.77, 95% CI 0.62–0.95; P = .01) but at the cost of manageable increased acute esophageal toxicity (relative risk [RR] 4.9, 95% CI 3.1–7.8; P < .001) (51).

A total of 6,325 locally advanced NSCLC patients aged ≥66 years and treated with chemo-radiotherapy were identified in the SEER database. A survival benefit was reported, but patients receiving concomitant chemo-radiotherapy experienced the greatest mortality risk, suggesting that a less aggressive strategy may be more appropriate for the elderly (52). Further retrospective analyses reported similar results but may suffer from selection bias, thus possibly rendering the conclusions not representative of the whole elderly population, but only of highly selected group of patients (53).

A prospective Phase III trial randomly assigned patients >70 years with unresectable Stage III NSCLC to either radiotherapy alone or radiotherapy and concurrent daily carboplatin. This trial was stopped early because of four deaths due to treatment toxicity (one on the radiotherapy alone arm and three on the radiotherapy plus carboplatin arm). Only 46 patients were treated reporting an OS of 14.3 months with radiotherapy versus 18.5 months with chemotherapy plus radiotherapy (54).

Thus, concomitant chemo-radiotherapy should be offered to elderly patients selected on the basis of performance status, comorbidities, and life expectancy due to the lack of specific prospective randomized trials and the higher risk of toxicity showed by available data. A sequential approach should be considered when the concurrent treatment is evaluated not feasible.

Metastatic Disease

Most NSCLC patients (40%) are diagnosed in Stage IV disease (19) when a systemic, palliative treatment is the standard of care with a 5-year survival rate less than 2% (20). The largest amount of clinical data for the treatment of elderly is available in this stage of disease.

First-Line Chemotherapy

Retrospective analyses showed that older patients were less likely to receive chemotherapy, however when they were treated the benefit of platinum-based doublets was greater than single-agent drug but with more adverse events, independently of comorbidities (55,56).

Two randomized Phase III trials evaluated the role of single-agent chemotherapy in patients aged ≥70 years (57,58). Vinorelbine was well-tolerated, and improved OS versus BSC (57) while when compared with docetaxel, the latter scored better in terms of objective response rate (ORR), progression-free survival (PFS) and, a trend not statistically significant, in terms of OS, the primary endpoint of the trial (58). Further two studies investigated a nonplatinum-based doublet, the combination of gemcitabine and vinorelbine, versus single-agent drug (59,60). The first study, involving 120 elderly patients, suggested the superiority of gemcitabine plus vinorelbine over single-agent vinorelbine in terms of ORR, OS, and QoL (59). However, a larger trial, randomizing nearly 700 older patients, concluded that the combination of gemcitabine and vinorelbine did not provide an OS benefit over single-agent vinorelbine or gemcitabine, and that the two-drug combination was more toxic than single-agent therapy (60). The discrepancies in the results reported by these last two trials may be ascribed to the different sample size. A meta-analysis assessed the efficacy and tolerability of a gemcitabine third-generation agent doublet versus single-agent treatment in elderly NSCLC patients. A significantly higher ORR was observed (OR 0.65; P < .001), but there was only a trend toward higher OS favoring the combination treatment (OR 0.78; P = 0.169). Toxicity was not significantly different, except for thrombocytopenia (61). Based on these available data, also the American Society of Clinical Oncology (ASCO) guidelines, 2003 update, recommended third-generation single-agent chemotherapeutic, that is, vinorelbine, gemcitabine, taxanes (docetaxel, paclitaxel), as a reasonable treatment choice in unselected elderly patients with advanced NSCLC (62). In clinical practice, the choice of the single agent should take into account the expected toxicity profile, pharmacokinetics, organ function, and comorbidities.

Third-generation platinum-based doublets represent the standard of care for advanced NSCLC in adult patients (63), but they are associated with significant toxicity, and the evaluation of the risk versus benefit ratio should be particularly strict in elderly patients due to the concerns discussed above. However, several retrospective analyses of large randomized trials found no differences in survival between elderly and younger patients, with a small increase in toxicity in the elderly, suggesting that advanced age alone should not preclude platinum-based chemotherapy. Nevertheless, these trials may be biased due to the enrollment of elderly patients considered by investigators to be eligible for aggressive treatment and thus not representative of the whole elderly population but rather of a small subgroup (64). Consequently, any extrapolation of these results to the general elderly population should be made with caution. Two prospective randomized Phase III trials investigated platinum-based regimens versus single-agent therapy in patients aged ≥70 years (65,66). Single-agent gemcitabine or vinorelbine was compared with the combination of carboplatin plus weekly paclitaxel in 451 elderly patients. Primary endpoint was OS, which was significantly longer for patients treated with combination chemotherapy (10.3 vs. 6.2 months; HR 0.64, 95% CI 0.52–0.78; *P* < .0001). The 1-year survival rate was 44.5% for the doublet and 25.4% for the monochemotherapy with a median PFS of 6.0 versus 2.8 months, respectively (HR 0.51, 95% CI 0.42–0.62; *P* < .0001), while ORR was 27.1% versus 10.2%, respectively. However, Grade 3 to 4 hematologic toxicities and treatment-related deaths were significantly more frequent in patients treated with doublet than single-agent therapy. At week 6 and week 18, the QoL was similar in the two arms (65). The second study randomized 276 elderly patients to receive 3-weekly docetaxel or weekly cisplatin plus docetaxel. The study failed to reach the primary endpoint, that is, OS. In fact, at the first interim analysis, OS was 17.3 months for the docetaxel and 13.3 months for the doublet (HR 1.557, 99.99% CI 0.624–3.884; *P* = .969). The predictive probability that the doublet could be superior to docetaxel at the final analysis was 0.996%, so the study was stopped. The updated OS was 13.3 months for the doublet and 14.8 for the single agent (HR 1.183, 95% CI 0.830–1.687; *P* = .824), PFS was 4.7 and 4.4 months (HR 0.924, 95% CI 0.714–1.197; *P* = .303) and ORR 34.4% and 24.6% (*P* = .101), respectively. Hematologic toxicities were higher in 3-weekly docetaxel, while nonhematologic toxicities were higher for the doublet arm. A subset analysis evaluated the OS of the patients aged <75 years (*n* = 62) and of those aged ≥75 years (*n* = 210), reporting no differences between the two arms of each group but a higher OS for the younger (66).

Another Phase III randomized trial compared, in 181 elderly patients, two doublets: carboplatin plus gemcitabine or plus paclitaxel. The main endpoint was QoL. Overall, Grade 3 to 4 toxicity occurred in 75% and 60% of patients treated with carboplatin plus gemcitabine or paclitaxel, respectively. Mean global QoL score at 18 weeks analysis did not differ between the two arms. The number of QoL responders (12% and 5% in carboplatin plus gemcitabine or paclitaxel, respectively) was not significantly different. A CGA was also carried out, with 38% and 25% of patients enrolled in the gemcitabine-based arm and the paclitaxel-based arm, respectively, reporting ≥2 comorbidities. Almost half of the patients had limitations in IADL, and more than a quarter had abnormal depression scores. The ORR was 27% and 19% with a median PFS of 4.7 and 4.5 months and an OS of 8.6 and 6.9 months, respectively (67).

The doses and schedules employed in these trials were similar to the ones generally administered in younger patients. Despite the data seem to favor the platinum-based combinations, the toxicities reported by the elderly should be strongly considered before standardizing this approach to the whole elderly population. In view of these considerations, of interest are the several Phase II studies investigating innovative third-generation platinum-based doublets modified with attenuated platinum doses or weekly schedules that would be more suitable in the elderly. Overall, these trials showed that these regimens could maintain the efficacy without increasing toxicity (64). A larger Phase I/II randomized trial evaluated the feasibility of cisplatin at attenuated doses combined with gemcitabine or vinorelbine in elderly patients with advanced NSCLC (68). In both arms, the treatments were active and feasible, but a better activity was reported by cisplatin plus gemcitabine, probably due to the higher cisplatin dose administered; thus, this regimen (cisplatin plus gemcitabine) is now being investigated versus single-agent gemcitabine in an ongoing Phase III randomized trial performed in patients aged ≥70 years (69). Smaller retrospective series demonstrate the feasibility and possible benefit of chemotherapy also in octogenarians (70).

Thus, in view of most of the last data shown, the ASCO guidelines, update 2009, recommend that the selection of a specific first-line chemotherapy drug or combination should no longer be based on age alone, as there is no evidence supporting this (63). However, platinum-based doublets should be reserved for fit older patients, with single-agent drug considered for the other elderly population. Table 2 summarizes the randomized Phase III trials performed in advanced NSCLC elderly patients.

Targeted Therapy

The major progresses in the understanding of lung cancer molecular abnormalities have led to the identification of genes involved in lung carcinogenesis which are being used as targets for the development of new biologic agents. Two pathways, studied in particular, provided specific inhibitors, which are currently in the clinical practice for the treatment of advanced NSCLC patients: the vascular endothelial growth factor (VEGF) and the epidermal growth factor receptor (EGFR).

A randomized Phase III trial showed that the addition of bevacizumab (15 mg/kg), an anti-VEGF monoclonal antibody, to the paclitaxel plus carboplatin doublet as first-line treatment of non-squamous NSCLC patients resulted in significant prolongation of PFS and OS. The squamous histology was excluded due to a higher incidence of pulmonary hemorrhage reported in this NSCLC histotype (71). A subgroup analysis performed in the 224 (26%) elderly patients (≥70 years) enrolled onto the trial showed no differences between young and elderly patients ($P = .34$). In the elderly population, there was no significant prolongation of OS, with a trend toward higher PFS in favor of the bevacizumab arm, which resulted in a significantly higher number of Grade ≥3 toxicities than in chemotherapy alone (72). Another retrospective analysis was performed in 304 elderly (≥65 years) out of 1,430 patients randomized to receive cisplatin plus gemcitabine alone or in combination with two doses of bevacizumab (7.5 or 15 mg/kg). The elderly patients receiving both doses of bevacizumab derived an improvement of ORR and PFS than placebo. OS was similar in all the treatment arms regardless of age. There were no safety signals of concern in older patients (73). Unfortunately, only retrospective data are available; therefore, bevacizumab should be used only in carefully selected advanced NSCLC elderly patients.

Gefitinib and erlotinib, two small-molecule EGFR tyrosine kinase inhibitors (TKIs), administered orally daily, were investigated in the elderly population. A large Phase II randomized trial compared gefitinib to vinorelbine as first-line treatment of unselected patients aged ≥70 years, showing similar efficacy with a lower toxicity profile and a better QoL favoring gefitinib (74). Also, erlotinib was investigated in 80 unselected elderly patients with previously untreated advanced NSCLC, reporting an interesting ORR of 10% and OS of 10.9 months with a significant improvement of key symptoms (dyspnoea, cough, fatigue, and pain) and a good tolerability (75). However, it

TABLE 2 Results from randomized Phase III trials in patients aged ≥70 years with advanced NSCLC

Author	Primary Endpoint	Treatment	No. of Patients	ORR (%)	PFS (months)	OS (months)	Toxicity	QoL
ELVIS (57)	QoL	VNR vs. BSC	76 78	20 NA	NR	6.5 4.8	Treatment was stopped in five patients due to Grade ≥3 constipation and Grade 2 heart toxicity	VNR better in functioning scales
Kudoh et al. (58)	OS	VNR vs. TXT	91 88	9.9 22.7	3.1 5.4	9.9 14.3	Grade ≥3 neutropenia and any grade alopecia more frequent in TXT than VNR arm ($P = .31$ and $P < .0001$, respectively)	No differences in QoL, but TXT significantly improved symptom score than VNR
Frasci et al. (59)	OS	VNR vs. VNR+GEM	60 60	15 22	NR	4.2 6.7	Two and one toxic deaths in doublet and single-agent arm. Treatment was stopped due to toxicity in seven and six patients, respectively	No QoL score impairment in 60% and 40% of patients in doublet and single-agent arm, respectively
Gridelli et al. (60)	OS	VNR or GEM vs. VNR+GEM	233 233 232	18 16 21	18[a] 17[a] 19[a]	8.3 6.5 6.9	Doublet reported more thrombocytopenia than VNR and more neutropenia, vomiting, fatigue, extravasation sequelae, cardiac toxicity, and constipation than GEM	Similar QoL across the three arms
Quoix et al. (65)	OS	VNR or GEM vs. CBDCA+PAC	226 225	10.2 27.1	2.8 6.0	6.2 10.3	Toxic death in 4.4% and 1.3% of doublet or single-agent arm, respectively. Grade 3 to 4 neutropenia, febrile neutropenia, thrombocytopenia, anemia, and sensory neuropathy were significantly more frequent in doublet arm	Global QoL was similar between the two arms at 6 and 18 weeks

(*Continued*)

TABLE 2 Results from randomized Phase III trials in patients aged ≥70 years with advanced NSCLC *(Continued)*

Author	Primary Endpoint	Treatment	No. of Patients	ORR (%)	PFS (months)	OS (months)	Toxicity	QoL
Abe et al. (66)	OS	TXT vs. CDDP+TXT	137 139	24.6 34.4	4.4 4.7	14.8 13.3	Grade ≥3 neutropenia in 89% and 10% of patients in TXT and doublet arm, respectively. Grade ≥3 febrile neutropenia in 15% and 0% of patients, respectively	Symptom score was more favorable in TXT than doublet arm
Biesma et al. (67)	QoL	CBDCA+GEM vs. CBDCA+PAC	90 91	27 19	4.7 4.5	8.6 6.9	Grade ≥3 toxicity reported in 75% and 60% of patients in CBDCA+GEM and CBDCA+PAC arm, respectively. Grade ≥2 neuropsychiatric toxicity was reported in 25% of patients in both arms	No difference in QoL score from baseline to week 18

ORR = objective response rate; PFS = progression-free survival; OS = overall survival; QoL = quality of life; ELVIS = Elderly Lung cancer Vinorelbine Italian Study; VNR = vinorelbine; BSC = best supportive care; NA = not applicable; NR = not reported; TXT = docetaxel; GEM = gemcitabine; CBDCA = carboplatin; PAC = paclitaxel; CDDP = cisplatin.

[a]Time to progression in weeks.

has been largely proven that the EGFR-TKIs are particularly active in patients affected by NSCLC-harboring EGFR-activating mutations. These data come from randomized Phase III trials demonstrating that first-line EGFR-TKIs scored better than standard chemotherapy in terms of ORR and PFS in advanced NSCLC patients selected by clinical features (adenocarcinoma histology, never smoker status, female gender, and Asian ethnicity) known to be related to a higher frequency of EGFR mutations or by biologic characteristic, that is, the presence of an activating EGFR mutation (76). These trials were not specifically addressed to elderly patients, but since the EGFR-TKI recognizes a specific target, the results could be generalized to all populations which harbor the EGFR mutations. In addition, the EGFR-TKIs also seem to be a viable treatment option in patients older than 80 years (70). Table 3 summarizes the results of the main trials performed in advanced NSCLC elderly patients with new biologic agents.

Overall, the availability of these new biologic agents and of pemetrexed, a new chemotherapeutic which, due to its specific greater effectiveness, is licensed only for the treatment of nonsquamous NSCLC histology (77), underlined an important topic: the need of an adequate amount of cancer tissue to perform the diagnosis of the type of NSCLC histology and the biomolecular analyses, in order to better address the treatment.

Second-Line Therapy

In clinical practice, two chemotherapeutics, docetaxel and pemetrexed (only for nonsquamous NSCLC histology), and one targeted agent, erlotinib, are registered for second-line treatment of the general population, while only erlotinib is licensed also for third-line therapy (63).

This issue was addressed in the elderly patients (≥70 years) by two retrospective analyses (78,79). The first was performed in 86 elderly out of a total of 571 patients enrolled in a randomized Phase III trial comparing second-line pemetrexed to docetaxel. The outcomes were similar between the elderly and their younger counterpart. Pemetrexed produced a more favorable toxicity profile with less febrile neutropenia (2.5% vs. 19%; $P = .025$) than docetaxel, and no toxic deaths (one treatment-related death was reported in the docetaxel arm) (78). The second was performed in 163 elderly patients out of 731 randomized to receive erlotinib or placebo. The elderly treated with erlotinib gained survival and QoL benefits similar to younger patients, but experienced greater toxicity (79).

A prospective Phase II trial investigated a modified schedule of docetaxel given as second-line therapy to 33 elderly patients. ORR was 21.2%, with Grade 3 hematologic and nonhematologic toxicities reported in less than 10% of patients (80) (Table 4).

Unfortunately, there is lack of data regarding the role of second-line treatment in the elderly NSCLC population. Considering the available results, age alone should not prevent the administration of second-line therapy, which should be chosen on the basis of life expectancy, expected benefit, comorbidities, and patient's preferences.

■ SMALL CELL LUNG CANCER

Approximately 15% of all new lung cancer cases are small cell lung cancer (SCLC), whose incidence has decreased during the last two decades probably as a result of decreased tobacco use (20). In an analysis of the SEER database, while SCLC represents about 14% to 16% of all lung cancer cases in patients with age <70 years and in those 70 to 79 years old, the proportion falls to only 9% to 11% in patients aged ≥80 years, with a 5-year survival rates of 7.1%, 3.9%, and 2.2%, respectively ($P < .0001$) (5). According to the two-stage system of the Veterans Administration Lung Cancer Group, more than two-thirds of patients are diagnosed as having an extensive disease (ED), while the remaining part as limited disease (LD) (81). However, the International Association for the Study of Lung Cancer staging project showed that tumor, node, metastasis (TNM) staging is also applicable to SCLC (82).

TABLE 3 Results from the main studies performed in advanced NSCLC elderly patients with new biologic agents

Author	Setting	Type of Study	Age	Treatment	No. of Patients	ORR (%)	PFS (months)	OS (months)	Toxicity
Ramalingam et al. (72)	Retrospective	III	≥70	CBDCA+PAC+BEV 15[a]	111	29	5.9	11.3	Toxic deaths 6.8% and 1.8% in BEV and placebo arms, respectively. Elderly experienced higher toxicity with BEV than younger counterpart
				vs.					
				CBDCA+PAC	113	27	4.9	12.1	
Leighl et al. (73)	Retrospective	III	≥65	CDDP+GEM+BEV 7.5[a]	89	40	HR 0.71	HR 0.84	Only Grade >3 thrombocytopenia was more frequent in BEV-containing arms than placebo. No toxicity differences between elderly and younger patients
				or					
				CDDP+GEM+BEV 15[a]	103	29	HR 0.84	HR 0.88	
				vs.					
				CDDP+GEM	112	30	–	–	
Crinò et al. (74)	Prospective	II randomized	≥70	GEF	97	3.1	2.7	5.9	Grade ≥3 toxicity in 12.8% and 41.7% of patients in GEF and VNR group, respectively
				vs.					
				VNR	99	5.1	2.9	8.0	
Jackman et al. (75)	Prospective	II	≥70	ERL	80	10	3.5[b]	10.9	ILD in 5% of patients with one toxic death

ORR = objective response rate; PFS = progression-free survival; OS = overall survival; CBDCA = carboplatin; PAC = paclitaxel;
BEV = bevacizumab; CDDP = cisplatin; GEM = gemcitabine; GEF = gefitinib; VNR = vinorelbine; ERL = erlotinib; ILD = interstitial lung disease.

[a]mg/kg.

[b]Time to progression.

TABLE 4 Available results of second-line therapy in elderly patients with advanced NSCLC

Author	Setting	Type of Study	Age	Treatment	No. of Patients	ORR (%)	PFS (months)	OS (months)	Toxicity
Weiss et al. (78)	Retrospective	III	≥70	Pemetrexed	47	5.0	4.6[a]	9.5	The presence of febrile neutropenia was slightly greater in the elderly than in the younger. Elderly patients receiving docetaxel had more toxicity than those treated with pemetrexed
				vs.					
				Docetaxel	39	5.6	2.9[a]	7.7	
			<70	Pemetrexed	224	9.8	3.0[a]	7.8	
				vs.					
				Docetaxel	238	9.2	3.9[a]	8.0	
Wheatley-Price et al. (79)	Retrospective	III	≥70	Erlotinib	112	7.6	3.0	7.6	Grade ≥3 were significantly more frequent in elderly than younger ($P < .001$). Elderly discontinued therapy more frequently than younger ($P < .0001$)
				vs.					
				Placebo	51	NR	2.1	5.0	
			<70	Erlotinib	376	9.3	2.1	6.4	
				vs.					
				Placebo	192	NR	1.8	4.7	
Tibaldi et al. (80)	Prospective	II	≥70	Docetaxel	33	21.2	4.0[a]	6.0	Grade ≥3 was reported in less than 10% of patients

ORR = objective response rate; PFS = progression-free survival; OS = overall survival; NR = not reported.
[a]Time to progression.

Three options can be identified for the treatment of SCLC elderly patients: (a) to use the same chemotherapy as in the younger counterpart, although the relevant toxicity shown by retrospective analyses would make it inadvisable; (b) to empirically reduce drug doses (usually of about 25%), but this may be criticized too because certain drugs, such as anthracyclines or cisplatin, are absolutely contraindicated in the cases of relevant cardiac or renal comorbidities; and (c) to design specific active and well-tolerated regimens for the elderly—the approach considered the most acceptable. Unfortunately, most of the prospective trials enrolled both LD- and ED-SCLC elderly patients, reporting results not always divided for each group, resulting in a difficult interpretation of the data (83).

Limited Disease

The standard of care for patients with good performance status and LD-SCLC is concurrent chemo-radiotherapy with four to six cycles of platinum-based regimen (CAV: cyclophosphamide, doxorubicin, and vincristine; PE: platinum and etoposide) and early (with cycle 1 or 2) thoracic radiotherapy. Prophylactic cranial irradiation (PCI) is indicated in patients who obtain a remission of disease. This intensive approach appears to be superior to sequential chemo-radiotherapy and yields higher OS, but (84) its feasibility is an important issue to be taken into account in the treatment of the elderly.

A meta-analysis showed that the survival advantage reported by thoracic radiotherapy in the general population was not observed in patients aged ≥70 years (85). However, retrospective analyses showed that also elderly LD-SCLC patients benefited from this approach even though with higher percentage of severe adverse events (86,87). Concerning the role of PCI, the increase in survival reported by a meta-analysis was not influenced by age (88). However, clinical trials have shown that PCI could be potentially related to neuropsychological impairments (89). In this view, neurological examinations and the use of tools in order to evaluate the mental status of the elderly could be useful.

A Phase II trial enrolled 55 patients aged >70 years to receive one cycle of CAV and one cycle of PE plus radiotherapy. ORR was 89% with a complete response in 51% of patients. The OS was 12.6 months. Despite overall toxicity was not pronounced, three treatment-related deaths were reported (90). In another Phase II trial, 72 elderly patients received only two courses of carboplatin and oral etoposide and accelerated hyperfractionated radiotherapy. ORR was 75% with complete response observed in 57% of patients. The OS was 15 months. Treatment was well tolerated with Grade 4 thrombocytopenia observed in one patient (91) (Table 5).

To sum up, chemo-radiotherapy in LD-SCLC elderly patients is still questionable and must be studied within trials specifically addressed to this subgroup of patients, while PCI should be accurately evaluated and not generally advised in elderly patients, considering most likely preexisting neurocognitive problems.

Extensive Disease

Systemic chemotherapy represents the standard treatment for patients affected by ED-SCLC, and radiotherapy plays a local palliative role (84). Single-agent chemotherapy, that is, oral etoposide, epidoxorubicin, and teniposide, is largely used for the treatment of ED-SCLC elderly patients, but resulted inferior to polychemotherapy; hence, single-agent drug should not be an "a priori" planned strategy in this subgroup of patients (83).

Several prospective trials investigated in the elderly the combination of carboplatin plus etoposide, the latter given orally or intravenously or plus teniposide at the same dose employed in younger patients, reporting an interesting activity (ORR, 59–81%; OS, 7.9–11.6 months), albeit with increased, prevalently hematologic toxicity (83).

TABLE 5 Results from main studies performed in elderly patients with SCLC

Author	Type of Study	Stage of Disease	Treatment	No. of Patients	ORR (%)	OS (months)	Toxicity
Murray et al. (90)[a]	II	LD	CAV (one cycle)+CE (one cycle)+RT	55	89	12.6	Toxicity was not pronounced, except for three treatment-related deaths
Jeremic et al. (91)	II	LD	cPE (two cycles)+RT	72	75	15	Grade 3 leukopenia (8.3%), esophagitis (2.8%), respectively. Only one patient experienced Grade 4 thrombocytopenia
Ardizzoni et al. (92)	II randomized	LD–ED	Low-dose CE	28	39.3	7.7	Grade ≥3 hematological and nonhematological toxicities (10% vs. 0% and 10% vs. 4%) more common in the full-dose cohort, with one treatment-related death
			vs.				
			full-dose CE+G-CSF	67	68.7	10.2	
Gridelli et al. (93)	I/II randomized	ED	GEM+VNR	31	36.7	23[b]	All of the four GEM-based regimens were well tolerated, reporting the expected toxicity
			GEM+VP-16	10	10	40[b]	
			GEM+CDDP	12	16.7	22[b]	
			GEM+CBDCA	26	61.5	37[b]	
Okamoto et al. (94)[c]	III	ED	cPE	102	73	10.8	Grade ≥3 leukopenia, neutropenia, and thrombocytopenia, in 54%, 95%, and 56% for cPE arm and 51%, 90%, and 16% in CE group, respectively
			vs.				
			SCE	100	73	10	

ORR = objective response rate; OS = overall survival; LD = limited disease; ED = extensive disease; RT = radiotherapy; CAV = cyclophosphamide + doxorubicin + vincristine; CE = cisplatin + etoposide; SCE = split doses of CE; cPE = carboplatin + etoposide; G-CSF = granulocyte-colony stimulating factor; GEM = gemcitabine; VNR = vinorelbine; CDDP = cisplatin; CBDCA = carboplatin.

[a]Plus infirm or noncompliant patients.

[b]Weeks.

[c]Included also 18 unfit patients <70 years.

In a randomized Phase II trial, 95 elderly ED-SCLC patients received two different doses (full vs. low) of cisplatin plus etoposide with G-CSF support in the full-dose arm. The accrual was stopped due to low activity and impaired survival in the low-dose arm, with an ORR of 39.3% and 1-year survival of 18%, compared with 68.7% and 39%, respectively, for the full-dose arm (92). A Phase I/II study investigated four different gemcitabine-based doublets (plus vinorelbine, or etoposide, or carboplatin, or cisplatin) in 78 eligible patients. Three of the doublets failed to progress beyond Phase I due to lack of acceptable clinical activity. Only gemcitabine plus carboplatin ($n = 26$) reported an ORR of 61.5% with a PFS of 25 weeks and OS of 37 weeks, resulting the only combination that may be worth further investigation (93). A Phase III study compared the efficacy and the safety of carboplatin plus etoposide versus split doses of cisplatin plus etoposide with G-CSF support in 220 elderly (≥70 years in 92% of cases) or poor-risk patients (<70 years with performance status 3). No significant differences in ORR, OS, or major toxicities were observed between the two groups, except for Grade 3 to 4 thrombocytopenia, which was higher in the carboplatin receiving cohort (56% vs. 16%; $P < .01$) (94) (Table 5).

Amrubicin was administered in 27 patients, either ≥75 years or with a performance status ≥2, reporting an ORR of 70% with an OS, in the elderly, of 9.0 months (95). Carboplatin plus amrubicin was investigated in 21 patients reporting an ORR of 89% with an OS of 12.8 months (96). The amrubicin therapy was well tolerated, and despite it is classified as an anthracycline cardiac, toxicity was not reported in these trials. To date, amrubicin is approved for use only in Japan.

Overall, based on the available results, fit elderly ED-SCLC patients should receive as first-line therapy a PE regimen paying attention to adverse events.

Second-Line Therapy

Despite high initial response rates, SCLC patients relapse frequently because of the rapid selection of a small number of residual tumor in sensitive cells or stem cells. The prognosis is very poor indeed: median OS is 2 to 3 months for individuals who do not receive second-line therapy. However, while second-line chemotherapy results in tumor regression, in the majority of patients this response tends to be short-lived, and OS, even in treated patients, is rarely greater than 6 months (84).

Topotecan is currently the only approved drug for the second-line treatment of SCLC patients. Generally, in clinical practice, sensitive patients who relapsed ≥90 days after a response to first-line therapy may be re-treated with the same induction regimen, usually PE (97). The amrubicin monotherapy was investigated in 31 relapsed SCLC patients (22 ≥ 70 years old), ORR and toxicities did not significantly differ between age groups (98). Hence, it is mandatory that an adequate patient selection should drive the second-line therapy of SCLC elderly.

■ CONCLUSIONS

Much of the data presented are limited by small sample size, selection bias, and the retrospective nature of the analyses. Categorizing patients by chronologic age alone is to some degree arbitrary but, although general agreement exists that patient selection is important, no data are available on the optimal methods to assess fitness in the elderly for all therapies.

Since, as stated earlier, the majority of data are available for metastatic NSCLC patients, it is specifically for this subgroup that recommendations can be drawn. Unfortunately, for early-stage and locally advanced NSCLC disease, due to lack of adequate trials, the therapeutic approach should be based on the evaluation of the general condition of every single patient. This last consideration should be applied also to elderly SCLC patients. In fact, all the studies addressing this issue have, up to now, enrolled only few elderly, making it difficult to draw any conclusion. Although very little data exist on octogenarians, there are small case series indicating that the specific therapy might be safe in selected patients and may be of benefit in terms of relieving symptoms and improving outcomes.

In conclusion, the treatment of elderly patients is still a challenge. Future progress in defining appropriate treatment options for this rapidly growing population will require carefully designed prospective trials in which important prognostic variables, such as performance status and comorbidities, are fully accounted for through a CGA at baseline, in order to select the best treatment to be administered to individual elderly patients.

■ REFERENCES

1. Yancik R. Population aging and cancer: a cross-national concern. *Cancer J.* 2005;11(6):437–441.
2. Yancik R, Ries LA. Cancer in older persons: an international issue in an aging world. *Semin Oncol.* 2004;31(2):128–136.
3. Ferlay J, Shin HR, Bray F, Forman D, Mathers C, Parkin DM. Estimates of worldwide burden of cancer in 2008: GLOBOCAN 2008. *Int J Cancer.* 2010;127(12):2893–2917.
4. Howlader N, Noone AM, Krapcho M, et al. SEER Cancer Statistics Review, 1975–2008, National Cancer Institute. Bethesda, MD, based on November 2010 SEER data submission, posted to the SEER web site, 2011. http://seer.cancer.gov/csr/1975_2008/. Accessed September 15, 2011.
5. Owonikoko TK, Ragin CC, Belani CP, et al. Lung cancer in elderly patients: an analysis of the surveillance, epidemiology, and end results database. *J Clin Oncol.* 2007;25(35):5570–5577.
6. Wingo PA, Cardinez CJ, Landis SH, et al. Long term trends in cancer mortality in the United States. *Cancer.* 2003;97(suppl 12):3133–3275.
7. Balducci L. Geriatric oncology: challenges for the new century. *Eur J Cancer.* 2000;36(14): 1741–1754.
8. Hutchins LF, Unger JM, Crowley JJ, Coltman Ca Jr, Albain KS. Underrepresentation of patients 65 years of age or older in cancer-treatment trials. *N Engl J Med.* 1999;341(27):2061–2067.
9. Townsley CA, Selby R, Siu LL. Systematic review of barriers to the recruitment of older patients with cancer onto clinical trials. *J Clin Oncol.* 2005;23(13):3112–3124.
10. Basche M, Baron A, Eckhardt SG, et al. Barriers to enrollment of elderly adults in early-phase cancer clinical trials. *J Oncol Pract.* 2008;4(4):162–168.
11. Janssen-Heijnen MLG, Smulders S, Lemmens VEPP, Smeenk FW, van Geffen HJ, Coebergh JW. Effect of comorbidity on the treatment and prognosis of elderly patients with non-small cell lung cancer. *Thorax.* 2004;59(7):602–607.
12. Balducci L, Extermann M. Management of cancer in the older person: a practical approach. *Oncologist.* 2000;5(3):224–237.
13. Jatoi A, Hillman S, Stella P, et al. Should elderly non-small-cell lung cancer patients be offered elderly-specific trials? Results of a pooled analysis from the North Central Cancer Treatment Group. *J Clin Oncol.* 2005;23(36):9113–9119.
14. Extermann M, Hurria A. Comprehensive geriatric assessment for older patients with cancer. *J Clin Oncol.* 2007;25(14):1824–1831.
15. Carreca I, Balducci L, Extermann M. Cancer in the older person. *Cancer Treat Rev.* 2005;31(5):380–402.
16. Fried LP, Tangen CM, Walston J, et al. Frailty in older adults: evidence for a phenotype. *J Gerontol A Biol Sci Med Sci.* 2001;56(3):M146–M156.
17. Saliba D, Elliott M, Rubenstein LZ, et al. The Vulnerable Elders Survey: a tool for identifying vulnerable older people in the community. *J Am Geriatr Soc.* 2001;49(12):1691–1699.
18. Govindan R, Page N, Morgensztern D, et al. Changing epidemiology of small-cell lung cancer in the United States over the last 30 years: analysis of the Surveillance, Epidemiologic, and End Results database. *J Clin Oncol.* 2006;24(28):4539–4544.
19. Morgensztern D, Ng SH, Gao F, Govindan R. Trends in stage distribution for patients with non-small cell lung cancer: a National Cancer Database survey. *J Thorac Oncol.* 2010;5(1):29–33.
20. Goldstraw P, Crowley J, Chansky K, et al. The IASLC lung cancer staging project: proposals for the revision of the TNM stage groupings in the forthcoming (seventh) edition of the TNM classification of malignant tumours. *J Thorac Oncol.* 2007;2(8):706–714.

21. Pallis AG, Gridelli C, van Meerbeeck JP, et al. EORTC elderly task force and lung cancer group and International Society for Geriatric Oncology (SIOG) experts' opinion for the treatment of non-small cell lung cancer in an elderly population. *Ann Oncol.* 2010;21(4):692–706.
22. Myrdal G, Gustafsson G, Lambe M, Horte LG, Stahle E. Outcome after lung cancer surgery. Factors predicting early mortality and major morbidity. *Eur J Cardiothorac Surg.* 2001;20(4):694–699.
23. Dyszkiewicz W, Pawlak K, Gasiorowski L. Early post-pneumonectomy complications in the elderly. *Eur J Cardiothorac Surg.* 2000;17(3):246–250.
24. Igai H, Takahashi M, Ohata K, et al. Surgical treatment for non-small cell lung cancer in octogenarians–the usefulness of video-assisted thoracic surgery. *Interact Cardiovasc Thorac Surg.* 2009;9(2):274–277.
25. Mun M, Kohno T. Video-assisted thoracic surgery for clinical stage I lung cancer in octogenarians. *Ann Thorac Surg.* 2008;85(2):406–411.
26. Yamamoto K, Padilla Alarcon J, Calvo Medina V, et al. Surgical results of stage I non-small cell lung cancer: comparison between elderly and younger patients. *Eur J Cardiothorac Surg.* 2003; 23(1):21–25.
27. Sawada S, Komori E, Nogami N, et al. Advanced age is not correlated with either short-term or long-term postoperative results in lung cancer patients in good clinical condition. *Chest.* 2005;128(3):1557–1563.
28. Yazgan S, Gursoy S, Yaldiz S, Basok O. Outcome of surgery for lung cancer in young and elderly patients. *Surg Today.* 2005;35(10):823–827.
29. Cerfolio RJ, Bryant AS. Survival and outcomes of pulmonary resection for nonsmall cell lung cancer in the elderly: a nested case-control study. *Ann Thorac Surg.* 2006;82(2):424–429.
30. Sigel K, Bonomi M, Packer S, Wisnivesky J. Effect of age on survival of clinical stage I non-small-cell lung cancer. *Ann Surg Oncol.* 2009;16(7):1912–1917.
31. Sullivan V, Tran T, Holmstrom A, et al. Advanced age does not exclude lobectomy for non-small cell lung carcinoma. *Chest.* 2005;128(4):2671–2676.
32. Van Cleave JH, Egleston BL, McCorkle R. Factors affecting recovery of functional status in older adults after cancer surgery. *J Am Geriatr Soc.* 2011;59(1):34–43.
33. Wisnivesky JP, Halm E, Bonomi M, Powell G, Bagiella E. Effectiveness of radiation therapy for elderly patients with unresected stage I and II non-small cell lung cancer. *Am J Respir Crit Care Med.* 2010;181(3):264–269.
34. Gauden SJ, Tripcony L. The curative treatment by radiation therapy alone of Stage I non-small cell lung cancer in a geriatric population. *Lung Cancer.* 2001;32(1):71–79.
35. Hayakawa K, Mitsuhashi N, Katano S, et al. High-dose radiation therapy for elderly patients with inoperable or unresectable non-small cell lung cancer. *Lung Cancer.* 2001;32(1):81–88.
36. Pignon T, Gregor A, Schaake Koning C, Roussel A, Van Glabbeke M, Scalliet P. Age has no impact on acute and late toxicity of curative thoracic radiotherapy. *Radiother Oncol.* 1998;46(3):239–248.
37. Berman AT, Rengan R. New approaches to radiotherapy as definitive treatment for inoperable lung cancer. *Semin Thorac Cardiovasc Surg.* 2008;20(3):188–197.
38. Gridelli C, Maione P, Rossi A. Treatment of stage I-III non-small-cell lung cancer in the elderly. *Oncology (Williston Park)* 2006;20(4):373–380.
39. Haasbeeck CJA, Lagerwaard FJ, Antonisse ME, Slotman BJ, Senan S. Stage I nonsmall cell lung cancer in patients aged ≥ 75 years: outcomes after stereotactic radiotherapy. *Cancer.* 2010;116(2):406–414.
40. Cesaretti JA, Pennathur A, Rosenstein BS, Swanson SJ, Fernando HC. Stereotactic radiosurgery for thoracic malignancies. *Ann Thorac Surg.* 2008;85(2):S785–S791.
41. Pignon JP, Tribodet H, Scagliotti GV, et al. Lung Adjuvant Cisplatin Evaluation: a pooled analysis by the LACE Collaborative Group. *J Clin Oncol.* 2008;26(21):3552–3559.
42. Pisters KM, Evans WK, Azzoli CG, et al. Cancer Care Ontario and American Society of Clinical Oncology adjuvant chemotherapy and adjuvant radiation therapy for stages I-IIIA resectable non small-cell lung cancer guideline. *J Clin Oncol.* 2007;25(34):5506–5518.
43. Pepe C, Hasan B, Winton T, et al. Adjuvant vinorelbine and cisplatin in elderly patients: National

Cancer Institute of Canada and Intergroup Study JBR.10. *J Clin Oncol.* 2007;25(12):1553–1561.
44. Fruh M, Rolland E, Pignon JP, et al. Pooled analysis of the effect of age on adjuvant cisplatin-based chemotherapy for completely resected non-small-cell lung cancer. *J Clin Oncol.* 2008;26(21):3573–3581.
45. Wisnivesky JP, Smith CB, Packer S, et al. Survival and risk of adverse events in older patients receiving postoperative adjuvant chemotherapy for resected stages II-IIIA lung cancer: observational cohort study. *BMJ.* 2011;343:d4013.
46. PORT Meta-Analysis Trialists Group. Postoperative radiotherapy in non-small cell lung cancer: systematic review and meta-analysis of individual patient data from nine randomised controlled trials. *Lancet.* 1998;352(9124):257–263.
47. Burdett S, Stewart L. Postoperative radiotherapy in non-small-cell lung cancer: update of an individual patient data meta-analysis. *Lung Cancer.* 2005;47(1):81–83.
48. Douillard JY, Rosell R, De LM, et al. Adjuvant vinorelbine plus cisplatin versus observation in patients with completely resected stage IB-IIIA non-small-cell lung cancer (Adjuvant Navelbine International Trialist Association [ANITA]): a randomised controlled trial. *Lancet Oncol.* 2006; 7(9):719–727.
49. Le Pechoux C, Dunant A, Pignon JP, et al. Need for a new trial to evaluate adjuvant postoperative radiotherapy in non-small-cell lung cancer patients with N2 mediastinal involvement. *J Clin Oncol.* 2007;25(7):e10–e11.
50. Gilligan D, Nicolson M, Smith I, et al. Preoperative chemotherapy in patients with resectable non-small cell lung cancer: results of the MRC LU22/NVALT 2/EORTC 08012 multicentre randomised trial and update of systematic review. *Lancet.* 2007;369(9577):1929–1937.
51. Auperin A, Le Pechoux C, Rolland E, et al. Meta-analysis of concomitant versus sequential radiochemotherapy in locally advanced non-small-cell lung cancer. *J Clin Oncol.* 2010;28(13): 2181–2190.
52. Davidoff AJ, Gardner JF, Seal B, Edelman MJ. Population-based estimates of survival benefit associated with combined modality therapy in elderly patients with locally advanced non-small cell lung cancer. *J Thorac Oncol.* 2011;6(5):934–941.
53. Gridelli C, Maione P, Rossi A, Ciardiello F, Raben D. Treatment of locally advanced non-small cell lung cancer in the elderly. *Curr Opin Oncol.* 2005;17(2):130–134.
54. Atagi S, Kawahara M, Tamura T, et al. Standard thoracic radiotherapy with or without concurrent daily low-dose carboplatin in elderly patients with locally advanced non-small cell lung cancer: a phase III trial of the Japan Clinical Oncology Group (JCOG9812). *Jpn J Clin Oncol.* 2005;35(4):195–201.
55. Chrischilles EA, Pendergast JF, Kahn KL, et al. Adverse events among the elderly receiving chemotherapy for advanced non-small-cell lung cancer. *J Clin Oncol.* 2010;28(4):620–627.
56. Davidoff AJ, Tang M, Seal B, Edelman MJ. Chemotherapy and survival benefit in elderly patients with advanced non-small-cell lung cancer. *J Clin Oncol.* 2010;28(13):2191–2197.
57. The Elderly Lung Cancer Vinorelbine Italian Study Group. Effects of vinorelbine on quality of life and survival of elderly patients with advanced non small cell lung cancer. *J Natl Cancer Inst.* 1999;91(1):66–72.
58. Kudoh S, Takeda K, Nakagawa K, et al. Phase III study of docetaxel compared with vinorelbine in elderly patients with advanced non-small-cell lung cancer: results of the West Japan Thoracic Oncology Group trial (WJOG 9904). *J Clin Oncol.* 2006;24(22):3657–3663.
59. Frasci G, Lorusso V, Panza N, et al. Gemcitabine plus vinorelbine versus vinorelbine alone in elderly patients with advanced non-small-cell lung cancer. *J Clin Oncol.* 2000;18(13):2529–2536.
60. Gridelli C, Perrone F, Gallo C, et al. Chemotherapy for elderly patients with advanced non-small-cell lung cancer: the Multicenter Italian Lung Cancer in the Elderly Study (MILES) phase III randomized trial. *J Natl Cancer Inst.* 2003;95(5): 362–372.
61. Russo A, Rizzo S, Fulfaro F, et al. Gemcitabine-based doublets versus single agent therapy for elderly patients with advanced nonsmall cell lung cancer: a literature-based meta-analysis. *Cancer.* 2009;115(9):1924–1931.

62. Pfister DG, Johnson DH, Azzoli CG, et al. American Society of Clinical Oncology treatment of unresectable non-small-cell lung cancer guideline: update 2003. *J Clin Oncol.* 2004;22(2): 330–353.
63. Azzoli CG, Baker S Jr, Temin S, et al. American Society of Clinical Oncology Clinical Practice Guideline update on chemotherapy for stage IV non-small-cell lung cancer. *J Clin Oncol.* 2009;27(36):6251–6266.
64. Gridelli C, Maione P, Rossi A. Therapy for elderly patients with advanced non-small cell lung cancer. Paper presented at: 47th Annual Meeting of American Society of Clinical Oncology Educational Book, June 3–7, 2011; Chicago, IL; 300–304.
65. Quoix E, Zalcman G, Oster JP, et al. Carboplatin and weekly paclitaxel doublet chemotherapy compared with monotherapy in elderly patients with advanced non-small-cell lung cancer: IFCT-0501 randomised, phase 3 trial. *Lancet.* 2011;378(9796):1079–1088.
66. Abe T, Yokoyama A, Takeda K, et al. Randomized phase III trial comparing weekly docetaxel (D)-cisplatin (P) combination with triweekly D alone in elderly patients (pts) with advanced non-small cell lung cancer (NSCLC): an intergroup trial of JCOG0803/WJOG4307L. *J Clin Oncol.* 2011;29(15S):478s. Abstract 7509.
67. Biesma B, Wymenga ANM, Vincent A, et al. Quality of life, geriatric assessment and survival in elderly patients with non-small-cell lung cancer treated with carboplatin-gemcitabine or carboplatin-paclitaxel: NVALT-3 a phase III study. *Ann Oncol.* 2011;22(7):1520–1527.
68. Gridelli C, Maione P, Illiano A, et al. Cisplatin plus gemcitabine or vinorelbine for elderly patients with advanced non small-cell lung cancer: the MILES-2P studies. *J Clin Oncol.* 2007; 25(29):4663–4669.
69. ClinicalTrials.gov. MILES-3: cisplatin in combination with gemcitabine for elderly patients with lung cancer. http://clinicaltrials.gov/ct2/show/NCT01405586. Accessed September 15, 2011.
70. Blanchard EM, Arnaoutakis K, Hesketh PJ. Lung cancer in octogenarians. *J Thorac Oncol.* 2010;5(6):909–916.
71. Sandler A, Gray R, Perry MC, et al. Paclitaxel-carboplatin alone or with bevacizumab for non-small-cell lung cancer. *New Engl J Med.* 2006; 355(24):2542–2550.
72. Ramalingam SS, Dahlberg SE, Langer CJ, et al. Outcomes for elderly, advanced-stage non small-cell lung cancer patients treated with bevacizumab in combination with carboplatin and paclitaxel: analysis of Eastern Cooperative Oncology Group Trial 4599. *J Clin Oncol.* 2008;26(1):60–65.
73. Leighl N, Zatloukal P, Mezger J, et al. Efficacy and safety of bevacizumab-based therapy in elderly patients with advanced or recurrent non-squamous non-small cell lung cancer in the phase III BO17704 study (AVAiL). *J Thorac Oncol.* 2010;5(12):1970–1976.
74. Crinò L, Cappuzzo F, Zatloukal P, et al. Gefitinib versus vinorelbine in chemotherapy-naive elderly patients with advanced non-small-cell lung cancer (INVITE): a randomized, phase II study. *J Clin Oncol.* 2008;26(26):4253–4260.
75. Jackman DM, Yeap BY, Lindeman NI, et al. Phase II clinical trial of chemotherapy-naïve patients ≥ 70 years of age treated with erlotinib for advanced non-small-cell lung cancer. *J Clin Oncol.* 2007;25(7):760–766.
76. Dienstmann R, Martinez P, Felip E. Personalizing therapy with targeted agents in non-small cell lung cancer. *Oncotarget.* 2011;2(3):165–177.
77. Scagliotti G, Hanna N, Fossella F, et al. The differential efficacy of pemetrexed according to NSCLC histology: a review of two phase III studies. *Oncologist.* 2009;14(3):253–263.
78. Weiss GJ, Langer C, Rosell R, et al. Elderly patients benefit from second-line cytotoxic chemotherapy: a subset analysis of a randomized phase III trial of pemetrexed compared with docetaxel in patients with previously treated advanced non-small-cell lung cancer. *J Clin Oncol.* 2006;24(27):4405–4411.
79. Wheatley-Price P, Ding K, Seymour L, et al. Erlotinib for advanced non-small-cell lung cancer in the elderly: an analysis of the National Cancer Institute of Canada Clinical Trials Group Study BR.21. *J Clin Oncol.* 2008;26(14):2350–2357.
80. Tibaldi C, Bernardini I, Chella A, et al. Second-line chemotherapy with a modified schedule of

docetaxel in elderly patients with advanced-stage non-small-cell lung cancer. *Clin Lung Cancer.* 2006;7(6):401–405.

81. Patel AM, Dunn WF, Trastek VF. Staging systems of lung cancer. *Mayo Clin Proc.* 1993;68(5): 475–482.
82. Vallieres E, Shepherd FA, Crowley J, et al. The IASLC Lung Cancer Staging Project: proposals regarding the relevance of TNM in the pathologic staging of small cell lung cancer in the forthcoming (seventh) edition of the TNM classification for lung cancer. *J Thorac Oncol.* 2009;4(9):1049–1059.
83. Rossi A, Maione P, Colantuoni G, et al. Treatment of small cell lung cancer in the elderly. *Oncologist.* 2005;10(6):399–411.
84. Jackman DM, Johnson BE. Small-cell lung cancer. *Lancet.* 2005;366(9494):1385–1396.
85. Pignon JP, Arriagada R, Ihde DC, et al. A meta-analysis of thoracic radiotherapy for small-cell lung cancer. *N Engl J Med.* 1992;327(23):1618–1624.
86. Schild SE, Stella PJ, Brooks BJ, et al. Results of combined-modality therapy for limited-stage small cell lung carcinoma in the elderly. *Cancer.* 2005;103(11):2349–2354.
87. Janssen-Heijnen MLG, Maas HAAM, van de Schans SAM, Coebergh JW, Groen HJ. Chemotherapy in elderly small-cell lung cancer patients: yes we can, but should be do it? *Ann Oncol.* 2011;22(4):821–826.
88. Auperin A, Arriagada R, Pignon JP, et al. Prophylactic cranial irradiation for patients with small-cell lung cancer in complete remission. *N Engl J Med.* 1999;341(7):476–484.
89. Crossen JR, Garwood D, Glatstein E, Neuwelt EA. Neurobehavioral sequelae of cranial irradiation in adults: a review of radiation induced encephalopathy. *J Clin Oncol.* 1994;12(3):627–642.
90. Murray N, Gratt C, Shah A, et al. Abbreviated treatment for elderly, infirm or noncompliant patients with limited-stage small-cell lung cancer. *J Clin Oncol.* 1998;16(10):3323–3328.
91. Jeremic B, Shibamoto Y, Acimovic L, Milisavljevic S. Carboplatin, etoposide and accelerated hyperfractionated radiotherapy for elderly patients with limited small lung carcinoma. *Cancer.* 1998;82(5):836–841.
92. Ardizzoni A, Favaretto A, Boni L, et al. Platinum-etoposide chemotherapy in elderly patients with small-cell lung cancer: results of a randomized multicenter phase II study assessing attenuated-dose or full-dose with lenograstim prophylaxis – a Forza Operativa Nazionale Italiana Carcinoma Polmonare and Gruppo Studio Tumori Polmonari Veneto (FONICAP-GSTPV) study. *J Clin Oncol.* 2005;23(3):569–575.
93. Gridelli C, Gallo C, Morabito A, et al. Phase I-II trial of gemcitabine-based first line chemotherapies for small cell lung cancer in elderly patients with performance status 0–2: the G-Step trial. *J Thorac Oncol.* 2012;7:233–242.
94. Okamoto H, Watanabe K, Kunikane H, et al. Randomised phase III trial of carboplatin plus etoposide vs split doses of cisplatin plus etoposide in elderly or poor-risk patients with extensive disease small-cell lung cancer: JCOG 9702. *Br J Cancer.* 2007;97(2):162–169.
95. Igawa S, Ryuge S, Fukui T, et al. Amrubicin for treating elderly and poor-risk patients with small-cell lung cancer. *Int J Clin Oncol.* 2010;15(5):447–452.
96. Inoue A, Ishimoto O, Fukumoto S, et al. A phase II study of amrubicin combined with carboplatin for elderly patients with small-cell lung cancer: North Japan Lung Cancer Study Group Trial 0405. *Ann Oncol.* 2010;21(4):800–803.
97. Stahel R, Thatcher N, Fruh M, et al. 1st ESMO consensus conference in lung cancer; Lugano 2010: small-cell lung cancer. *Ann Oncol.* 2011;22(9): 1973–1980.
98. Nakao M, Oguri T, Suzuki T, et al. Amrubicin monotherapy for elderly patients with previously treated lung cancer. *Intern Med.* 2010;49(17): 1857–1862.

Emerging Cancer Therapeutics

Surgical Approaches to Early-Stage Lung Cancer

Rodney J. Landreneau*

Professor of Surgery, Department of Cardiothoracic Surgery, University of Pittsburgh, Pittsburgh, PA

ABSTRACT

This chapter provides a brief perspective on the evolution of the surgical management of early-stage lung cancer over the last century. It then describes the current clinical considerations that influence the surgical plan for each patient with early-stage, non-small cell lung cancer (NSCLC). At one time, surgeons believed that radical pneumonectomy was the best treatment for all lung cancer, but in the 1960s, it became evident that lobectomy was sufficient for early-stage NSCLC. Since then, the morbidity, mortality, and oncologic efficacy of lesser resections have been explored. Sublobar resections are associated with oncologic outcomes that are comparable to lobectomy in subcentimeter Stage IA NSCLC. However, for larger lesions, particularly those greater than 3 cm in size, several surgical series have suggested that lobectomy results in the best long-term survival. Additionally, in younger patients with Stage I NSCLC, survival may to be enhanced with lobectomy as the resective procedure. Although the use of computed tomography scanning has improved the staging of NSCLC, it is important for the physician to recognize the frequency of clinical upstaging following pathologic review of the resected specimen, and modify the patient's treatment plan accordingly.

Keywords: non-small cell lung cancer, Stage I, lobectomy, segmentectomy, thoracic surgery, history

INTRODUCTION

The surgical management of early-stage non-small cell lung cancer (NSCLC) has continued to evolve as our understanding of the biologic nature of lung cancer matures. Similarly, a more accurate estimate of the clinical stage of the tumor as "early" and regionally confined allows us to more accurately identify those patients who may benefit from surgical resection of their primary lung cancer. Like most areas of medicine, the evolution of surgical care of lung cancer has been largely empirical in nature (1). This is not necessarily a bad thing; however, refinement of the care of the patient is enhanced and expedited with steadfast attention

*Corresponding author, Department of Cardiothoracic Surgery, University of Pittsburgh, Pittsburgh, PA
E-mail address: landreneaurj@upmc.edu

Emerging Cancer Therapeutics 3:1 (2012) 95–110.

DOI: 10.5003/2151–4194.3.1.95

to an honest, objective enquiry into the relative benefit of various surgical (or ablative) approaches being used for the management of "early-stage" lung cancer.

In this chapter, a brief perspective of the evolution of surgical management of early-stage lung cancer over the last century is provided. In addition, the clinical considerations at play today that influence the surgical plan for an "individual" patient with presumed early-stage lung cancer are described.

■ HISTORICAL PERSPECTIVE RELATED TO PERFORMING THORACOTOMY FOR LUNG DISEASE

The first successful resection of a "lung tumor" was accomplished by a rural Georgia surgeon Milton Anthony in 1823 (2). This surgery involved the removal of a two-pound suppurative tumor involving the chest wall and lung from the unfortunate patient who was eased his pain only through the effects of "strong spirits" as local anesthetics, and general anesthetics were yet to be a reality for the surgical patient. It was not until the end of the 19th century that the use of general anesthesia, achieved through inhalational ether and chloroform, allowed surgeons to contemplate and eventually perform open thoracotomy to manage benign and malignant problems (3).

Other problems that retarded the surgical approach to thoracic disease, and lung cancer in particular, were the result of misconceptions regarding the importance of closed chest drainage following thoracotomy and delay in implementing endotracheal intubation with positive pressure ventilation during the operation. Jules Emil Pean is believed to be the first to perform open thoracotomy and cautery excision of a peripheral lung tumor in 1861. He sutured the lung edge to the thoracic incisional wound to avoid pulmonary collapse and pneumothorax after the lung resection (4). Davies is credited with the first anatomic lobectomy for lung cancer in 1912, but his patient died from pulmonary insufficiency and pneumonia, which was related to the lack of closed chest drainage, and resultant pulmonary collapse a week after his surgery (5,6). Lilienthal saw similarly poor results, greater than 40% mortality with pulmonary resection, even though he recognized the importance of positive pressure ventilation during surgery, as he also neglected the use of closed chest drainage following thoracotomy (7). Although many primarily acclaim Evarts Graham with the performance of the first single-staged pneumonectomy in 1933, an accomplishment independently performed by five other surgeons in the same year (8,9), possibly Graham's most important contribution to the field of thoracic surgery was his identification of the importance of closed chest drainage of streptococcal emypema (10,11). It was not until Brunn demonstrated success with pulmonary lobectomy using closed chest drainage of the pleural space following pulmonary lobectomy that the basic strategies for pulmonary resection necessary to achieve success in the management of lung cancer were realized (12).

Certainly, improvement in perioperative management of the patient with suspected lung cancer, including enhanced clinical staging, blood transfusion (13,14), enhanced anesthetic management, introduction and acceptance of minimally invasive surgical approaches (15,16), and intensive care strategies for the high-risk patient have made surgical resection of the early-stage lung cancer the standard of care. Now, rather than having a "coin toss" for survival between surgical resection and death as a result of the primary lung cancer, the patient and the surgeon must choose from a variety of surgical and nonsurgical image-guided ablative approaches for the cure of early-stage lung cancer.

■ CLINICAL PERCEPTIONS OF CANCER AND "ADEQUATE SURGERY FOR CURE"

It has long been appreciated that total removal of a malignant neoplasm is the only effective surgical therapeutic option. Indeed, the great John Hunter, anatomist and leading surgical educator of the 18th century, stated plainly that partial removal of the tumor was as good as not approaching the tumor at all surgically (17). The concept of total removal of the tumor and affected organ became the standard of surgical oncologic practice for most of the 19th century, as well as into the mid-20th century. The surgical treatment of breast cancer is a good example of philosophy of most surgeons during this period.

The radical mastectomy popularized by William Halsted was the "poster child" for surgical management of all cancers. It was believed that the malignancy spread as a spilt can of paint from primary site to conjoining tissues without interruption. The only effective surgical treatment was to remove the entire breast and its associated lymphatic bed. Contiguous organs potentially affected by the cancer would also have to be extirpated even if it meant the loss of the ipsilateral upper extremity (18). Surgeons recognized that they could offer little help to their cancer patients beyond local control of the disease. They fully realized that the patient's fate was usually sealed due to the eventual systemic progression of the malignancy. Certainly, the late presentation of most breast cancer patients usually meant that the disease was locally advanced and local control would necessarily require a radical resection. As the results of mastectomy improved, more patients sought surgical care at an earlier clinical stage of disease. As more "cures" were observed with the total mastectomy being employed, the mindset of mid-20th century surgeons was that if even more radical surgery was performed, the cure rate should also improve. This latter assumption of improved survival with even greater radicality of resection was not realized.

Thoracic surgeons of this era were similarly influenced by this "Halstedian" surgical oncologic concept, and most believed that total pneumonectomy was the only appropriate therapy for lung cancer even though the surgical mortality and morbidity in reported series were high (19–22). Again, most lung cancers were diagnosed and resected when they were symptomatic and advanced locally. Like breast cancer, the late presentation of lung cancer also affected decision making regarding the extent of pulmonary resection required to completely extirpate the malignancy.

The morbidity of mastectomy and the mortality associated with pneumonectomy inspired a natural aversion toward these procedures by many patients and thoracic surgeons alike. It was not until the experience with safer and more appealing lesser resections demonstrated equivalent cancer-related survival that radical mastectomy and pneumonectomy were generally abandoned as the standard of care for the "early" cancer patient (23,24). The contrast in surgical morbidity between pneumonectomy and lobectomy and the steady shift toward lobectomy as the preferred operation for small peripheral cancers was clearly noted in 1962 in a comparison of surgical outcomes between the Ochsner clinic where radical pneumonectomy remained the standard of care and the New England Deaconess Hospital where lobectomy was being favored for early lung cancer (Figure 1) (24). This study demonstrated long-term survival equivalent to radical pneumonectomy when lobectomy was used for cancer localized to the lung and completely resected by this lesser, less morbid approach rather than by pneumonectomy. Although even lesser resections for primary early lung cancer were explored (25,26), by the mid-1960s anatomic lobectomy with mediastinal nodal dissection had become the standard of care for early-stage lung cancer (27).

Jensik and Read independently explored the utility of anatomic segmentectomy in the 1970s as the primary anatomic surgical resection for small, peripheral lung cancer (28,29). Their clinical results with anatomic segmentectomy appeared equivalent to those of lobectomy or pneumonectomy for appropriate clinical circumstances. The controversy regarding the most appropriate resection for the small peripheral lung cancer became even more acute after Erret's report of equivalent long-term survival among his patients with poor pulmonary function who underwent wedge resection only for early, Stage I lung cancer as compared

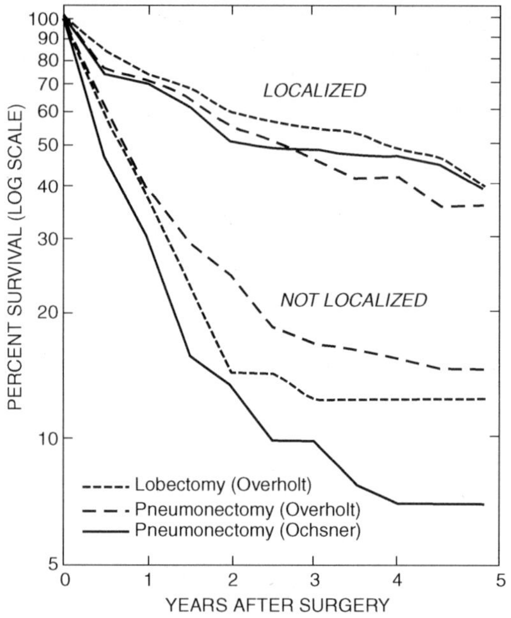

FIGURE 1
Relative survivals between pneumonectomy and lobectomy at Ochsner and Overholt clinics reported in 1962.

Source: Reprinted from Ref. (24). Copyright Mosby (1962).

with his patients with superior cardiopulmonary reserve with Stage I lung cancer for whom he chose lobectomy to manage their disease (30).

Consequently, the Lung Cancer Study Group (LCSG) initiated and completed a randomized study of lobectomy compared with sublobar resection of Stage I NSCLC, which resulted in a mixed review of the points of discussion (31). Note that the trial was limited to resection of T1 tumors (a tumor less than 3 cm in diameter without visceral pleural invasion) and the confirmation of the absence of mediastinal and hilar lymph node involvement by intraoperative frozen section analysis was required prior to randomization to either lobectomy or sublobar resection. Interestingly, no significant difference in 5-year survival between lobectomy and sublobar resection was noted; however, an important increased incidence in local recurrence (6% vs. 17% $P = .008$) was noted among patients who underwent sublobar resection. Landreneau et al., representing the emerging minimally invasive thoracic surgical era, reported similar outcomes the following year for Stage I NSCLC patients chosen for sublobar resection because of impairment in cardiopulmonary function compared with good-risk patients who underwent lobectomy. Again, no difference in survival was seen between resection groups; however, local recurrence was significantly more common among the sublobar resection group (all sublobar resection patients underwent wedge resection in this series) (32). The general conclusions for the surgical management of the early-stage NSCLC by the thoracic surgical community by the middle of the 1990s were therefore, "Wedge resection, done by open thoracotomy or video-assisted techniques, appears to be a viable "compromise" surgical treatment of Stage I (T1N0M0) NSCLC for patients with cardiopulmonary physiologic impairment. Because of the increased risk for local recurrence, anatomic lobectomy remains the surgical treatment of choice for patients with Stage I NSCLC who have adequate physiologic reserve" (32).

With the influx of patients with severe emphysema referred for lung volume reduction surgery (LVRS) in the mid-1990s (33,34), many patients coming in for evaluation for LVRS were found to have incidental lung cancers. Pigula et al. from the University of Pittsburgh reported a prevalence of 10 lung cancers found among 125 patients initially referred for lung volume reduction (35).

Additionally, the increased number of patients with significant emphysema having surprisingly satisfactory outcomes following LVRS, particularly those procedures done by video-assisted thoracoscopic surgery (VATS), encouraged thoracic surgeons that sublobar resection of malignant peripheral nodules identified in such patients could be safely accomplished. The scourge of local recurrence continued to be an issue for patients with Stage I NSCLC who had undergone sublobar resection. External beam radiation therapy had been reported by Hatcher and Miller as "postage stamp" adjuvant radiation following sublobar resection of peripheral cancers by open thoracotomy in physiologically impaired patients (36). They identified a reduction in local recurrence; however, the reproducible benefits in overall control and pulmonary function preservation with this external beam radiation approach were tempered by the difficulty in radiation treatment planning along the serpiginous arrangement of wedge resection staple lines commonly resulting in significant local radiation damage to the lung parenchyma and associated loss of pulmonary reserve. The addition of intraoperative radiobrachytherapy immediately following sublobar resection began to be explored as a means of reducing this local recurrence problem. Hilaris, Martini, and their associates at Memorial Sloan Kettering had reported on the use of intraoperative brachytherapy to manage advanced lung cancer with close or positive margins following surgical resection (37). They reported an improvement in local control for these advanced stage patients but with no improvement in survival. Of note, d'Amato et al. were the first to report the use of intraoperative, radioactive I-125 brachytherapy as an adjunct to VATS resection of peripheral Stage I NSCLC to reduce local recurrence in these otherwise curable lung cancers identified in functionally impaired patients (38). Santos expanded upon d'Amato's results when he reported an extended experience with intraoperative I-125 brachytherapy following sublobar resection in 99 consecutive patients from the same institution. In the report, Santos reported a postoperative local recurrence rate of 1%, which faired favorably against the reported local recurrence of nearly 20% in earlier series (39). The group at Boston University also reported a similar reduction in local recurrence following sublobar resection with intraoperative I-125 brachytherapy (40).

The results of these two retrospective clinical investigations led the American College of Surgeons Oncology Group (ACOSOG) to conduct a study of over 200 Stage I NSCLC patients with impaired cardiopulmonary reserve randomized to undergo sublobar resection alone or sublobar resection with intraoperative brachytherapy (Z4032). Patient accrual to this study has been completed, but the results are still pending. Hopefully, this study will give us insight into proper patient selection for the use of adjuvant brachytherapy among high-risk patients chosen for sublobar resection of peripheral Stage I NSCLC.

■ CLINICAL IMPORTANCE OF SURVEILLANCE AND IMPACT ON SURGICAL APPROACHES

So with the historical background and the general concepts of "adequacy of resection" described above, how is it that the general pattern of resection for many cancers has changed from "radical" to less extensive and parenchymal preserving?

A great deal of the credit for this trend relates to cancer surveillance measures leading to early, subclinical diagnosis of suspected malignancy for the disease screened. Using breast cancer as the primary model, we see that historically breast cancer presented at an advanced stage where only radical extirpation of the breast and matted lymph nodes of the axilla could have any chance for local control and the faintest possibility of cure. The concept of self-breast examination was not a popular practice during the conservative Victorian age and the thought of undergoing a horrific deforming operation with little if any anesthesia was certainly a fearful thought. William Halsted must be credited with turning the tide toward surgery for this awful disease of the time through the use of the now available "ether" general anesthesia, meticulous surgical technique, and the championing of strict antiseptic surgical principles. His surgical concepts of complete extirpation of the involved organ and its lymphatic drainage gained popularity throughout the surgical culture, and indeed these concepts are still honored today. As surgical success defined primarily by local control was more commonly realized, super radical mastectomy was also advocated by some surgeons aiming to effectuate a greater cure rate from the cancer (3).

As would naturally occur, with the identification of smaller, minimally symptomatic lesions, local control and cure were seen more commonly; however, the morbidity, deformity, and psychological trauma related to radical mastectomy remained an important negative characteristic of breast cancer treatment. Nonsurgical alternatives and lesser surgery were certainly a tempting possible alternative for many patients and physicians.

Radiographic examination of the breast, mammography, was introduced by the German surgeon Albert Salomon in 1913 who used radiography to study the pathologic spread of breast cancer to regional lymph nodes (41). We must credit Robert L. Egan a radiologist who graduated from the University of Pittsburgh and was recruited to MD Anderson Cancer Center, in the 1950 and 1960s, who "spread the gospel of mammography." He coined the term "occult carcinoma" as mammographically, "one which remains totally unsuspected following examination by the usual methods used to examine the breast by an experienced and competent physician." To qualify for this definition, no symptoms or signs should be present (42). These advances in identifying small, truly early breast cancers, and the advent of more effective systemic therapy for breast cancer ultimately encouraged breast surgeons, radiation oncologists, and medical oncologist to explore the use of lesser surgery and expanded the use of nonsurgical options for breast cancer (23).

The diagnosis of lung cancer and this disease's therapy have followed a similar pathway. In 1951, Overholt was early in recommending surgical treatment of "silent lung disease" identified by radiographic examination serendipitously or associated with minimal symptoms (43). At that time, the incidence of primary lung cancer was dramatically rising across the world with growing tobacco exposure. In an effort to identify lung cancer at a potentially more curable state that could also be handled with lesser resections than pneumonectomy, he recommended close attention to radiographic findings and aggressive surgical removal of suspicious lesions. This strategy of early intervention ultimately led the way to more frequent use of lobectomy and anatomic segmentectomy for the definitive management of smaller lesions that could be completely removed by these parenchymal sparing, less morbid surgeries (25–30,32,44,45).

Now, computed tomography (CT) scan surveillance is coming to fore as a potential means of identifying even more lung cancers at a highly curable stage. Although overdiagnosis bias and lead-time bias are considerations, the recent results of the National Lung Screening Trial and the International Early Lung Cancer Action Program suggest that lung cancers can be identified at an early curable stage and that a significant reduction in lung cancer-related deaths and deaths from all causes may be affected with routine CT surveillance of patients at high risk for lung cancer (older smokers with impaired pulmonary reserve) (46,47). Investigators at the University of Pittsburgh have identified similar clinical findings (48).

With the identification of small peripheral tumors, easily resected by generous wedge resection or anatomic segmentectomy with generous parenchymal margins of resection, the debate over the necessity of lobectomy in this clinical setting has reemerged (Figures 2 and 3). With national chest CT surveillance in place for several decades in Japan, surgical investigators there have led the way in exploring this clinical issue (49–51). The remaining aspects of this discussion will explore the information at hand today regarding the management of the Stage I NSCLC in this era of enhanced diagnostics and minimally invasive surgical approaches to resection.

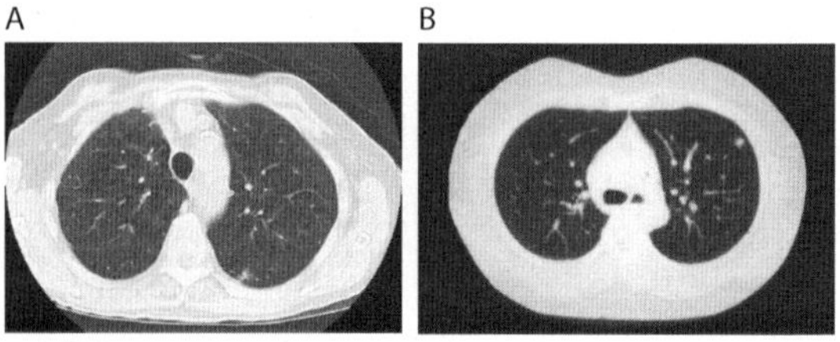

FIGURE 2
CT images of subcentimeter lung nodules identified by screening CT.

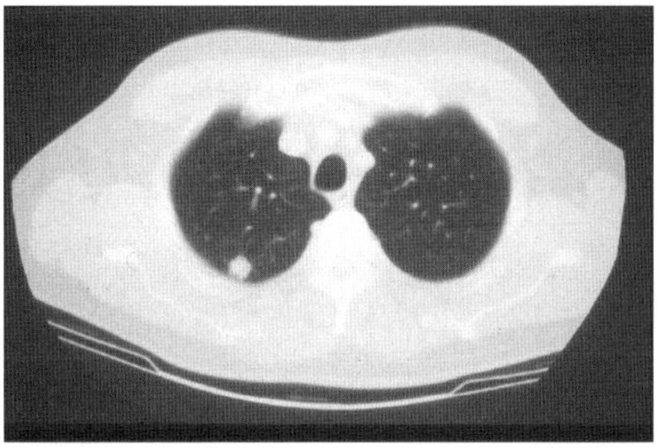

FIGURE 3
CT image of small peripheral nodule amenable to complete resection with clear margins by anatomic segmentectomy or extended wedge resection.

■ PHYSIOLOGIC CONSIDERATIONS

As discussed earlier, sublobar resection may often be the only surgical approach that can be safely considered for patients with impaired cardiopulmonary reserve or advanced age. Mery et al. examined the clinical outcomes of 14,555 patients with Stage I or II NSCLC whose records were present within the national Surveillance, Epidemiology, and End Results (SEER) database to identify various parameters associated with long-term survival related to the surgical approach used to primarily manage the patients' lung cancer (52). The primary message of their analysis was that cancer-related and overall survival for older patients (> 75 years of age) was the same regardless of whether the patient had undergone lobectomy or sublobar resection. This message has been supported by the work of other investigators (53–55). For younger patients, survival appeared to be enhanced with lobectomy as the resective procedure (52). These results were predictable among older patients due to associated comorbidities contributing to postoperative survival time. Intrinsic biases that would be hard to extract from the limited data available in the SEER database leave questions open as to why the survivorship was greater among younger patients undergoing lobectomy. Selection bias due to comorbidity among younger patients who underwent sublobar resection may have affected overall results with this lesser procedure (Figures 4 and 5). These results, and the overall analysis of the role of any surgery for cancer, may also be a result of an "overtreatment" bias related to removal of biologically indolent cancers that would not have an impact on the patient's survival. This "overtreatment" bias associates salutary cancer treatment effects for patients who may "die with" but not "die from" their cancer, such as some breast, prostate, and thyroid malignancies.

Our group has also explored the effects of age upon postoperative morbidity and long-term

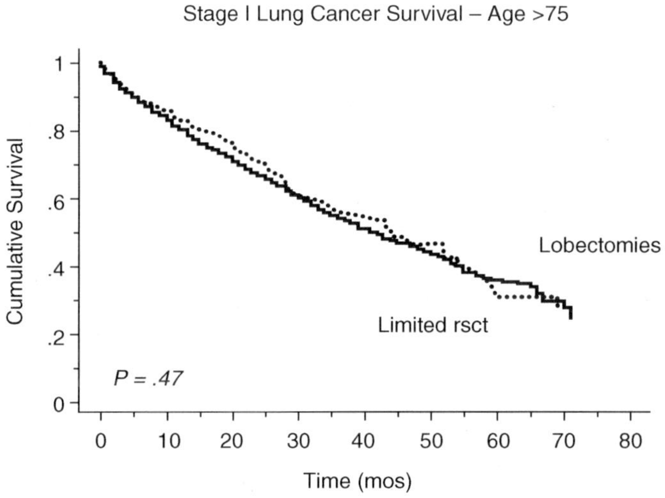

FIGURE 4
Survival differences among early lung cancer patients older than 75 years of age: sublobar resection versus lobectomy.

Source: Reproduced with permission from the American College of Chest Physicians. From Ref. (52).

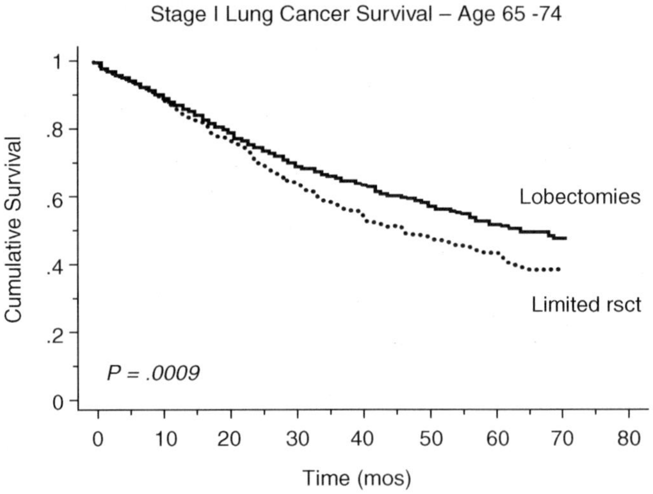

FIGURE 5
Survival differences among early lung cancer patients younger than 75 years of age: sublobar resection versus lobectomy.

Source: Reproduced with permission from the American College of Chest Physicians. From Ref. (52).

survival following resection of Stage I NSCLC by either lobectomy or sublobar resection (56). As discussed earlier, sublobar resection appears to be a reasonable compromise procedure when approaching the patient with impaired cardiopulmonary reserve (32,38,39). Several other investigators have also looked at the utility of anatomic segmentectomy compared to lobectomy for the management of the elderly patients with Stage I NSCLC (56–59). The clinical outcomes of 184 patients who underwent surgery (78 segmentectomy; 106 lobectomy) from 2002 through 2007 with equivalent mean age of 78 years were analyzed. Surgical mortalilty and morbidty were significantly less among elderly patients undergoing segmentectomy compared to lobectomy, and there was no difference in long-term survival between the surgical groups (Figure 6).

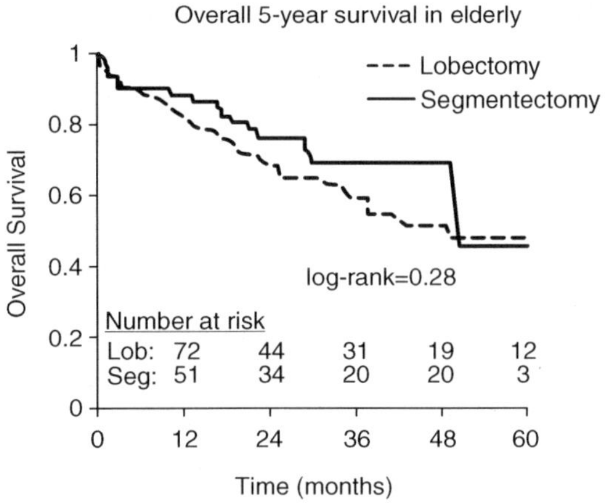

FIGURE 6
Survival among elderly (average age = 78) early cancer patients: anatomic segmentectomy versus lobectomy.

Source: Reprinted from Ref. (56). Copyright (2009) with permission from The Society of Thoracic Surgeons/ Elsevier.

■ ANATOMIC/PATHOLOGIC CONSIDERATIONS

Size matters, among other things! As we further analyze the results with surgical resection of early-stage NSCLC, we come to find that several pathologic tumor characteristics affect prognosis depending upon the nature of the surgical resection performed. Okada et al. have been leaders in the investigation of the most appropriate surgical approach to peripheral lung cancer (57). These investigators retrospectively reviewed their surgical outcomes among 1,272 patients with early-stage NSCLC based upon tumor size and type of resection used (Table 1). The results of this analysis demonstrated that for Stage I tumors

TABLE 1 Differential survival by tumor size between resective approaches used for early-stage NSCLC

Tumor Size	Segmental Resection	Lobectomy	Wedge Resection
20 mm or less	96.7	92.4	85.7
20–30 mm	84.6	87.4	39.4
More than 30 mm	62.9	81.3	0

Source: Adapted from Ref. (57).

TABLE 2 Distribution of Stage IA NSCLC cancers resected by anatomic segmentectomy or lobectomy

	Anatomic Segmentectomy (*n* = 182)	Lobectomy (*n* = 246)
Stage IA	109 (60%)	114 (46%)
Mean Tumor Size (cm)	1.7	1.9

less than 2 cm in diameter, survival was equivalent between lobectomy and anatomic segmentectomy. Indeed for lesions of this size, wedge resection in their experience was also appeared to be a reasonable surgical option. However, for larger lesions, particularly those greater than 3 cm, it appeared that lobectomy provided the best long-term survival rates (57). Schuchert and colleagues demonstrated similar results with anatomic segmentectomy compared to lobectomy for Stage IA NSCLC (58) (Table 2 and Figure 7).

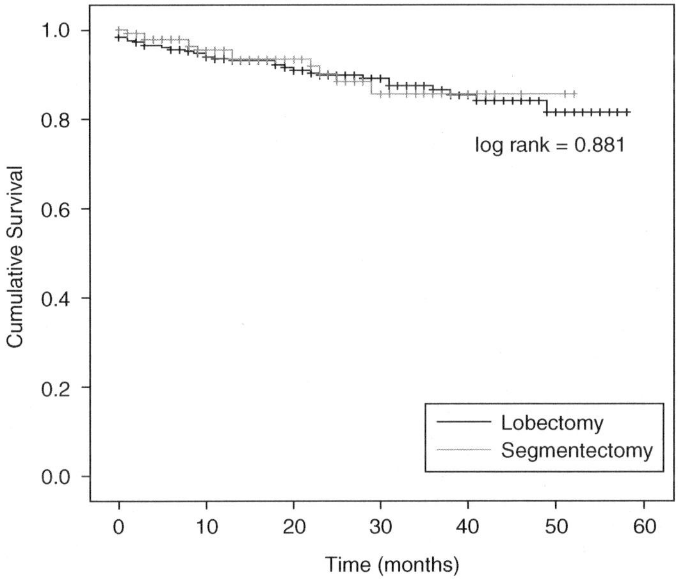

FIGURE 7
Survival among Stage IA NSCLC patients undergoing anatomic segmentectomy or lobectomy.

Source: Reprinted from Ref. (58). Copyright (2007) with permission from The Society of Thoracic Surgeons/Elsevier.

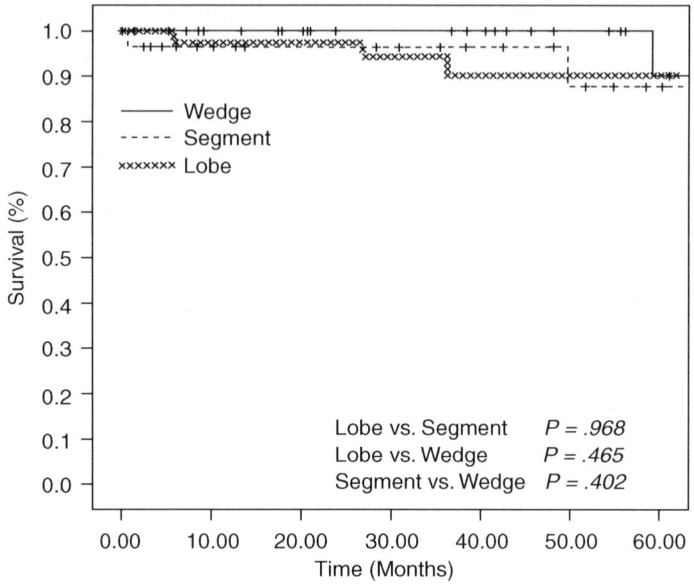

FIGURE 8
Recurrence-free survival of patients undergoing sublobar resection of subcentimeter peripheral nodules (wedge vs. segmentectomy vs. lobectomy).

Source: Reprinted from Ref. (59). Copyright (2011) with permission from The Society of Thoracic Surgeons/ Elsevier.

Schuchert and associates have also looked at the survival among patients with subcentimeter lung cancers treated by sublobar resection or lobectomy (59). The outcomes of 104 patients with this most favorable Stage IA disease who underwent lobecotomy (n=32) segmentectomy (n=40), or extended wedge resection (n=35) were analyzed for long-term survival (Figure 8). The conclusions of this work were "Sublobar resections are associated with oncologic outcomes that are comparable to lobectomy in subcentimeter Stage IA NSCLC, suggesting that they may be appropriate surgical interventions in this patient cohort." These conclusions have also been supported by others (60–62).

The presence of visceral pleural invasion is also another important clinical parameter, which may portend a differential prognosis dependent upon the surgical resection chosen for early-stage lung cancer. Visceral pleural invasion and angiolymphatic invasion by the tumor are commonly associated and both have been associated with a generally less optimistic prognosis for otherwise localized node negative lung cancer (63).

Indeed, Schuchert and associates recently published their clinical results in the management of 524 Stage I NSCLC patients undergoing surgical resection by lobectomy (n=285) or anatomic segmentectomy (n=239) (63). Survival was significantly improved with the use of lobectomy when angiolymphatic invasion and pleural invasion were present compared to segmentectomy (Figure 9). Horne et al. have also noted the association of tumor infiltrating lymphocytes within Stage IA NSCLC and long-term survival. When angiolymphatic invasion is absent in the surgical specimen, the association with lymphatic infiltration appears to provide even further improvement in early cancer prognosis irrespective of the extent of surgical resection performed (64).

In addition to these pathologic features of the primary tumor, the surgeon must also be focused on the adequacy of the surgical margin of resection so as to reduce the likelihood of local recurrence. The resected marginal distance from the tumor should be at least equivalent to the diameter of the tumor (58,65,66). Accordingly, a 2 cm tumor should have a 2 cm parenchymal margin of

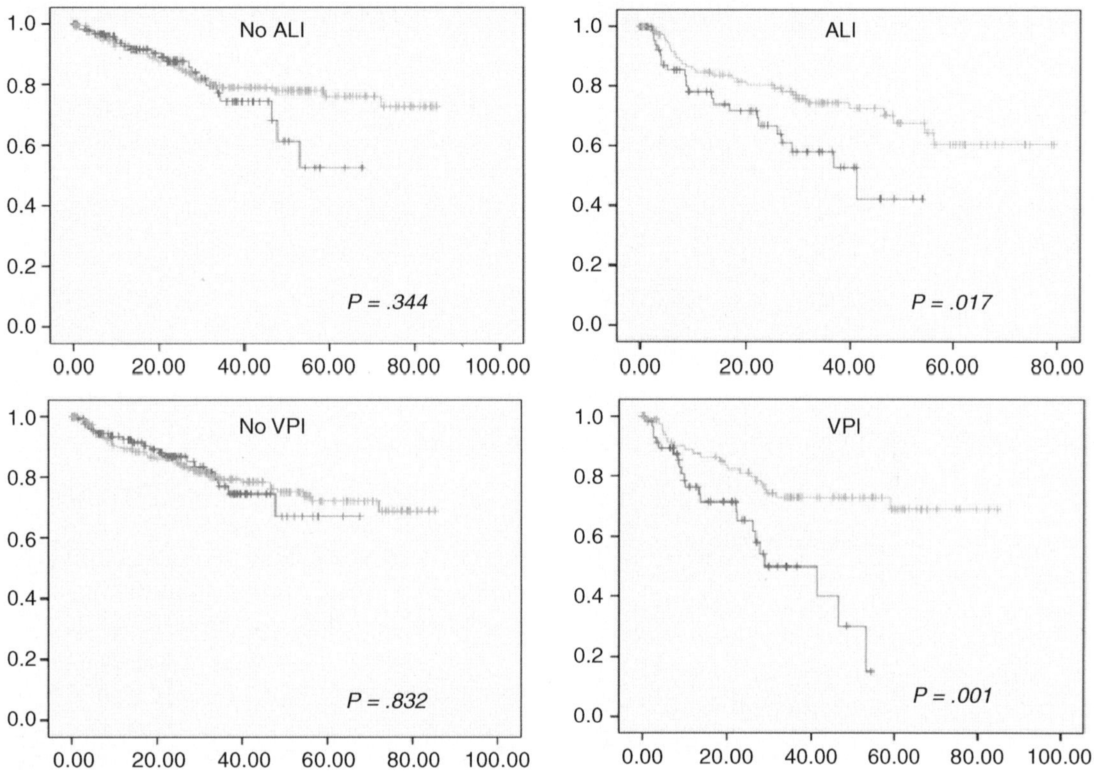

FIGURE 9
Effect of angiolymphatic (ALI) and visceral pleural (VPI) invasion on recurrence-free survival among resected early-stage NSCLC based upon segmental resection (black/dark gray on plots) versus lobectomy (light gray on plots).

resection to optimize the local control status following sublobar resection. When these parameters cannot be met, consideration for adjuvant brachytherapy may be considered if the cardiopulmonary reserve of the patient is in question, or lobectomy should be performed if the patient's functional reserve can tolerate this resection.

All of this information has led the thoracic surgical community to engage in the present intergroup trial initiated by Cancer and Leukemia Group B (CALGB 140503) led by Nasser Altorki, in which sublobar resection by extended wedge resection or segmentectomy is being compared with lobectomy for Stage Ia NSCLC (tumors > 2 cm with node negativity determined before randomization intraoperatively—similar to the earlier mentioned LCSG trial).

■ SURGICAL MORBIDITY AND MORTALITY

When the primary care physician is considering a patient with a newly diagnosed early-stage lung cancer for surgical resection, there are several parameters that should be considered. The physician should make the patient and their family aware of the standard of care for early-stage lung cancer in the United States and internationally. The physician should also be aware of the standard of care regarding preoperative staging by noninvasive means (CT scans, PET scans, etc), endoscopic staging measures (i.e., bronchoscopy and endoscopic bronchial ultrasound), and surgical staging (i.e., mediastinoscopy and VATS diagnostic evaluation). The physician should make the patient aware of the national standards related to accepted morbidity and mortality for the procedure in question and accordingly weigh the risk-benefits of the procedure versus cancer risk to the patient. Allen et al., representing ACOSOG, have recently published new standards for surgical morbidity and mortality for Stage I NSCLC based upon the outcomes of over 1,100 early-stage lung cancer patients involved in clinical trials supported by ACOSOG (67). In this large national series, operative mortality for anatomic lung resection was less than 2% and significant perioperative morbidity was less than 15%. This work by ACOSOG has set the standard of care for the early-stage lung cancer patient. Our group has independently noted clinical results related to improved morbidity and mortality among patients who undergo segmentectomy for early-stage NSCLC (58,68,69).

■ CLINICAL STAGING AND TREATMENT PLANNING

Finally, in this age of adjuvant therapy following resection of "surprise" node-positive NSCLC identified in clinically early-stage disease, it is important for the physician to recognize the frequency of clinical upstaging following pathologic review of the resected specimen. Schuchert et al. recently presented their occurrence among clinically Stage I NSCLC patients at the University of Pittsburgh. Among 1,300 patients who underwent definitive resection following modern preoperative clinical staging (PET/CT, bronchoscopy, mediastinoscopy), clinical upstaging was noted in approximately 30% of patients (70). This finding is similar to previous authors reporting of this subject (71).

Certainly, physicians managing lung cancer patients must be aware of these issues and ensure that the surgeon caring for their patients perform adequate preoperative and intraoperative staging of the patient's disease so as to avoid loss of recognition of this upstaging, which would potentially prevent the patient from receiving the benefits of adjuvant chemotherapy should hilar or mediastinal node positivity be identified in pathologic review.

■ SURGICAL RESECTION OR IMAGE-GUIDED ABLATIVE TREATMENT

To date, there has been no objective review of image-guided ablative procedures compared with surgical resection for early-stage NSCLC. Such protocols are being contemplated for high-risk patients with otherwise resectable NSCLC.

In this era of increasing emphasis upon individualized therapy for the NSCLC patient, "tissue remains the issue." There are several advantages of surgical resection over image-guided ablative techniques (stereotactic body radiation therapy (SBRT) or radiofrequency ablation (RFA)) for the patient with peripheral lung cancer patient in a potentially early stage. Parenchymal/pulmonary functional preservation with the use of anatomic segmentectomy over lobectomy is a consideration for those small peripheral lesions anatomically amenable to this approach. Certainly, surgical resection provides clear delineation of the adequacy of the margins of extirpation of the malignancy as compared with the mystery associated with image-guided ablations. Complete mediastinal and hilar nodal sampling/dissection is done to identify those patients with more advanced pathologic disease in whom adjuvant systemic therapy may be considered. Finally, pathologic assessment and pharmacogenomic testing of the malignant tissue and surrounding lung tissue to assess individualized future therapy for the high-risk patient for recurrent cancer are made available.

■ REFERENCES

1. Conner CF. *A People's History of Science: Miners, Midwifes, and Low Mechanicks*. New York: Nation Books; 2005.
2. Brewer LA. Historical notes on lung cancer before and after Graham's successful pneumonectomy in 1933. *Am J Surg.* 1982;143:650–659.
3. Imber G. *Genius on the Edge: The Bizarre Double Life of Dr. William Stewart Halsted*. New York: Kaplan Publishing; 2010.
4. Pean JE. Chirurgie des poumons. Congres Francais de Chirurgie. 1895;9:Session 72.
5. Meyer JA. Hugh Morriston Davies and lobectomy for cancer, 1912. *Ann Thorac Surg.* 1988;Oct; 46(4):472–474.
6. Davies, HM. Recent advances in surgery of the lung and pleura. *Br.J. Surg.* 1913;1:228–258.
7. Lilienthal H. Resection of the lung for suppurative infections with a report based on 31 operative cases in which resection was done or intended. *Ann Surg.* 1922;75:257–320.
8. Mountain CF, Hermes KE. Surgical treatment of lung cancer. Past and present. *Methods Mol Med.* 2003;75:453–487.
9. Ellis H. The first pneumonectomies for lung cancer. *J Perioper Pract.* 2008;18:130–131.
10. Aboud FC, Verghese AC. Evarts Ambrose Graham, empyema, and the dawn of clinical understanding of negative intrapleural pressure. *Clin Infect Dis.* 2002;34:198–203.
11. Graham EA. *Some Fundamental Considerations in the Treatment of Empyema Thoracis*. St. Louis, MO: CV Mosby; 1925.
12. Brunn H. Surgical principles underlying one stage lobectomy. *Arch Surg.* 1929;180:490.
13. Katz J. George Washington Crile, anoci-association, and pre-emptive analgesia. *Pain.* 1993;53(3): 243–245.
14. MacLean LD, Entin MA. Norman Bethune and Edward Archibald: Sung and unsung heroes. *Ann Thorac Surg.* 2000;70:1746–1752.
15. Landreneau RJ, Hazelrigg SR, Ferson PF, et al. Thoracoscopic resection of 85 pulmonary lesions. *Ann Thorac Surg.* 1992;54:415–419.
16. Landreneau RJ, Mack MJ, Hazelrigg SR, et al. Video-assisted thoracic surgery: Basic technical concepts and intercostal approach strategies. *Ann Thorac Surg.* 1992;54:800–807.
17. Wendy Moore. *The Knife Man. Blood, Body Snatching, and the Birth of Modern Surgery*. New York: Broadway Books of the Doubleday Broadway Publishing group; 2005.
18. Halsted WS. *The results of operations for the cure of cancer of the breast performed at the Johns Hopkins Hospital from June, 1899, to January, 1894*. The Johns Hopkins Hospital Reports 4:297.
19. Graham EA, Singer JJ. Successful removal of an entire lung for carcinoma of the bronchus. *JAMA.* 1933;101:1371–1374.
20. Ochsner A, DeBakey M. Significance of metastasis in primary carcinoma of the lung. *J Thor Surg.* 1942;11:357–387.
21. Graham EA. Indications for total pneumonectomy. *Dis. Chest.* 1944;10:87–94.
22. Brock R, Whytehead LL. Radical pneumonectomy for bronchialcarcinoma. *Br J Surg.* 1955;43:8–24.
23. Fisher B, Anderson SJ. The breast cancer alternative hypothesis. Is there evidence to justify replacing it? *JCO.* 2010;28:366–374.
24. Shimkin MB, Connelly BS, Marcus BS, Cutler SJ. Pneumonectomy and lobectomy in bronchogenic carcinoma. *J Thorac Cardiovasc Surg.* 1962;44:503–519.
25. Churchill ED, Belsey R. Segmental pneumonectomy in bronchiectasis; lingula segment of the left upper lobe. *Ann Surg.* 1939;109:481–499.
26. Overholt, A. A new technique for pulmonary segmental resection. *Surg Gyn Obst.* 1947;84,257–268.
27. Churchill ED, Sweet RH, Scannell JG, Wilkins EW Jr. Further studies in the surgical management of carcinoma of the lung: A further study of the cases treated at the Massachusetts General Hospital from 1950 to 1957. *J Thorac Surg.* 1958;36:301–308.
28. Jensik RJ, Faber LP, Milloy FJ, Monson DO. Segmental resection for lung cancer: a fifteen year experience. *J Thorac Cardiovasc Surg.* 1973;63: 433–438.
29. Read RC, Yoder G, Schaeffer RC. Survival after conservative resection for TINOMO non-small cell lung cancer. *Ann Thorac Surg.* 1990;49:242–247.
30. Erret LE, Wilson J, Chiu RC-J, Munro DD. Wedge resection as an alternative procedure for peripheral

bronchogenic carcinomas in poor-risk patients. *J Thorac Cardiovasc Surg.* 1985;90:656–661.
31. Ginsberg RJ, Rubinstein LV. Randomized trial of lobectomy versus limited resection for T1 N0 non-small cell lung cancer. Lung Cancer Study Group. *Ann Thorac Surg.* 1995;60:615–622.
32. Landreneau RJ, Sugarbaker DJ, Mack MJ, et al. Wedge resection versus lobectomy for stage I (T1NOMO) non-small cell lung cancer. *J Thorac Cardiovasc Surg.* 1997;113:691–700.
33. Keenan RJ, Landreneau RJ, Sciurba FC, et al. Unilateral thoracoscopic surgical approach for diffuse emphysema. *J Thorac Cardiovasc Surg.* 1996; 111:308–316.
34. Sciurba FC, Rogers RM, Keenan RJ, et al. Improvement in pulmonary function and elastic recoil after lung-reduction surgery for diffuse emphysema. *New Engl J Med.* 1996;334: 1095–1099.
35. Pigula FA, Keenan RJ, Ferson PF, Landreneau RJ. Unsuspected lung cancer found in work-up for lung reduction operation. *Ann Thorac Surg.* 1996;61:174–176.
36. Miller JI, Hatcher CR. Limited resection of bronchogenic carcinoma in the patient with marked impairment of pulmonary function. *Ann Thorac Surg.* 1987;44:340–343.
37. Hilaris BS, Martini N.The current state of intraoperative interstitial brachytherapy in lung cancer. *Int J Radiat Oncol Biol Phys.* 1988;15(6): 1347–1354.
38. d'Amato TA, Galloway M, Szydloski G, et al. Intraoperative brachytherapy following thoracoscopic wedge resection of stage I lung cancer *Chest.* 1998;114(4):1112–1115.
39. Santos R, Colonias A, Parda D, et al. Comparison between sublobar resection and 125 Iodine brachytherapy after sublobar resection in high-risk patients with Stage I non-small-cell lung cancer. *Surgery.* 2003;134:691–697.
40. Ketchedjian A, DiPetrillo TA, Daly B, Fernando HC. Role of adjuvant radiation (external beam/ brachytherapy) for stage I NSCLC. *Thorac Surg Clin.* 2007;17(2):273–278.
41. Gold RH, Bassett LW, Widoff BE. Highlights from the history of mammography. *Radiographics.* 1990;10:1110–1131.
42. Egan R. Fifty three cases of carcinoma of the breast, occult until mammography. *AJR.* 1962;88: 1095–1101.
43. Overholt RH. The value of exploration in silent lung disease. *Dis Chest.* 1951;20:111–125.
44. Bonfils-Roberts EA, Clagett OT. Contemporary indication for pulmonary segmental resections. *J Thorac Surg.* 1972;63:433.
45. Lewis RJ. The role of video-assisted thoracic surgery for carcinoma of the lung: Wedge resection to lobectomy by simultaneous individual stapling. *Ann Thorac Surg.* 1993;56:762–768.
46. The International Early Lung Cancer Action Program Investigators. Survival of patients with stage I lung cancer detected on CT screening. *N Engl J Med.* 2006;355:1763–1771.
47. McLoud TC. Initial results of the National Lung Cancer Screening Trial Cancer Imaging. 2011;3(11):S85.
48. Wilson DO, Weissfeld JL, Fuhrman CR, et al The Pittsburgh Lung Cancer Screening Study (PLuSS): Outcomes within three years of a first computed tomography scan. *Am J Respir Crit Care Med.* 2008;178:956–961.
49. Yoshikawa K, Tsubota N, Kodama K, et al. Prospective study of extended segmentectomy for small lung tumors: The final report. *Ann Thorac Surg.* 2002;73:1055–1059.
50. Koike T, Yamato Y, Yoshiya K, et al. Intentional limited pulmonary resection for peripheral TINOMO small-sized lung cancer. *J Thorac Cardiovasc Surg.* 2003;125:424–928.
51. Okada M, Yoshikawa K, Hatta T, et al. Is segmentectomy with lymph node assessment an alternative to lobectomy for non-small cell lung cancer of 2 cm or smaller? *Ann Thorac Surg.* 2001;71: 956–961.
52. Mery CM, Pappas AN, Bueno R, et al. Similar long-term survival of elderly patients with non-small cell lung cancer treated with lobectomy or wedge resection within the surveillance, epidemiology, and end results database. *Chest.* 2005;128(1):237–245.
53. Osaki T, Shirakusa T, Kodate M, Nakanishi R, Mitsudomi T, Ueda H. Surgical treatment of lung cancer in the octogenarian. *Ann Thorac Surg.* 1994;57:188–192.

54. Yancik R. Population aging and cancer: a cross-national concern. *Cancer J.* 2005;11:437–441.
55. Castillo MD, Heerdt PM. Pulmonary resection in the elderly. *Curr Opin Anaesthesiol.* 2007;20:4–9.
56. Kilic A, Schuchert MJ, Pettiford BL, et al. Anatomic segmentectomy for stage I non-small cell lung cancer in the elderly. *Ann Thorac Surg.* 2009;87(6):1662–1666; discussion 1667–1668.
57. Okada M, Nishio M, Sakamoto T, et al. Effect of tumor size on prognosis in patients with non-small cell lung cancer: the role of segmentectomy as a type of lesser resection. *J Thorac Cardiovasc Surg.* 2005;129:87–93.
58. Schuchert MJ, Pettiford BL, Keeley S, et al. Anatomic segmentectomy in the treatment of stage 1 non-small cell lung cancer. *Ann Thorac Surg.* 2007;84:926–932.
59. Schuchert MJ, Kilic A, Pennathur A, et al. Oncologic outcomes after surgical resection of subcentimeter non-small cell lung cancer. *Ann Thorac Surg.* 2011;91(6):1681–1687.
60. Ketchedjian A, Daly B, Landreneau R, Fernando H. Sublobar resection for the subcentimeter pulmonary nodule. *Sem Thorac Cardiovasc Surg.* 2005;17:128–133.
61. Kondo D, Yamada K, Kitayama Y, Hoshi S. Peripheral lung adenocarcinomas: 10 mm or less in diameter. *Ann Thorac Surg.* 2003;76:350–355.
62. Okada M, Koike T, Higashiyama M, Yamato Y, Kodama K, Tsubota N. Radical sublobar resection for small-sized nonsmall cell lung cancer: a multicenter study. *J Thorac Cardiovasc Surg.* 2006;132:769–775.
63. Schuchert MJ, Schumacher L, Kilic A, et al. Impact of angiolymphatic invasion on outcomes following resection of stage I non-small cell lung cancer. *Ann Thorac Surg.* 2011;91:1059–1065.
64. Horne ZD, Jack R, Gray ZT, et al. Increased levels of tumor-infiltrating lymphocytes are associated with improved recurrence-free survival in stage 1A non-small-cell lung cancer. *J Surg Res.* 2011;171(1):1–5.
65. Sawbata N, Ohta M, Matsumura A, et al. Optimal distance of malignant negative margin excision of non-small cell lung cancer: a multicenterprospective study. *Ann Thorac Surg.* 2004;77(2):415–420.
66. El-Sherif A, Gooding WE, Santos R, et al. Outcomes of sublobar resection versus lobectomy for stage I non-small cell lung cancer: A 13-year analysis. *Ann Thorac Surg.* 2006;82(2):408–415.
67. Allen MS, Darling GE, Pechet TT, et al Morbidity and mortality of major pulmonary resections in patients with early-stage lung cancer: initial results of the randomized, prospective ACOSOG Z0030 trial *Ann Thorac Surg.* 2006;81:1013–1019.
68. Keenan RJ, Landreneau RJ, Maley RH Jr, et al. Segmental resection spares pulmonary function in patients with stage I lung cancer. *Ann Thorac Surg.* 2004;78:228–233.
69. Fernando HC, Santos R, Benfield JR, et al. Lobar and sublobar resection with and without brachytherapy for small stage IA non-small cell lung cancer. *J Thorac Cardiovasc Surg.* 2005;129: 261–267.
70. Schuchert MJ, Abbas G, Pennathur A, et al. Anatomic lung resection for clinical stage I non-small cell lung cancer (NSCLC): equivalent outcomes following anatomic segmentectomy and lobectomy. *Proceedings of the The American College of Chest Physicians*, Vancouver, BC, Canada, November 4, 2010.
71. Stiles BM, Servais EL, Lee PC, Port JL, Paul S, Altorki NK. Clinical stage IA non–small cell lung cancer determined by computed tomography and positron emission tomography is frequently not pathologic IA non–small cell lung cancer: The problem of understaging. *J Thorac Cardiovasc Surg.* 2009;137:13–19.

Advances in First- and Second-Line Therapy of Small Cell Lung Cancer

Shir Kiong Lu,[1†] Patrizia Giannatempo,[2†] Mary O'Brien[3*]

[1]*Royal Marsden NHS Foundation Trust, London, UK*

[2]*Fondazione Istituto di Ricovero e Cura a Carattere Scientifico, Istituto Nazionale dei Tumori, Milano, Italy*

[3]*Royal Marsden NHS Foundation Trust, Downs Road, Sutton, UK*

[†]*The authors have contributed equally*

ABSTRACT

Small cell lung cancer (SCLC) accounts for up to 20% to 25% of lung cancer. It is an aggressive subtype and carries a poor prognosis. Over the past years, there have been numerous research and clinical trials looking into improving the survival of patients with SCLC. However, there has been little progress made beyond the discovery of use of platinum plus etoposide chemotherapy, which is the standard chemotherapy treatment in Europe. Other modalities that have established survival benefit include modification in thoracic radiation in limited disease (LD) SCLC patients and the role of prophylactic cranial irradiation in reducing intracranial relapses in both LDSCLC and extensive disease (ED) SCLC. SCLC is one of the most complex genetic human cancers, and its cell's molecular biology remains poorly understood. To date, in the era of targeted therapy, there is still no agent that has been approved in the treatment of SCLC. This review aims to focus on the advances made, current knowledge, and progress made in the treatment of SCLC, which improves the survival of patients with this lethal disease.

Keywords: small cell lung cancer, advances, chemotherapy, targeted therapy

*Corresponding author, Royal Marsden NHS Foundation Trust, Downs Road, Sutton, UK

E-mail address: mary.obrien@rmh.nhs.uk

Emerging Cancer Therapeutics 3:1 (2012) 111–128.

DOI: 10.5003/2151–4194.3.1.111

demosmedpub.com/ecat

■ INTRODUCTION

Small cell lung cancer (SCLC) is a classic smoking induced lung cancer. Its incidence has decreased in the last 30 years; in the United States, SEER database and U.K. database (LUCADA), SCLC now accounts for 13% to 15% of all lung cancers. However, there are reports of increasing incidence in China, and there appears to be a trend to increasing incidence in young women with female smoking in Western countries. Currently, the majority of patients are elderly men; however, if the incidence in this group continues to decrease and we begin to see SCLC in young individuals then the public health need will increase (1,2).

SCLC is a subtype of lung cancer characterized by neuroendocrine features, rapid growth and doubling time, and early development of widespread metastases. Nowadays, SCLC is distinguished morphologically by small cells, morphological features like hyperchromatic nuclear staining, crush artifact, and an immunohistochemistry pattern of staining for nonspecific enolase and CD56 (N-CAM). Thyroid transcription factor 1 (TTF1) can also be positive in SCLC patients but EGFR mutations are not present (3,4).

The Veteran's Administration Lung Cancer Study Group study, which was revised in 1989 by the International Association for the Study of Lung cancer, staged patients as having LD or ED. This may be replaced by the seventh edition of the TNM classification (5). Clinical staging with conventional radiology often underestimates the severity of NSCLC, and fluorodeoxyglucose–positron emission tomography (FDG PET) imaging appears reliable but more work is needed to define

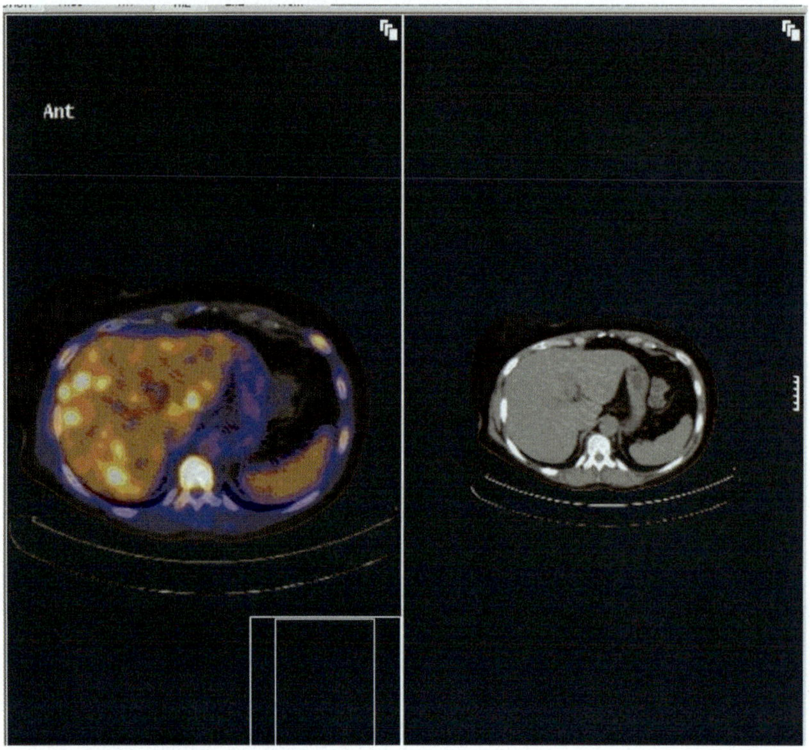

FIGURE 1
Transaxial PET (left) with corresponding CT (right) images showing intense FDG-avid disease in the liver which was negative on CT.

the role of FDG PET in staging of this disease (6). Figure 1 shows the report of a patient with SCLC with liver metastasis detected only with FDG PET and negative at CT scan.

Chemotherapy Treatment of SCLC

The prognosis remains very poor and despite a relatively robust initial response to chemotherapy, a high percentage of patients develop refractory disease. The median survival time for patients with ED and LD is approximately 9 months and 18 months, respectively.

In the last 10 years, significant improvements have been achieved in the treatment of LDSCLC, thanks to a multidisciplinary treatment approach: better staging, platinum-based chemotherapy, and use of prophylactic cranial irradiation (PCI). Surgery is not considered very often, but there is a small subset of patients with small peripheral tumors and LD (T1–2, N0) who could be considered for surgical resection, given the good outcome of these patients in the reported series. However, with better staging, these patients would probably do well with chemotherapy and radiotherapy, and a trial to address this question would be a recruitment challenge (7).

Etoposide plus cisplatin (EP) or carboplatin (EC) are the chemotherapy regimens commonly used in SCLC treatment. The superiority in terms of overall survival (OS) of the EP combination as first-line standard treatment over anthracycline-based regimes has been hard to demonstrate with only one randomized trial showing a clear benefit in LD and a trend in ED (8). The Cochrane review in SCLC failed to show significant difference between platinum-based and non-platinum-based chemotherapy regimens in LD or ED in terms of survival and overall tumor response, but it showed an improvement in complete response rate with the platinum-based combination. Toxicity was higher in the platinum-based treatment in terms of nausea, vomiting, anemia, and thrombocytopenia, while the anthracyclines caused more mucositis, myelosuppression, and cardiopulmonary toxicity (9) The advantages of the platinum-based regimens are the ability to give them safely with concomitant radiotherapy and the fact that four courses of platinum-based regimen is equivalent to six courses of the anthracycline treatment in ED (10).

Although advances in the treatment of SCLC have been limited, advanced made in other areas of oncology and supportive care are helping patients with SCLC. The EORTC 2010, ESMO 2007, and ASCO 2006 guidelines recommend prophylactic G-CSF or pegylated filgrastim in patients receiving a chemotherapy regimen with high risk of febrile neutropenia (age, performance status, and chemotherapy regimens associated with febrile neutropenia in 10%–20% of patients). Most treatments for SCLC fit these criteria, but despite this, there are varying uptakes of these guidelines in institutions and countries.

Despite the high response rate in patients with ED, the relapse rate is still high and the overall prognoses remain poor, probably caused by rapidly development of drug resistance. Little is known about the mechanism of drug resistance in SCLC or indeed if it is any different from the mechanisms of drug resistance in other tumors.

The topoisomerase II alpha gene in the context of HER 2/neu amplification may be a predictor of efficacy of anthracyclines in breast cancer (11). This data needs to be validated, but this approach may be useful in picking up SCLC patients who would preferentially benefit from anthracyclines over platinum-based treatments.

Other drugs (antifolates, taxane, and camptothecins) and strategies have been investigated in the treatment of extensive-stage SCLC, including dose intensification, maintenance treatment, extending treatment cycle number, intensive weekly therapy, and high-dose chemotherapy, without major breakthroughs (12,13).

Irinotecan and topotecan are topoisomerase 1 inhibitors. Irinotecan with cisplatin was reported as superior to EP in SCLC patients in a Japanese Phase III trail in 2002. This trial showed higher response rate (84% versus 68%), longer median survival (12.8 versus 9.4 months) and higher 2-year survival rate (19% versus 5%), but these results were not confirmed in two successive trial from the United States, Australia, and Canada and the S0124 trial of Southwest Oncology group (SWOG) (14,15). A recent study from Norway reported a moderate benefit of treatment with carboplatin and irinotecan compared with EC, but doses were not standard in either arm and therefore the clinical relevance is not clear (16). Pharmacogenomic differences between study populations—in particular, genetic differences of metabolic enzyme UGT as already described for toxicity—may be relevant for irinotecan (17,18).

Topotecan has been tested in several Phase II and III trial for ES-SCLC in comparison with standard treatment in first- and second-line, and it has shown significant antitumor activity and symptom palliation in relapsed SCLC patients, but, as it is not superior in activity and has a difficult intravenous administration schedule, it has not been widely adopted as first-line treatment (19). Oral topotecan with cisplatin has also been tested and again is not superior to a standard EP regimen in the first-line setting (20). However, oral topotecan is the first drug to be licensed for the treatment of relapsed SCLC as it gave both improved survival and symptom control when it was compared with best supportive care (21).

Pemetrexed with cisplatin was compared in a Phase III trial with EP, which gave inferior results; however, no thymidylate synthetase (TS) expression data has been presented, and high predicted levels in SCLC may have contributed to the failure of this regimen, as an association is now recognized between low TS expression and improved outcomes with pemetrexed (22,23).

Paclitaxel is active in SCLC patients; however, of the three trials done to date, none of them have replaced EP or EC as a standard treatment. Again, no biomarker data on taxane sensitivity was available. Gemcitabine (G) in combination with Carboplatin (C) was tested to find a less toxic and better-tolerated treatment (24). The G–C combination has a lower grade of alopecia and nausea but higher rate of haematological toxicity Grade 3 and 4. In conclusion, the GC regimen is noninferior compared with EP, and it could be an alternative option for patients with mixed small cell and non-small cell, and for the patients for whom alopecia is a real problem.

The most recent first-line contender has been amrubicin, a third generation synthetic anthracycline agent that does not appear to cause anthracycline-related cardiomyopathy. It has shown comparable response rate as a single agent (61%) to cisplatin/etoposide (63%) and a promising response of 77% in combination with cisplatin (25). Toxicity was largely myelosuppression in all three arms. New combinations in SCLC patients must show a survival advantage over cisplatin/etoposide unless there is a significantly different toxicity profile.

Maintenance Therapy

Maintenance therapy is being revisited in NSCLC and may well be useful in SCLC. A recent meta-analysis of all reported trials (11 trial employing chemotherapy, 6 interferon, and 4 other biological agents) analyzed 3,688 patients and suggested a small increase in OS in the maintenance arm with chemotherapy (less than 1 month) and an absolute improvement in survival (9% at 1 year) (26). Maintenance therapy with intravenous topotecan versus observation was associated with improved progression-free survival (PFS) (3.6 versus 2.3 months, $P < .001$) but not OS (8.9 versus 9.3 months, $P = .43$) (27). It is unlikely that oral topotecan would be different from the intravenous, but the oral schedule may improve compliance.

Radiotherapy

Research continues on optimizing the use of radiotherapy in the treatment of SCLC. Timing of radiotherapy has been addressed in eight different trials. Thirty day after the beginning of the chemotherapy is considered the cut-off to distinguish early from late. A recent meta-analysis reported a significant improvement in 3- to 5-year survival (absolute benefit of 5.7%–7.7%) in patients with good compliance to chemotherapy in favor of early radiotherapy over late. The advantages of early RT was most impressive when the trials using non-platinum-based chemotherapy were excluded (5-year survival rate of 20.2 % for early versus 13.8% for late). The toxicities related to treatment (anemia, esophageal, and cardiac) were worse in patients treated with early radiotherapy (28). Improved 5-year survival rates of greater than 20% were observed when the interval was less than 30 days from day one of chemotherapy (29). The advantage of twice-daily compared with once-daily RT need further data from ongoing trials like the CONVERT randomized trial in United Kingdom and Europe.

Prophylactic Cranial Irradiation

Brain metastasis are common in SCLC; approximately 14% to 24% of SCLC patients have brain metastasis at the time of diagnosis, and over the next two years, it will emerge into about 50% to 60% of patients, and 20% to 30% of these metastasis will be the sole site disease recurrence.

SCLC patients with no progression on first-line chemotherapy with either limited or ED have a survival benefit with PCI as it reduces the risk of brain metastases at first year by 26% versus 15% without PCI. In the study of PCI in ED, the quality of life analysis of the study showed that the irradiated group had more prolonged hair loss and increased fatigue but a trend to improved overall global health (30). Further studies on dose did not confirm a dose response and therefore the recommendation remains at 20 to 25 Gy in 10 fractions. In these later studies, age at baseline and the PS were predictors of neurocognitive decline which took the form of mild deterioration in communication, weakness of legs, intellectual deficit and memory deterioration (31).

Relapsed SCLC

Despite high initial response rates to chemotherapy (45%–75% CR) was reported in patients with LD and 20% to 30% in patients with ED, the duration of response is usually short with PFS time of 4 months for patients with ED and 12 months for patients with LD. At the time of suspected first recurrence of cancer, it still is unclear whether biopsy confirmation has to be performed to confirm the diagnosis or to look for new molecular mutation, but this is an area for further exploration.

Patients who relapse within 3 months of completion of first-line treatment are called refractory, and patients who relapse after 3 months are called sensitive. However, these definitions have been called into questions as with active second-line agents; responses can be seen in both categories (21). Patients with sensitive relapses can be treated with the same induction regimen used initially, and we do not know if current second lines are superior, but on balance, we assume there is equivalence. Patients with early relapse are treated with non-cross-resistant combination chemotherapy or single agents.

The only approved drug for second-line SCLC is topotecan, which is available in both intravenous and oral formulation. Randomized studies have suggested that the activity on single agent intravenous topotecan is similar to an anthracycline combination, but the patients treated with topotecan had greater improvement of the symptoms, dyspnoea, anorexia, fatigue, insomnia, and energy levels (32). The overall response rate was 2% to 7% with 45% to 23% of patients achieving SD as a best response. This is a low response rate and therefore its meaning has been investigated by a trial comparing oral topotecan to no topotecan in patients with performance status 0 to 2. In the oral topotecan group, the OS was significantly longer (median survival 25.9 versus 13.9 weeks), and the QoL and symptoms control were significantly improved. A survival advantage for oral topotecan was seen in all subgroups including the refractory patients.

There are other active drugs in the second-line setting: gemcitabine had only modest activity against refractory relapses (response rate, 0–13%) and paclitaxel plus carboplatin for second line after EP or CDE (cyclophosphamide, doxorubicin and etoposide) had a 25% response rate but similar OS as other drugs (33,34).

Picoplatinum is a cisplatinum analogue designed to avoid the development of platinum resistance, but recent data presented at ASCO 2011 showed no statistical significance survival benefit in picoplatin compared with placebo in the second-line setting (35). There was a suggestion of activity in the primary refractory patients in a subgroup analysis.

Amrubicin is a third generation synthetic anthracycline agent, which does not appear to cause anthracycline-related cardiomyopathy. The ACT-1 Phase III randomized trial enrolled 637 patients with ED SCLC including sensitive and resistant relapse disease randomized in amrubicin or topotecan regimen. The OS were similar in both arms, but amrubicin had improved response rates and PFS, and achieved symptom control with acceptable toxicity. Amrubicin appears to have a modest advantage OS in refractory patients compared with topotecan (median OS of 6.2 mo versus 5.7 mo respectively), but not in sensitive patients, and amrubicin improved survival after 6 months in the refractory subgroup (36).

Temozolomide is a cytotoxic agent that is currently in use for the treatment of brain cancers and melanoma. A Phase II nonrandomized trial is ongoing for relapsed sensitive or refractory SCLC with collection of circulating tumor cells (CTCs) to study the biology of these patients (37).

Ones to Watch For in the Future

Nanotechnology is presently contributing scientifically to the progress of medical science, as it can target tumor tissues and deliver water-insoluble drugs, and thus give enhanced activity. Drugs such as SN-38 (the biologically active metabolite of irinotecan), Abraxane (containing paclitaxel), and obatoclax are in early clinical trials. A Phase II trial was performed by Spiegal et al. to evaluate NK012 (delivering SN-38) in 40 patients with sensitive SCLC relapse (38). This study showed the activity of NK012 with a 22% overall response rate and 68% disease control rate (DCR); the treatment was generally well tolerated, and the most common side effects were myelotoxicity and diarrhea. Abraxane is the nanoparticle albumin-bound formulation of paclitaxel, which has efficacy in breast cancer and also shown activity with carboplatin in SCLC (39).

This leads us into the era of new treatment development for SCLC, and obatoclax will be discussed with other antiapoptotic agents.

Current Cancer Biology as Applicable to SCLC

Figure 2 shows the signaling pathways that are therapeutic targets or potentially could be targeted in SCLC. Table 1 lists some of the members in the cell-survival pathways that are involved in carcinogenesis and that have shown therapeutic activities in SCLC and other tumor types when targeted.

Better understanding of SCLC's molecular biology and oncogenic drivers will require more tissue from repeat biopsies at diagnosis and at relapse. However, rebiopsies are rare or not possible in most SCLC cases, and the tissues obtained are frequently inadequate to perform molecular profiling. CTCs may fill this tissue gap and serum biomarkers could potentially have diagnostic, prognostic, and predictive values in SCLC. CTCs are detected in SCLC, and higher numbers have been shown to be associated with poorer prognosis (40). They are currently being incorporated into the clinical studies with temozolomide (above) and PARP inhibitors (below). The "magic number" of 5 seems also to be applicable to SCLC as a prognostic cut-off for CTCs (37). Studies have shown that cell death biomarkers, M30 and M65, and CTC number are prognostic for survival in patients with SCLC (41). Nucleosomal DNA and M30 levels are associated

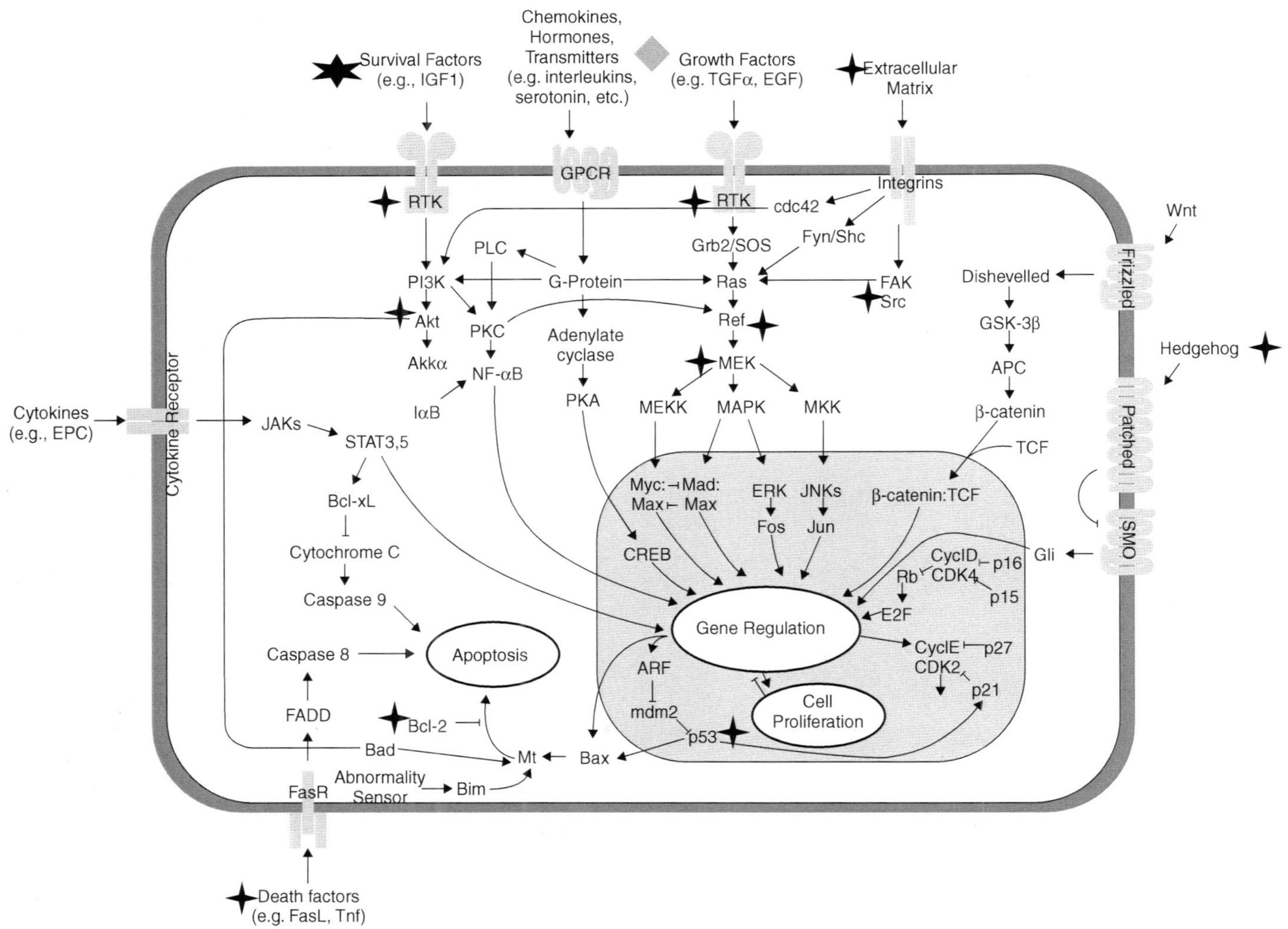

FIGURE 2
Signalling pathways that may be involved in carcinogenesis and potential therapeutic targets in SCLC.

TABLE 1 Cell survival pathways shown to be upregulated in SCLC

Targets	SCLC (in vitro)	SCLC (in vivo)	NSCLC	Others
P53	+	+	+	+
K-Ras mutation	NK	NK	+	+
Raf mutation	NK	NK	+	+
Akt	NK	NK	+	+
PTEN loss/mutation	+	NK	+	+
C-Kit	+	+	+	+
IGF	+	NK	+	+
C-met	+	+	+	+
Her 2	–	–	+	+
VEGF	+	+	+	+
EGFR	+	+	+	+
FGF	+	+	+	+
Alk	NK	NK	+	+
Hedgehog	+	+	+	+
Bcl 2	+	+	+	+

+ Positive antitumor activity.
– Negative antitumor activity.
NK = Not known.

with early response to chemotherapy and severe toxicity, respectively (42). Other novel biomarkers that have been recently indentified include pro-opiomelanocortin, a precursor of ACTH, and microRNA, miR-92–2 that are associated with chemoresistance and decreased survival (43,44).

Antiapoptotic Inhibitors

One of the characteristics of SCLC tumors is the substantial alterations in its apoptotic system. High levels of anti-apoptotic protein such as Bcl-2, bcl-xL, and survivin are characteristic of many SCLC tumors. Chemotherapy including platinum compounds and topoimerase II inhibitors exert their cytotoxic effects by inducing apoptosis via the intrinsic pathway regulated by Bcl-2. Upregulation of antiapoptotic proteins results in resistance to chemotherapy in vitro and in vivo. Oblimersen (G3139) is an antisense nucleotide and is the first targeted Bcl-2 inhibitor that has demonstrated synergistic efficacy with chemotherapy in preclinical models (45). A randomized Phase II study on carboplatin and etoposide with or without oblimersen was conducted, and, disappointingly, it showed no difference in response rate; instead patients receiving oblimersen had worse survival outcome (46).

The Bcl-2 antagonist, obatoclax, inhibits BCL-2 proteins and in combination with topotecan have shown activity in relapsed SCLC, but failed to show improvement in response rate compared with topotecan alone (47). However, in newly diagnosed ED-SCLC, a randomized Phase II study involving 155 patients treated with EC with or without obatoclax was presented at meetings in 2011 (48). EC plus obatoclax versus EC demonstrated an improvement in terms of response rate (64.9% versus 53.8%), PFS (6 versus 5.4 months, HR = 0.795, P = .08) and OS (10.5 versus 9.8 months, HR = 0.724, P = .05), and therefore a confirmatory Phase III trial is planned.

Navitoclax, another inhibitor of Bcl-2, has shown preliminary efficacy data on SCLC, with one patient with PR lasting more than 2 years and 8 patients having SD. This drug is well tolerated with dose-dependent thrombocytopenia seen as the major toxicity (49).

AT-101 is an oral BH3 (subfamily of proapoptotic) mimetic that mimics the natural antagonists of prosurvival proteins, and its functions include inhibiting the heterodimerization of antiapoptotic proteins, upregulating the proapoptotic proteins, and inhibiting angiogenesis. It has shown good responses in combination with cisplatin/etoposide in NSCLC and high-grade neuroendocrine tumor patients and is now recruiting treatment-naive EDSCLC patients into the MTD expansion cohort (50).

Borrtezomib blocks the activity of the ubiquitin–proteosome, which is responsible for the degradation of the vast majority of intracellular proteins including p21; p27; p53; cyclins D,E, and A; and nuclear factor kB and members of Bax family, thus affecting multiple signaling pathways within cells. Bortezomib is the first proteasome inhibitor to be evaluated in human studies and is approved for use in multiple myeloma. Bortezomib in relapsed SCLC patients did not show sufficient efficacy (only 1 patient had partial response in platinum refractory and none in platinum sensitive) in the Phase II SWOG 0327 study (51). Bortezomib in combination with topotecan is currently underway in the second-line setting.

Vaccine/Immunotherapy

Immunotherapy makes a comeback every 10 years creating excitement and hope in many tumors including SCLC. The last big trial was with BEC2, an anti-idiotypic monoclonal antibody (MAb) that mimics GD3 (a ganglioside involved in cell growth regulation and cell adhesion), and it has been tested in combination with BCG as adjuvant therapy in Phase 3 trial in LDSCLC patients. Despite the promising Phase II result, there was no survival advantage compared with observation alone (52). Chemotherapy with or without a suspension of heat-killed *Mycobacterium vaccae* (SRL 172) showed no survival benefit for the combination, but there was no added toxicity, and QOL was improved (53). Another mycobacterium is being tested in combination with chemotherapy in NSCLC in India and has resulted in survival benefit (54).

Ipilimumab is a new class of fully humanized MAb that potentiates the immune system by inhibiting cytotoxic T lymphocyte-associated antigen 4 (CTLA-4, which is in itself a T cell suppressor antigen). It is the first agent to improve survival in advanced melanoma. SCLC was one of the subgroups treated in the large Phase II studies of the addition of ipilimumab to a standard regimen as first line treatment (55). Data on SCLC patients showed sequenced ipilimumab in combination with paclitaxel/carboplatin resulted in statistically significant benefit in immune-related PFS of 6.4 months ($P = .03$) and improvement in OS of 12.9 months ($P = .13$) compared with concurrent regimen. This data supports investigation of ipilimumab in SCLC in a Phase III setting.

CD56 (NKH-1; neural cell adhesion molecule [NCAM]) antigen is expressed on the surface of virtually all SCLC cases. Conjugated MAbs have been developed to target specifically the epitopes of CD56. BB-10901 is a chimeric humanized anti-CD56 MAb that is conjugated to a maytansinoid toxin (DM1), as in T (trastuzumab)-DM1 which is being tested in Her2 positive breast cancer. Once bound to CD56, the conjugate is internalized and releases DM1. DM1 then inhibits tubulin polymerization and microtubule assembly, causing cell death. Clinical response has been observed in SCLC patients (and Merkel cell tumor patients) in the Phase I and II trials (56). The agent will now be combined with chemotherapy and taken to Phase III.

Angiogenesis

Vascular endothelial growth factor (VEGF) expression is present in 80% of SCLC patients, and overexpression is a poor prognostic factor for survival in SCLC (57).

Thalidomide, a nonspecific, multitargeted antiangiogenic agent, has been tested in combination with chemotherapy in first-line treatment of EDSCLC and as maintenance therapy. A large Phase III study by Lee et al. reported no survival benefit but increased toxicity with the addition of thalidomide to chemotherapy (58).

Bevacizumab, an anti-VEGF-A MAb, has been tested in a few Phase II trials in combination with a doublet chemotherapy backbone (cisplatin/irinotecan, cisplatin/etoposide, cisplatin or carboplatin/etoposide) in untreated EDSCLC. The results, in particular the randomized Phase II (SALUTE), showed no major superiority in efficacy compared with the same regimen without bevacizumab (59). Paclitaxel added to bevacizumab in relapsed SCLC gave an overall response rate of 18.1%, median PFS 14.7 weeks (equivalent to historical controls) and median OS 30 weeks (60). It is unlikely that bevacuzimab will have a major impact on the treatment of SCLC.

Aflibercept, another angiogenesis inhibitor, has been developed to bind to VEGF-A and VEGF-B, thereby preventing the ligand binding to cell receptors. A Phase II trial testing topotecan with aflibercept is recruiting patients with platinum-treated EDSCLC (NCT00828139).

Fibroblast growth factors (FGF) are mitogens, which are involved in neoangiogenseis in vivo. FGF receptor-1 amplification is present in smoking-related lung cancer and is amplified in 20% of squamous cell cancer and SCLC and can be sought to select patients for targeted treatments. FGF-2 has been found to increase antiapoptotic proteins and result in chemoresistance in SCLC. FGFR inhibitors have been developed and undergoing clinical trials in advanced solid tumors and leukemia and could potentially be active in SCLC.

Tyrosine Kinase Inhibitors

Multikinase inhibitors, which target not only angiogenesis but also tumor proliferation, have also been evaluated. Cediranib, a potent inhibitor of VEGFR-1/2, c-kit, platelet-derived growth factor (PDGF)-beta showed good activity in combination with cisplatin and etoposide with a median PFS observed of 8 months but Grade 3 to 4 toxicities observed (61). Vandetanib, another oral inhibitor of VEGFR-2/3, rearranged during transfection (RET) and epidermal growth factor receptor (EGFR) used as maintenance therapy showed no advantage compared with placebo (62).

Sunitinib a multitargeted inhibitor of VEGFR-1/2/3, PDGFR alpha/beta, Flt 3, c-kit, RET, in combination with cisplatin/etoposide in EDSCLC resulted in prolonged haematological toxicity and treatment-related mortality (63). A Phase II trial using carboplatin/irinotecan and sunitinib 25 mg od in treatment-naive EDSCLC is ongoing. Clearly, all these agents are difficult to combine with chemotherapy at current recommended doses in SCLC patients who may be less robust than renal patients. As monotherapy in second-line treatment for relapsed or refractory SCLC, sunitinib has anecdotally given responses in an EORTC second line-study (personal communication, O'Brien, Royal Marsden Hospital, UK). A small randomized Phase II maintenance study after response to platinum plus etoposide chemotherapy in 12 patients was aborted because of toxicity (64). Sunitinb at 50 mg od was discontinued in half of the patients due to Grade 3 or 4 toxicities or patients' request. There were 31% of patients with Grade 3 or 4 thrombocytopenia, but dose reductions were reported in only 6% to 13% of patients. In another trial, sunitinib, 25 mg od, as maintenance therapy after response to platinum-doublet chemotherapy, was better tolerated with no Grade 3 or 4 toxicities in more than one patient and an encouraging 1 year OS of 54% (65). This is a drug which has some activity if the dose is right but predicting which patients will benefit remains a challenge.

Sorafenib, a multikinase inhibitor of Raf, VEGFR 2,3, and PDGFR, has shown an overall response rate of 36% (4% had partial response) in relapsed SCLC patients. Median survival was 7 months in platinum-sensitive and 5 months in platinum-refractory patients, which are comparable to or better than historical controls receiving salvage chemotherapy (66). In light of this, a Phase

1 trial on sorafenib in combination with weekly four topotecan in relapsed patients, and a Phase II study of maintenance sorafenib in patients achieving CR or PR after induction chemotherapy are under way in the Far East (NCT01159327).

Pazopanib is a new ATP-competitive tyrosine kinase inhibitors of VEGFR-1/2/3, PDGFR alpha/beta and c-kit. Preliminary data from Phase I and II studies have demonstrated antitumor activity in subjects with a variety of malignancies including renal cell cancer, soft tissue sarcoma, breast cancer, ovarian cancer, and lung cancer. Pazopanib has shown single agent activity in preoperative early-stage NSCLC (67). This compound is now being tested as monotherapy in a Phase II trial for relapsed or refractory SCLC patients (NCT01253369).

C-kit

Elevated expression of c-kit and its ligand stem cell factor (SCF) is present in 30% to 70% of SCLC patients. C-kit encodes a transmembrane receptor kinase of PDGF receptor subfamily and upon SCF binding, c-kit homodimerizes and initiates an intracellular signalling cascade, including the phosphoinositide-dependent kinase-1–Akt–mammalian target of rapamycin (PI3K/Akt/mTOR) pathway. Phase II studies of imatinib, a small-molecule c-kit inhibitor, in combination with chemotherapy in first-line treatment of EDSCLC failed to show improvement in survival rates compared with chemotherapy alone (68). It is also surprising that in patients with c-kit expressing SCLC, imatinib failed to show any clinical activity in relapsed SCLC patients or as maintenance therapy (69,70). This may suggest that c-kit expression is not adequate or a main driver in SCLC survival and proliferation.

Phosphoinositide-Dependent Kinase-1–Akt–Mammalian Target of Rapamycin Pathway

PI3K is constitutively active in SCLC cells, thereby promoting anchorage-independent proliferation. Multiple mechanisms can contribute to activation of the PI3K/Akt/mTOR pathway in SCLC patients including mutations in PTEN gene, expression of specific P13K isoforms, secretion and activity of cytokines or growth factors including SCF that activates tyrosine kinase kit, and insulin-like growth factor (IGF), and adhesion to extracellular matrix (ECM). This pathway has a biomarker, and targeted treatments are in Phase I studies but should be developed in SCLC.

ECM-mediated activation of the PI3K/Akt/mTOR pathway confers resistance to standard and novel therapeutic agents including doxorubicin, etoposide, and cisplatin. Laminin-mediated (an ECM component) activation of PI3K/Akt pathway promotes resistance to cisplatin, etoposide as well as tyrosine kinase inhibitor of c-kit, imatinib (71). This may be one of the reasons for the negative results seen with imatinib and future studies combining Akt/mTOR inhibitor with imatinib, chemotherapy or other agents may be effective in SCLC.

The mTOR is downstream of the PI3K/Akt pathway, which is involved in cell growth, proliferation, cell motility, survival, protein synthesis, and transcription. The mTOR inhibitors, temsorilimus and evirolimus, have been tested in SCLC patients with disappointing results. Temsorilimus was tested in a randomized Phase II studies with 2 different doses and showed an overall median survival of 2 months, and 1-year PFS rate was 5%, which were similar in the two treatment arms (72). Two Phase II trials evaluated evorolimus in EDSCLC failed to show any benefits in the relapsed or maintenance setting (73,74).

Insulin-Like Growth Factor

Another common molecular abnormality is overexpression of IGF-1 and its receptor. IGF-1 is also an important regulator of VEGF expression and angiogenesis in SCLC. Inhibition of IGF receptors with MAbs in combination with chemotherapy is in trials in NSCLC and other tumors with limited success and some toxicity to date. As described above, the PI3K/Akt pathway is also mediated by c-kit. Therefore, a dual inhibition of both c-kit and

IGF-1R may be an effective therapy with additional antiproliferative and proapoptotic effects.

Others

P53

P53, the guardian of the genome, functions as a tumor-suppressor gene that maintains genomic stability, thereby preventing genome mutation that leads to tumorigenesis. P53 gene is mutated in approximately 90% of SCLC. Preclinical studies using mouse models and an ex-vivo human culture model have shown that the induction of an anti-p53 CTL response selectively killed tumor cells and spared normal cells (75). New cancer vaccine consisting of dendritic cells transduced with wild-type p53 gene delivered via an adenoviral vector in patients with EDSCLC showed that 57% of patients mounted a T-cell response, and this group of patients were found to have a higher response rate to chemotherapy than those who did not (76). A Phase II trial on dendritic vaccine therapy to immunize EDSCLC patients in combination with chemotherapy with or without all-trans retinoic acid is underway (NCT00617409).

Targeting Telomerase

Telomerase is an enzyme that is essential to maintaining telomere length and cell immortality, and its expression is silenced in terminally differentiated cells but frequently activated in malignant cells resulting in unlimited proliferative capacity. The RNA component of telomerase is upregulated in 98% of SCLC, thus representing a target for directed inhibition or as a tumor antigen (77). Synthetic peptide vaccines, telomerase-specific oncolytic virus, and telomerase inhibitors have been developed and are undergoing preclinical evaluation in advanced solid tumors.

Heat Shock Protein 90 Inhibitor

Heat shock protein (Hsp) 90 is a molecular chaperone protein that has crucial role in signaling pathway necessary for the growth, survival, and limitless replicative potential of most tumors. Ganetespib (STA-9090), an Hsp 90 inhibitor, is able to induce cell cycle arrest of SCLC cells at G2/M checkpoint (78). An ongoing Phase II study is underway in SCLC (NCT01173523). Geldanamycin not only is an Hsp 90 inhibitor but also has shown to affect c-met expression (below) resulting in reduced growth and viability of SCLC cell lines (79).

Targeting Hedgehog

Hedgehog (Hh) pathway is an essential embryonic signaling cascade that regulates the differentiation of stem and progenitor cells, thus regulating tumorigenesis. The membrane spanning receptor, Smoothened (Smo), is involved in the malignant activation of the Hh pathway resulting in cell differentiation, migration and proliferation. This has provided a new insight into the progression and recurrence of cancer and could provide an alternative means for targeting tumor growth.

Preclinical study on SCLC cell lines showed that Smo localized to primary cilium in a subpopulation of tumor cells and blocking the pathway inhibited the self-renewing capacity of SCLC cells in vitro. GDC-0449 is the first-in-human, potent systemic inhibitor of Hh signal pathway. It has shown impressive efficacy in basal cell carcinoma (55% clinical response with 2 complete remissions). A randomized Phase II study (E1508) that include three-arms is currently recruiting in SCLC. This trial compares cisplatin plus etoposide with and without the Hh inhibitor GDC-0449 or IGF-1R MAb A12 (cixutumumab).

C-Met/Hepatocyte Growth Factor

The c-Met receptor tyrosine kinase and its ligand hepatocyte growth factor have been shown to be involved in angiogenesis, cellular motility, growth, invasion, and differentiation. The overexpression of c-Met mRNA has been found in SCLC tissues. There are numerous clinical trials looking at c-Met pathway antagonists including tyrosine kinase inhibitors, MAb blocking receptor/ligand interaction and blockade of the receptor/effector interaction.

Poly ADP Ribase Polymerase

Poly ADP ribase polymerase (PARP) inhibitors represent a new therapeutic option in oncology in potentiating the effects of chemotherapy and radiotherapy and overcoming drug resistance. Tumors with breast cancer tumour suppressor gene (BRCA), mutations have deficient homologous recombination repair leading to accumulation of unrepaired double-strand breaks (DSB) that confers cancer susceptibility through genomic instability. Inhibition of PARP leads to inability to repair DSB in BRCA deficient cells, and therefore cell death. BRCA mutations are not normally associated with SCLC. PARP inhibitors also sensitize and have therapeutic activity in tumors without BRCA1/2 mutations as they exploit mutations in DNA repair pathways that are plentiful in SCLC cells. Olaparib, with intravenous topotecan, was toxic in combination (80). Olaparib at doses up to 400 mg bd as monotherapy is generally well tolerated and has given positive results as maintenance therapy in ovarian cancer (ASCO 2011), and currently, a randomized Phase II trial is underway in the United Kingdom testing single-agent olaparib as maintenance in chemoresponsive SCLC with PFS at 4 months as the primary endpoint (STOMP trial).

■ CONCLUSION

Clinical trials in SCLC can be done rapidly as the disease is still relatively common in some countries, the median survival in ED is short, and the second-line options are limited. There should be advances in the coming years as the molecular drivers of this malignant tumor are unraveled and targeted.

■ REFERENCES

1. Arnold M, Razum O, Coebergh JW. Cancer risk diversity in non-western migrants to Europe: An overview of the literature. *Eur J Cancer.* 2010; 46 (14): 2647–2659.
2. Boniol M, Autier P. Prevalence of main cancer lifestyle risk factors in Europe in 2000. *Eur J Cancer.* 2010;46(14):2534–2544.
3. Kitamura H, Yazawa T, Sato H, et al. Small Cell Lung Cancer: Significance of RB alterations and TTF-1 expression in its carcinogeniesis, phenotyphe, and biology. *Endocr Pathol.* 2009;20(2):101–107.
4. Tatematsu A, Shimizu J, Murakami Y, et al. Epidermal Growth Factor Receptor Mutations in Small Cell Lung Cancer. *Clin Cancer Res.* 2008;14: 6092.
5. Shepherd FA, Crowley J. The International Association for the Study of Lung Cancer lung cancer staging project: Proposals regarding the clinical staging of small cell lung cancer in the forthcoming (seventh) edition of the tumor, node, metastasis classification for lung cancer. *J Thorac Oncol.* 2007;2(12):1067–1077.
6. Kamel EM, Zwahlen D. Whole-body (18) F-FDG PET improves the management of patients with small cell lung cancer. *J Nucl Med.* 2003;;44(12):1911–1917.
7. Lim E, Belcher E, Yap YK, et al. The Role of Surgery in the Treatment of Limited Disease Small Cell Lung Cancer: Time to Reevaluate. *J Thoracic Oncol.* 2008;3(11):1267–1127
8. Sundstrom S, Bremnes RM, Kaasa S, et al. Norwegian Lung Cancer Study Group. Cisplatin and etoposide regimen is superior to cyclophosphamide, epirubicin, and vincristine regimen in a small-cell lung cancer: Results from a randomized phase III trial with 5 years' follow-up. *J Clin Oncol.* 2002:20(24):4665–4672.
9. Amarasena IU, Walters JA, Wood-Baker R, Fong K. Platinum versus non-platinum chemotherapy regimens for small cell lung cancer. *Cochrane Database Sysr Rev.* 2008;issue 8: CD006849.
10. Roth BJ, Johnson DH, Einhorn LH, et al. Randomized study of cyclophosphamide, doxorubicine, and vincristine versus etoposide and cisplatin versus alternation of these two regimens in extensive small-cell lung cancer: a phase III trial of Southeastern Cancer Study Group. *J Clin Oncol.* 1992;10(2):1632–1638.
11. Tanner M, Isola J, Wiklund T, et al. Topoisomerase IIα gene amplification predicts

favorable treatment response to tailored and dose-escalated anthracycline-based adjuvant chemotherapy in HER-2/neu–amplified breast cancer: Scandinavian Breast Group Trial 9401. *JCO.*2006;24(16):2428–2436.
12. Popat S, O'Brien MER. Chemotherapy strategies in the treatment of small cell. *Anticancer Drugs.* 2005;16:361–372.
13. Puglisi M, Dolly S, Faria A, et al. Treatment options for small cell lung cancer—do we have more choice? *Br J Cancer.* 2010;102(4):629–638.
14. Sekine I, Nishiwaki Y, Noda K, et al. Randomized phase II study of cisplatin, irinotecan and etoposide combinations administered weekly or every 4 weeks for extensive small-cell lung cancer (JCOG9902-DI). *Ann Oncol.* 2003;14(5):709.
15. Hanna N, Bunn PA Jr, Langer C, et al. Randomized phase III trial comparing irinotecan/cispaltin with etoposide/cisplatin in patients with previously untreated extensive-stage disease small-cell lung cancer. *J clin Oncol.* 2006;24:2038–2043.
16. Hermes A, Bergam B, Bremnes R, et al. Irinotecan plus carboplatin versus oral etoposide plus carboplatinum in extensive small-cell lung cancer: A randomized phase III trial. *J Clin Oncol.* 2008;26:4261–4267.
17. Innocenti F, Undevia SD, Iyer L, et al. Genetic variants in the UDP-glucuronosyltransferase 1A1 gene predict the risk of severe neutropenia of irinotecan. *J Clin Oncol.* 2004;22(8):1382–1388.
18. Lara PN, Gandara DR. Common arm comparative outcomes analysis of phase 3 trials of cisplatin + irinotecan versus cisplatin + etoposide in extensive stage small cell lung cancer: final patient-level results from Japan Clinical Oncology Group 9511 and Southwest Oncology Group 0124. *Cancer.* 2010;116(24):5710–5715. doi: 10.1002/cncr.25532. Epub: 2010 Aug 24.
19. Heigener DF, Freitag L, Eschbach C, et al. Topotecan/cisplatin (TP) compared to cisplatin/etoposide (PE) for patients with extensive disease-small cell lung cancer (ED-SCLC): Final results of a randomized phase III trial. *J Clin Oncol.* 2008;26(15):7513.
20. Eckardt JR, von Pawel J, Papai Z, et al. Open-label, multicenter, randomized, phase III study comparing oral topotecan/ciplatin versus etoposide/cisplatin as treatment for chemotherapy-naïve patients with extensive-disease small-cell lung cancer. *J Clin Oncol.* 2006;24:2044–2051.
21. O'Brien MER, Ciuleanu T-E, Tsekov H, et al. Phase III Trial Comparing Supportive Care Alone With Supportive Care With Oral Topotecan in Patients With Relapsed Small-Cell Lung Cancer. *J Clin Oncol.* 2006;24(34):5441–5447.
22. Socinski MA, Smit EF, Lorigan P, et al. Phase III study of pemetrexed plus carboplatin (PC) versus etoposide plus carboplatin (EC) in chemonaive patients with extensive-stage disease small cell lung cancer (ED-SCLC): interim results. *J Clin Oncol.* 2008;26:400S.
23. Scagliotti G, Kaiser C, Biesma B, et al. Correlations of biomarker expression and clinical outcome in a large phase III trial of pemetrexed plus cisplatin or gemcitabine plus cisplatin in chemonaive patients with locally advanced or metastatic non-small cell lung cancer (NSCLC): C6–0. *J Thoracic Oncol.* 2007;2(8):S375
24. Lee SM, James LE, Qian W, et al. Comparison of Gemcitabine and Carboplatin versus cispatin and etoposide for patients with poor-prognosis small cell lung cancer. *Thorax.* 2009;64(1):75–80.
25. O'Brien MER, Konopa K, Lorigan P, et al. Randomised phase II study of amrubicin as single agent or in combination with cisplatin versus cisplatin etoposide as first line treatment in patients with extensive stage small cell lung cancer EORTC 08062. *Eur J Cancer.* 2011 Jun 16. [Epub ahead of print].
26. Rossi A, Garassino MC, Cinquini M, et al. Maintenance or consolidation therapy in small-cell lung cancer: A systematic review and meta-analysis. *Lung Cancer.* 2010;70(2) :119–128.
27. Schiller JH, Adak S, Cella D, et al. Topotecan versus observation after cisplatin plus etoposide in extensive-stage small-cell lung cancer: E7593—A Phase III trial of the Eastern Cooperative Oncology Group. *J Clin Oncol.* 2001;19(8):2114–2122.
28. De Ruysscher, Paris E, Le Péchoux C, et al. A Meta-Analysis of Randomised Trials using Individual Patient Data on the Timing of Chest Radiotherapy in Patients with Limited Stage Small Cell Lung Cancer. 14th world conference on lung cancer, Amsterdam, the Netherlands, July 3,7–2011.
29. De Ruysscher D, Pijls-Johannesma M, Bentzen SM, et al. Time Between the First Day of Chemotherapy

and the Last Day of Chest Radiation Is the Most Important Predictor of Survival in Limited-Disease Small-Cell Lung Cancer. *J Clin Oncol.* 2006;24(7):1057–1063.

30. Slotman BJ, Mauer ME, Bottomley A, et al. Prophylactic Cranial Irradiation in Extensive Disease Small-Cell Lung Cancer: Short-Term Health-Related Quality of Life and Patient Reported Symptoms, Results of an International Phase III Randomized Controlled Trial by the EORTC Radiation Oncology and Lung Cancer Groups. *J Clin Oncol.* 2009;27(1):78–84.
31. Le Pechoux C, Dunant A, Senan S, et al. Standard-dose versus higher-dose prophylactic cranial irradiation (PCI) in patients with limited-stage small-cell lung cancer in complete remission after chemotherapy and thoracic radiotherapy (PCI 99–01, EORTC 22003–08004, RTOG 0212, and IFCT 99–01): A randomised clinical trial. *Lancet Oncol.* 2009;10(5):467–474.
32. von Pawel J, Schiller JH, Shephard FA, et al. Topotecan versus cyclophospamide, doxorubicin, and vincristine for the treatment of recurrent small-cell lung cancer. *J Clin Oncol.* 1999;17:658–667.
33. Masters GA, Declerck L, Blanke C, et al. Phase II trial of gemcitabine in refractory or relapse small-cell lung cancer: Eastern Cooperative Oncology Group trial 1597. *J Clin Oncol.* 2003;21:1550–1555.
34. Kakolyris S, Mavroudis D, Tsavaris N, et al. Paclitaxel in combination with carboplatin as salvage treatment in refractory small-cell lung cancer (SCLC): A multicenter phase II study. *Ann Oncol.* 2001;12:193–197.
35. Ciuleanu T, Samarzjia M, Demidchik Y, et al. Randomized phase III study (SPEAR) of picoplatin plus best supportive care (BSC) or BSC alone in patients (pts) with SCLC refractory or progressive within 6 months after first-line platinum-based chemotherapy. *J Clin Oncol.* 2010;28:15s.
36. von Pawel J, Jotte R, Spigel DR, et al. Randomized phase 3 trial of amrubicin versus topotecan as second-line treatment for small cell lung cancer (SCLC). 14th world conference on lung cancer, Amsterdam, the Netherlands, July 3,7–2011.
37. Pietanza MC, Krug LM, Sima CS, et al. Measurement of Circulating Tumor Cells (CTCs) in Patients with Small Cell Lung Cancer (SCLC) during a Phase II Clinical Trial. Mini Oral Session, 14th World Conference on Lung Cancer, Amsterdam, the Netherlands, July 3,7–2011.
38. Spigel DR, Hainsworth J, Jeffrey R, et al. MO19.08 NK012 (a nanodevice formulation of SN-38) in patients with relapsed small-cell lung cancer. *J Thoracic Oncol.* 2011;6 abstr P3.273: 12:15–14:15.
39. Grilley-Olson J, Keedy V, Sandler A, et al. A randomized Phase II study of carboplatin and Abraxane with two different schedules, in patients with extensive stage small cell lung cancer (ES-SCLC). *J Thoracic Oncol.* 2011;6 abstr P3.272:12:15–14:15.
40. Hiltermann TJ, Liesker J, Schouwink H, et al. Circulating tumor cells (CTC) in small cell lung cancer (SCLC), a promising prognostic factor. *J Clin Oncol.* 2010;28(15s):suppl; abstr 7630.
41. de Haas EC, di Pietro A, Simpson KL, et al. Clinical evaluation of M30 and M65 ELISA cell death assays as circulating biomarkers in a drug-sensitive tumor, testicular cancer. *Neoplasia.* 2008;10(10):1041–1048.
42. Hou JM, Greystoke A, Lancashire L, et al. Evaluation of circulating tumor cells and serological cell death biomarkers in small cell lung cancer patients undergoing chemotherapy. *Am J Pathol.* 2009;175(2):808–816. Epub 2009 Jul 23.
43. Stovold R, Meredith S, Simpson K, et al. Pro-opiomelanocortin identifies SCLC cells negative for cytokeratin biomarkers. *Endo Rel Canc* 2010.
44. Ranade AR, Cherba D, Sridhar S,et al. MicroRNA 92a-2*: A biomarker predictive for chemoresistance and prognostic for survival in patients with small cell lung cancer. *J Thorac Oncol.* 2010;5(8):1273–1278.
45. Zangemeister-Wittke U, Schenker T, Luedke GH, et al. Synergistic cytotoxicity of bcl-2 antisense oligodeoxynucleotides and etoposide, doxorubicin and cisplatin on small-cell lung cancer cell lines. *Br J Cancer.* 1998;78(8):1035–1042. 25(18S).
46. Rudin CM, Salgia R, Wang X, et al. Randomized Phase II Study of Carboplatin and Etoposide With or Without the bcl-2 Antisense Oligonucleotide Oblimersen for Extensive-Stage Small-Cell Lung Cancer: CALGB 30103. *J Clin Oncol.* 2008;26(6): 870–876.
47. Paik PK, Rudin CM, Pietanza MC et al. A phase II study of obatoclax mesylate, a Bcl-2 antagonist,

plus topotecan in relapsed small cell lung cancer. *Lung Cancer.* 2011;74(3):481–485.

48. Langer C, Albert I, Kovacs P, et al. Randomized phase II Study of Carboplatin and etoposide with or without pan-BCL-2 antagonist Obatolclax in Extensive Stage Small-cell lung cancer (ES-SCLC). WLCO-14th world conference in lung cancer. *J Clin Oncol.* 2011;29: suppl; abstr 7001.
49. Gandhi L, Camidge DR, de Oliveira M R, et al. Phase I study of Navitoclax (ABT-263), a novel Bcl-2 family inhibitor, in patients with small-cell lung cancer and other solid tumors. *J Clin Oncol.* 2011;29(7):909–916. Epub 2011 Jan 31.
50. Leal TB, Schelman W, Traynor A, et al. A phase I study of R-(-)-gossypol (AT101) in combination with cisplatin (P) and etoposide (E) in patients with advanced solid tumors and extensive-stage small cell lung cancer (ES-SCLC). *J Clin Oncol.* 2009;27:suppl;abstr 13502.
51. Joel J, Chansky K, Lara PN, et al. The proteasome inhibitor PS341 (Bortezomib) in platinum (plat)-treated extensive-stage small cell lung cancer (E-SCLC): A SWOG (0327) phase II trial. ASCO Annual Meeting Proceedings. *J Clin Oncol.* 2005; 23(16S) Part I of II (June 1 Suppl):7047.
52. Giaccone G., Debruyne C., Felip E., et al. Phase III study of adjuvant vaccination with Bec2/Bacille Calmette-Guerin in responding patients with limited disease small-cell lung cancer (European Organisation for Research and Treatment of Cancer 08971–08971b; Silva Study). *J Clin Oncol.* 2005;23:6854–686
53. Assersohn L, Souberbielle BE, O'Brien ME, et al. A randomized pilot study of SRL172 (Mycobacterium vaccae) in patients with small cell lung cancer (SCLC) treated with chemotherapy. *Clin Oncol (R Coll Radiol).* 2002;14(1):23–27.
54. Belani CP, Desai D, Khamar BM. Open-label, randomized multicenter phase II clinical trial of a toll-like receptor-2 (TLR2) agonist mycobacterium w (Cadi-05) in combination with paclitaxel plus cisplatin versus paclitaxel plus cisplatin in advanced non-small cell lung cancer (NSCLC). *J Clin Oncol.* 2011;29:suppl; abstr 7501.
55. Reck M, Bondarenko I, Luft A, et al. Ipilimumab in combination with paclitaxel and carboplatin as first-line treatment in extensive disease-small cell lung cancer (ED-SCLC): Results from a phase II trial. Session info: Oral session, [O09] SCLC I. 14th World Conference on Lung Cancer, July 2011.
56. Fossella FV, Tolcher A, Elliott M, et al. Phase I trial of the monoclonal antibody conjugate, BB-10901, for relapsed/refractory small cell lung cancer (SCLC) and other neuroendocrine (NE) tumors. *Proc Am Soc Clin Oncol.* 2002;21:abstr 1232.
57. Zhan P, Wang J, Lv XJ, Wang Q, et al. Prognostic value of vascular endothelial growth factor expression in patients with lung cancer: a systematic review with meta analysis. *J Thorac Oncol.* 2009;4(9):1094–1103.
58. Lee S -M, Woll PJ, James LE, et al. A phase III randomised, double blind, placebo controlled trial of etoposide/carboplatin with or without thalidomide in advanced small cell lung cancer (SCLC): Prs-04. *J Thorac Oncol.* 2007;2:S306–S307.
59. Spigel DR, Townley PM, Waterhouse DM, et al. Randomized Phase II study of bevacizumab in combination with chemotherapy in previously untreated extensive-stage small-cell lung cancer: Results from the SALUTE trial. *J Clin Oncol.* 2011;29:2215–2222
60. Jalal S, Bedano P, Einhorn L, et al. Paclitaxel plus bevacizumab in patients with chemosensitive relapsed small cell lung cancer: a safety, feasibility,and efficacy study from the Hoosier Oncology Group. *J Thor Oncol.* 2010;5(12):2008–2011.
61. Ramalingam SS, Mack PC, Vokes EE, et al. Cediranib (Azd2171) for the treatment of recurrent small cell lung cancer (SCLC): a California Consortium phase II study (Nci # 7097). *J Clin Oncol (Meeting Abstracts).* 2008;26:8078–8078.
62. Arnold AM, Seymour L, Smylie M, et al. Phase II study of vandetanib or placebo in small-cell lung cancer patients after complete or partial response to induction chemotherapy with or without radiation therapy: National Cancer Institute of Canada Clinical Trials Group Study Br.20. *J Clin Oncol.* 2007;25:4278–4284.
63. Ready N, Dunphy F, Pang H, et al. Combination chemotherapy with sunitinib (IND 74019; NSC 736511) for untreated extensive-stage small cell lung cancer: CALGB 30504 phase IB safety results. *J Clin Oncol.* 2010;28(15s):suppl; abstr 7056.

64. Schneider B, Gadgeel SM, Ramnath N, et al. Phase II trial of sunitinib maintenance therapy after platinum-based chemotherapy in patients with extensive stage small cell lung cancer (ES SCLC). *J Clin Oncol.* 20410;28:suppl; abstr e18041.
65. Spigel DR, Hainsworth JD, Rubin MS, et al., Phase II Study of Sunitinib Monotherapy Following Irinotecan/Carboplatin as First-Line Treatment for Patients with Extensive-Stage Small-Cell Lung Cancer. OA2-Oral Abstract Session II. 20th Chicago Multidisciplinary symposium in thoracic oncology, 2010.
66. Gitlitz BJ, Glisson BS, Moon J., et al. Sorafenib in patients with platinum (plat) treated extensive stage small cell lung cancer (E-SCLC): A Swog (S0435) phase II trial. *J Clin Oncol (Meeting Abstracts).* 2008;26:8039–8039.
67. Altorki N, Lane ME, Bauer T, et al. Phase II proof-of-concept study of pazopanib monotherapy in treatment-naive patients with stage I/II resectable non-small-cell lung cancer. *J Clin Oncol.* 2010;28(19):3131–3137. Epub 2010 Jun 1.
68. Spigel DR, Hainsworth JD, Simons L, et al. Irinotecan, carboplatin, and imatinib in untreated extensive-stage small-cell lung cancer: A phase II trial of the Minnie Pearl Cancer Research Network. *J Thorac Oncol.* 2007;2(9):854–861.
69. Krug LM, Crapanzano JP, Azzoli CG, et al. Imatinib mesylate lacks activity in small cell lung carcinoma expressing c-kit protein: A phase II clinical trial. *Cancer.* 2005;103:2128–2131.
70. Schneider BJ, Gadgeel S, Ramnath N, et al. Phase II trial of imatinib maintenance therapy after irinotecan and cisplatin in patients with c-kit positive extensive-stage small cell lung cancer (ES SCLC). *J Clin Oncol (Meeting Abstracts).* 2006;24:17089–17089
71. Tsurutani J, West KA, Sayyah J, et al. Inhibition of the Phosphatidylinositol 3-Kinase/Akt/ Mammalian Target of Rapamycin Pathway but not the MEK/ERK Pathway Attenuates Laminin-Mediated Small Cell Lung Cancer Cellular Survival and Resistance to Imatinib Mesylate or Chemotherapy. *Cancer Res.* 2005;65:8423.
72. Pandya KJ, Dahlberg S, Hidalgo M, et al. A randomized, phase II trial of two dose levels of temsirolimus (cci-779) in patients with extensive-stage small-cell lung cancer who have responding or stable disease after induction chemotherapy: A trial of the eastern cooperative oncology group (E1500). *J Thorac Oncol.* 2007;2:1036–1041.
73. Tarhini A, Kotsakis A, Gooding W, et al. Phase II study of everolimus (RAD001) in previously treated small cell lung cancer. *Clin Cancer Res.* 2010;16(23):5900–5907. Epub 2010 Nov 2.
74. Owonikoko TK, Stoller RG, Petro D, et al. Phase II study of Rad001 (everolimus) in previously treated small cell lung cancer (SCLC). *J Clin Oncol (Meeting Abstracts).* 2008;26:19017–19017.
75. Yu E, Clark JI, van Beynen J, et al. Dendritic cell transduced with full-length wild-type p53 generate antitumor cytotoxic T lymphocytes from peripheral blood of cancer patients. *Clin Cancer Res.* 2001;7:127.
76. Gabrilovich DI, Mirza N, Chiappori A, et al. Initial results of a Phase II trial of patients with extensive stage small cell lung cancer (SCLC) immunized with dendritic cells (DC) transduced with wild-type p53. ASCO Annual Meeting Proceedings. *J Clin Oncol.* 2005;23(16S), Part I of II (June 1 Supplement):2543.
77. Sarvesvaran J, Going JJ, Milroy R, et al. Is small cell lung cancer the perfect target for anti-telomerase treatment? *Carcinogenesis.* 1999;20(8):1649–1651.
78. Lee D, Lai CH, Wang Y, et al. Mechanism(s) of action and potency of Hsp90 inhibitor STA-9090 in small cell lung carcinoma cells. 14th World Conference on Lung Cancer, Amsterdam, the Netherlands, July 3–7, 2011.
79. Maulik G, Kijima T, Patrick C. Ma, et al. Modulation of the c-Met/Hepatocyte Growth Factor Pathway in Small Cell Lung Cancer. *Clin Cancer Res.* 2002;8:620.
80. Samol J, Ranson M, Scott E, et al. Safety and tolerability of the poly (ADP-ribose) polymerase (PARP) inhibitor, olaparib (AZD2281) in combination with topotecan for the treatment of patients with advanced solid tumors: A phase I study. *Invest New Drugs.* 2011 May 18. [Epub ahead of print].

demos
MEDICAL

ECAT
Emerging Cancer
Therapeutics

Adjuvant Chemotherapy for Early-Stage Non-Small Cell Lung Cancer

Manali I. Patel[1*] and Heather A. Wakelee[2]

[1]*Department of Hematology/Oncology, Stanford University School of Medicine, Stanford, CA*

[2] *Department of Medicine, Thoracic Oncology, Stanford University School of Medicine, Stanford, CA*

■ ABSTRACT

Adjuvant chemotherapy has been used in many malignancies such as breast and colon cancers to improve survival after surgical resection. The use of adjuvant chemotherapy has more recently become a standard of care for patients with Stage II to IIIB non-small cell lung cancer. Evidence from many recent trials and meta-analyses supports the benefit of adjuvant chemotherapy with cisplatin-based regimens for patients with resected Stage II-IIIA non-small cell lung cancer, as well as for selected patients with Stage IB disease. Recent studies have also demonstrated the benefit of other non-cisplatin-based regimens including the uracil–tegafur (UFT) although this has only been extensively studied in Japan. Although the optimal regimen is still under consideration, the strongest data is with cisplatin–vinorelbine, although many newer cisplatin-doublet regimens may be equally efficacious. Further advances in the evaluation of biomarkers and targeted therapies are in development. These therapies are currently under investigation with hopes for continued future improvements in survival of patients with non-small cell lung cancer.

Keywords: lung cancer, adjuvant therapy, chemotherapy, patient selection

*Corresponding author, Department of Medicine, Division of Hematology/Oncology, Stanford University, School of Medicine, 136 Middlefield Road, Palo Alto, CA 94301
E-mail address: manalip@stanford.edu

Emerging Cancer Therapeutics 3:1 (2012) 129–140.

DOI: 10.5003/2151–4194.3.1.129

INTRODUCTION

Lung cancer, the most common cause of death from cancer worldwide, kills over 157,000 men and women each year in the United States (1). Of the two types of lung cancer, non-small cell lung cancer (NSCLC) comprises 80% to 90% of the total cases of lung cancer. The best possible treatment for NSCLC is surgery; however, only 20% to 25% of patients have resectable disease. Five-year survival rates for NSCLC despite optimal surgery are low at 50% to 60% for Stage IB, 40% to 50% for Stage II, and 20% to 30% for Stage III (1,2). The standard of care for resected Stage II to IIIA NSCLC now includes the use of chemotherapy based on the results of recent data from the past decade, which provide evidence for survival advantages in resected NSCLC. This chapter discusses the historical background of adjuvant therapy for NSCLC, the debate between platinum compounds, future ongoing trials evaluating molecular targets, and new directions in early-stage NSCLC treatment.

CHEMOTHERAPY EMERGES FOR THE ADJVUANT SETTING

The first adjuvant chemotherapy for NSCLC, cyclophosphamide, was used alone and in combination with other chemotherapeutics as early as the 1960s. Twenty years later, in the 1980s, the first randomized clinical trials were published, which evaluated the role of chemotherapy in the adjuvant setting. The Lung Cancer Study Group (LCSG) conducted two of the earliest randomized controlled clinical trials to evaluate adjuvant therapy for early-stage disease albeit with differing results. The first trial represented the earliest published indication of the beneficial effect of adjuvant chemotherapy in patients with resected lung cancer. In this trial, 130 patients with completely resected Stage II or III adenocarcinomas were randomized to either cyclophosphamide/doxorubicin/cisplatin (CAP) versus immunotherapy with Bacille Calmette-Guérin (bCG) or levamisole. The trial showed a statistically significant 6-month delay in median time to recurrence and most importantly a 15% survival advantage at 1 year favoring chemotherapy, whereas survival of the control immunotherapy group was similar to that of patients treated with surgery alone (3). The second LCSG study failed to replicate these results; however, the trial examined incompletely resected NSCLC, and therefore was not a true "adjuvant" trial. A total of 164 patients were randomly assigned to postoperative radiotherapy with or without six cycles of CAP. Although initial results seemed promising and demonstrated favorable findings with a 14% difference in survival and a longer progression free survival favoring the chemotherapy arm, the results were not significant ($P = .66$). Additionally, median survival was only marginally improved with chemotherapy, and there was no 5-year survival benefit (4).

The conflicting results of these two LCSG trials led to additional randomized controlled trials. In 1992, Niiranen et al. evaluated 6 cycles of CAP in Stage T1–3N0 (WHO stages 1991) in patients with surgically resected disease. Out of the 110 patients enrolled, 5-year survival rate was 67% in the chemotherapy group and 56% in the control group ($P = .050$). Of the patients in the chemotherapy group, there was a difference in survival rate among those who completed therapy versus those who did not (72.5% versus 50.3%) although not statistically significant ($P = .15$) (5).

These early trials demonstrated improved local control and disease-free survival, but overall survival benefits were marginal and not definitive. These earlier trials used potentially ineffective chemotherapy regimens and included only a small numbers of patients, and in the early 1990s, an international panel recommended against the use of adjuvant chemotherapy outside of clinical trials.

NSCLC Collaborative Meta-Analysis

The inconclusive results of earlier clinical trials led to the growing role and publication of meta-analyses, which were well powered to evaluate accurate survival differences. The best-known earlier meta-analysis was completed by the NSCLC Collaborative Group in 1995, which included a total of 9,387 patients in 52 randomized controlled trials. Subgroup analysis of 14 randomized trials that evaluated surgical resection versus adjuvant chemotherapy after surgical resection included over 4,000 patients (6). The meta-analysis demonstrated the trend of cisplatin-based regimens to provide overall survival benefit in NSCLC. Overall survival with cisplatin-based chemotherapy was associated with a 13% reduction in the risk of death and a 5% overall survival benefit at 5 years, though not statistically significant (P = .08). The trend of benefit was seen despite chemotherapy regimen chosen: platinum/vinca/etoposide (HR 0.94, P = .27) versus platinum/vinorelbine (HR 0.82, P = .02) or other platinum combinations (HR 0.90, P = .36). The benefit observed, only though a trend, and role of therapy in other malignancies prompted additional evaluation of chemotherapy in patients with resected lung cancer. The trials established after the 1995 meta-analysis utilized more modern chemotherapy regimens and have mostly shown a more significant survival improvements from adjuvant chemotherapy such that updated results in another meta-analysis by the NSCLC collaborative group (Medical Research Council) in 2010 demonstrated a statistically significant survival benefit of adjuvant chemotherapy for early-stage NSCLC in 34 trial comparisons (22 of which examined a cisplatin-based regimen), which included 8,447 patients (7). The trial demonstrated a median follow-up of 8 years and reiterated the benefit of adjuvant chemotherapy (HR 0.86, 95% CI: 0.81–0.92, P < .0001) on survival, conferring a 4% absolute increase in survival (95% CI: 3–6) at 5 years from 60% to 64%). A more detailed discussion of the key trials included in this updated meta-analysis follows.

ECOG 3590 Trial

In the ECOG 3590 trial, Keller et al. randomly assigned 488 patients with Stage IIA and IIIA disease to receive either radiation alone or radiation administered concurrently with four cycles of cisplatin and etoposide (8). Median survival was 39 months for the radiation-alone arm versus 38 months for the chemotherapy plus radiation arm (P = .56). Toxicity was more pronounced with the concurrent chemotherapy and radiation treatment. A major concern of the study pertained to the fact that concurrent therapy has been shown for bulky disease but not for treating minimal residual disease in the adjuvant setting.

Adjuvant Lung Project Italy Trial and Big Lung Trial

Two large studies completed after the 1990s (Table 1) with negative results include the Adjuvant Lung Project Italy (ALPI) Trial and the Big Lung Trial (BLT). The ALPI trial enrolled 1,209 patients between 1994 and 1999 with Stage I, II, or IIIA NSCLC (9). Patients were randomly assigned to receive surgery with or without adjuvant mitomycin, vindesine, or cisplatin dosed every 3 weeks for three cycles. At 5 years, there were no statistically significant differences in overall survival (HR 0.96, 95% CI: 0.81–1.13; P = .589) or disease-free survival (HR 0.89, 95% CI: 0.76–1.03; P = .128). The ALPI trial, however, was limited by poor compliance as only 69% patients received the full three cycles of chemotherapy likely due to the use of mitomycin C and this poor compliance could attribute to the negative results of the study.

Similarly, the BLT showed no advantage to adjuvant chemotherapy in early-stage disease (10). A total of 381 patients with Stage I, II, and III NSCLC were randomized to receive cisplatin-based chemotherapy with three cycles of 3-week therapy of cisplatin/vindesine, mitomycin/ifosfamide/cisplatin, mitomycin/vinblastine/cisplatin, or vinorelbine/cisplatin. Chemotherapy was administered before surgery in 3% of cases while the adjuvant setting represented 97% of cases. A total of 95% of cases achieved a complete remission but after a median follow-up period of 34.6 months there was

TABLE 1 Adjuvant chemotherapy trials after 1990s

Trial	Stage	Chemotherapy	Survival Benefit
ALPI (9)	I, II, IIIA	Cisplatin 100 mg/m^2 × 3 Mitomycin C 8 mg/m^2 × 3 Vindesine 3 mg/m^2 × 6	NA
BLT (10)	I, II, III	Cisplatin 80 mg/m^2 (biotherapies) or Cisplatin 50 mg/m^2 (tritherapies) Vindesine 3 mg/m^2 × 6 or Vinorelbine 30 mg/m^2 × 6 or Mitomycin 6 mg/m^2 × 3 and ifosfamide 3 g/m^2 × 3 or Mitomycin 6 mg/m^2 × 3 and vinblastine 6 mg/m^2 × 3	NA
IALT (11)	I, II, III	Cisplatin 100 or 120 mg/m^2 × 3 or Cisplatin 80 or 100 mg/m^2 × 4 Vindesine 3 mg/m^2 × 6–8 or Vinblastine 4 mg/m^2 × 6–8 or Vinorelbine 30 mg/m^2 weekly × 13 or Etoposide 100 mg/m^2 × 9–12	5 year; No benefit at 7 years
JBR.10 (13)	IB, II	Cisplatin 50 mg/m^2 × 2 Vinorelbine 25 mg/m^2 × 16	5 years; Benefit at > 9 years
ANITA (14)	I-IIIA	Cisplatin 100 mg/m^2 × 4 Vinorelbine 30 mg/m^2 × 16	5 years; Benefit at 7 years
CALGB (16,17)	IB	Carboplatin AUC 6 × 4 Paclitaxel 200 mg/m^2 × 4	4 years; No benefit at 57 and 74 months

no significant difference in overall survival (HR 1.02, 95% CI: 0.77–1.35; P = .90) or disease-free survival (HR 0.97, 95% CI: 0.74–1.26, P = .81).

IALT Trial

Despite the ALPI and BLT results, in the early 2000s, positive results were observed with adjuvant chemotherapy in other studies. The largest trial that has been conducted to date, the International Adjuvant Lung Cancer Collaborative Group Trial (IALT) enrolled a total of 1,867 patients with completely resected I, II, or IIIA lung cancer (11). Patients were randomly assigned to observation or to three or four cycles of an investigator chosen cisplatin-based chemotherapy of the four following regimens: cisplatin plus vindesine, etoposide, vinorelbine, or vinblastine. In this trial, more than 50% of patients in the treatment group received a combination of cisplatin plus etoposide. A total of 148 centers in 33 countries enrolled patients and the distribution by stage was 36% of patients with Stage I, 25% with Stage II, and 39% Stage III disease. Radiation was left to the discretion of the institution, but a consistent standard was maintained, and approximately 25% of patients received adjuvant radiation. Although the accrual target was 3,300 patients, the trial was closed after enrollment of 1,867 patients due to a planned interim analysis that revealed a significant benefit of adjuvant chemotherapy on survival (HR 0.86, 95% CI: 0.76–0.98; P < .03). Median OS improved from 44 months to 50 months, translating to a 4% improvement in OS at 5 years (44.5% versus 40.4%; P < .03). Disease-free survival rate was also higher in the chemotherapy arm than in the observation arm (HR 0.83, 95% CI: 0.74–0.94,

$P < .003$). These results were the first to demonstrate the very clear benefit of adjuvant platinum-based chemotherapy in the adjuvant early-stage setting for NSCLC. This trial was a pivotal trial in helping to lead the path for changing treatment standards. Recent subset analysis after a long-term follow-up in 2008 revealed no trend for benefit on either stage of disease or chemotherapy regimen chosen (12) and no significant effect of adjuvant chemotherapy on overall survival at 7 years (HR 0.91, 95% CI: 0.8–1.02; $P = .10$). Despite the long-term follow-up results, clearly the survival benefit observed at 5 years was significantly different and confirmed the effect of chemotherapy at least for the first 5 years after surgery.

JBR.10 Trial

Similar results emerged from the trial conducted by the North American Intergroup, led by the National Cancer Institute of Canada (13). The JBR.10 study included completely resected 1B or Stage II NSCLC patients with good performance status. Out of 482 patients enrolled, 45% had Stage I and 55% had Stage II disease with a median age of 61 years. Patients were randomly assigned to observation or four cycles of cisplatin 50 mg/m^2 on days 1 and 8 plus vinorelbine 25 mg/m^2 weekly (days 1,8,15, and 22) for a 28-day regimen for 16 weeks.. This trial demonstrated the most striking benefit to date of adjuvant therapy with an overall and relapse-free survival prolonged in the chemotherapy group relative to the observation group (94 versus 73 months, HR 0.69, CI: 0.52–0.91; $P = .04$; not reached vs. 46.7 months HR 0.60, 95% CI: 0.45–0.79; $P < .001$, respectively). Five-year survival rates were 69% and 54% in the adjuvant and control arms, respectively ($P = .03$), a 15% improvement in 5-year survival favoring chemotherapy. Toxicity of the regimen was as expected with chemo-related deaths in two patients. Recent updates in 2009 demonstrated the benefit of adjuvant therapy retained at >9 years (13).

ANITA Trial

A third large study, which also demonstrated the benefit of adjuvant chemotherapy in early NSCLC, was a large international study, the Adjuvant Navelbine International Trialist Association (ANITA). The trial investigated the benefit of the cisplatin–vinorelbine regimen in patients with Stage 1B-IIIA NSCLC (14). Patients were randomized to receive adjuvant chemotherapy consisting of four cycles of vinorelbine at 30 mg/m^2 on days 1,8,15, and 22 (16 doses) plus 100 mg/m^2 cisplatin ($n = 407$) on day 1 (4 doses) or observation ($n = 433$). Postoperative radiotherapy was optional and was initiated according to the policy of individual centers. A total of 301 patients had Stage IB (36%), 203 (24%) had Stage II disease, and 325 (39%) had Stage IIIA disease. After median follow-up of 76 months, median survival was 65.7 months in the chemotherapy group versus 43.7 months in the observation group (HR 0.80; $P = .017$). Chemotherapy improved overall survival at 5 years by 8.6% and this survival advantage was maintained at 7 years. Toxicity included neutropenia (92%) and seven (2%) toxic deaths. In this study, compliance was greater with cisplatin than with vinorelbine. The favorable impact of chemotherapy on survival was observed in Stages II and IIIA, but there was no benefit for overall survival in patients with Stage IB NSCLC.

LACE Meta-Analysis

Given the mixed results of the five large recent trials, ALPI, ANITA, BLT, IALT, and JBR.10, the Lung Adjuvant Cisplatin Evaluation (LACE) meta-analysis, the second largest meta-analysis, pooled individual patient data for evaluation of the benefit of adjuvant chemotherapy for NSCLC. The meta-analysis included 4,584 patients with a median follow-up of 5.1 years and demonstrated a positive overall HR of death of 0.89 (95% CI: 0.82–0.96; $P < .005$) corresponding to a 5-year absolute benefit of 4.2% with chemotherapy (15). The benefit varied with stage, with no benefit seen in Stage IA (HR 1.41, 95% CI: 0.96–2.09). All other stages, which were included in the clinical trials, however, demonstrated benefit. This was not statistically significant for Stage IB (HR 0.93, 95% CI: 0.78–1.10) but was statistically significant for the higher stages, including Stage II (HR 0.83, 95% CI: 0.73–0.95) and stage III (HR 0.83, 95% CI: 0.73–0.95). The benefit also varied with therapy used. Two studies exclusively examined cisplatin–vinorelbine combinations (JBR.10 and ANITA) while the other three (BLT, IALT, and ALPI) allowed investigator's choice of cisplatin-based regimens. Subgroup analyses in the LACE meta-analysis demonstrated a trend of superiority toward cisplatin paired with vinorelbine (HR 0.80, 95% CI: 0.70–0.91) versus with cisplatin/etoposide or cisplatin/vinca-alkaloid (HR 0.92, 95% CI: 0.80–1.06). Most of the positive studies used the cisplatin–vinorelbine combination, and 86% of these used a cisplatin dosing of greater than 300 mg/m^2. Cisplatin dosing of <300 mg/m^2 versus >300 mg/m^2 demonstrated a trend toward overall survival in favor of higher dosing (*P* = .10). (This is further discussed in Optimal Chemotherapy section.) Despite chemotherapy regimen used, the LACE meta-analysis further confirmed the role of cisplatin-based chemotherapy in adjuvant early-stage NSCLC, as was also demonstrated in the updated NSCLC collaborative group (Medical Research Council) meta-analysis in 2010.

CALGB9633 Trial

Unlike the studies discussed above, the CALGB 9633 trial conducted by the Cancer and Leukemia B group, RTOG and the North Central Cancer Treatment group exclusively evaluated the role of adjuvant chemotherapy in patients with resected stage IB. Unlike other studies that used a cisplatin-based backbone, this study randomized patients following complete resection to paclitaxel 200 mg/m^2 and carboplatin (area under the curve = 6) every 3 weeks for four cycles or observation. The total number of patients enrolled was 344 although the initial accrual target was 500. In 2004, preliminary results of the trial demonstrated a statistically significant improvement in disease-free and overall survival in patients receiving the chemotherapy with a 12% improvement in 4-year overall survival at a median follow-up of 34 months (*P* = .028) (16). Because of this planned interim analysis, the study was terminated by the Data Safety Monitoring Board. At 57 months, however, survival was not different between the arms (60% versus 58%; *P* = .32). Additionally, at a median follow-up of 74 months the significance of the first report could not be confirmed with overall survival of 60% versus 58% for the chemotherapy and observation groups, respectively (HR 0.83, 95% CI 0.64–1.08, *P* = .125) (17). Disease-free survival however favored chemotherapy in the intention to treat analysis (HR 0.74, *P* = .27) with a trend toward improvement in overall survival (HR 0.80; *P* = .10). An exploratory analysis demonstrated a significant survival difference though in favor of adjuvant chemotherapy for patients with tumors >4 cm in diameter (HR 0.69, 90% CI: 0.48–0.99; *P* = .043)

This negative trial highlighted the hazards of terminating a trial early based on short follow-up, the need for sufficient sample sizes to detect small but potentially significant improvements in survival, and the use of adequate chemotherapy regimens that had previously been proven significant in other stages. Regardless of the limitations of this study, current data do not support the use of chemotherapy in patients undergoing resection of stage IB NSCLC whose tumors are less than 4 cm in size. These results are similar to subset analyses observed in the JBR.10 study (18).

■ CISPLATIN VERSUS CARBOPLATIN

The advantage of cisplatin-based therapy on survival from NSCLC is evident for patients with Stage II and III cancer given that all three positive trials since 2003, IALT, JBR.10, and ANITA, used a cisplatin-based therapy (two with vinorelbine) for

4 cycles. Despite the pivotal role of cisplatin-based chemotherapy, treatment with cisplatin is associated with a number of serious side effects, which has led many clinicians to use the cisplatin analog, carboplatin. Most of the data demonstrating the role of carboplatin has been from the metastatic settings, but these studies have led to the use of carboplatin in the adjuvant setting for early-stage disease. Two North American Phase III trials in the advanced stage setting have evaluated carboplatin versus cisplatin and demonstrated equivalence in survival when combined with paclitaxel (19,20). The only large meta-analysis, however, although in the metastatic setting, the cisplatin versus carboplatin (CisCa) meta-analysis provides our strongest evidence of a trend of superiority of cisplatin over carboplatin (21). Among 2,968 patients analyzed in CisCa, cisplatin therapy was associated with improved response rates with chemotherapy (30%) compared with carboplatin (24%) (OR of 1.37, 95% CI: 1.16–1.62; $P < .001$). Carboplatin was associated with a statistically significant increase in mortality in subgroup analysis of patients with nonsquamous tumors and those treated with third generation chemotherapy, (HR 1.12, 95% CI: 1.01–1.23 and HR 1.11, 95% CI: 1.01–1.21, respectively). The trial showing the largest benefit for carboplatin over cisplatin was an outlier in that it was restricted to patients with squamous histology and used an older regimen and was comprised of primarily younger males with Stage III cancers compared with others studies included in the meta-analysis. Furthermore, the study used a higher carboplatin dosing (500 versus 325 or 300 mg/m^2) compared with other studies in the CisCa meta-analysis (22). When this trial was excluded from the meta-analysis, the test for heterogeneity no longer reached statistical significance, and the modified CisCa meta-analysis affirmed that cisplatin is the preferred platinum agent for treatment of NSCLC in advanced disease. A recent British study combining gemcitabine with either carboplatin or cisplatin though did not find a superiority for the cisplatin regimens and the debate over cisplatin versus carboplatin continues (23).

Our only data in early-stage disease with carboplatin comes from the CALGB9633 trial, which utilized carboplatin/paclitaxel for resected stage IB NSCLC and was discussed in detail earlier (16). This study failed to show a survival advantage in the population with the carboplatin regimen but was small and included only patients with Stage IB NSCLC, and therefore the results may not be solely attributable to the superiority of cisplatin. The current guidelines from the National Comprehensive Cancer Network, a professional organization of 21 of the world's largest leading cancer centers, recommend adjuvant chemotherapy using a cisplatin-based regimen (24). Given the current evidence to date, as there are no future studies planned to evaluate carboplatin versus cisplatin in the adjuvant setting cisplatin is the favored platinum of choice. The substitution of carboplatin is a frequent practice, however, especially in the elderly (as discussed in the section on chemotherapy in the elderly below) and those with contraindications to cisplatin such as renal impairment.

■ OPTIMAL ADJUVANT CISPLATIN-BASED REGIMEN

Although the role of adjuvant therapy in early-stage NSCLC became standard of care in the past 10 years, there is a paucity of data regarding the best cisplatin-based regimen. Although the NCCN guidelines recommend any combination cisplatin-based therapy with previously studied third-generation agents such as vinorelbine, vincristine, and etoposide, the guidelines also suggest combinations with other, newer agents that have not been thoroughly and extensively tested in the adjuvant setting such as gemcitabine, docetaxel, or pemetrexed. The NSCLC Meta-analysis Collaborative Group, which analyzed randomized control clinical trials from 1965 onward, demonstrated little variation depending on the chosen chemotherapy regimen. Although there was no significant difference in effect between chemotherapy categories in the first meta-analysis, the use of older platinum combinations with a vinca-alkaloid or etoposide had a slightly lower effect (HR 0.94; P = .27) than the trials that used platinum with vinorelbine (HR 0.82; P = .02). Similarly, data from the LACE meta-analysis show a marginal trend of superiority when using cisplatin/vinorelbine combinations compared with other cisplatin combinations (P = .04) and the trial with the most positive outcome used cisplatin/vinorelbine. The results of these trials, however, may have more do to with the delivery and higher dosing intensity of the regimen as opposed to the superiority of the actual cisplatin–vinorelbine regimen. For instance, cisplatin–vinorelbine was dosed at a higher cisplatin dosing (> 300 mg/m^2) in 86% of patients who received this regimen suggesting that the dose intensity of cisplatin may account for the benefit observed compared to the other regimens. In the adjuvant setting, there are many modern drugs that have not been studied, and because the only definitive data exists in the metastatic setting, the questions about which is the best regimen remain unanswered in the adjuvant setting. Despite the lack of data in the adjuvant setting, however, many different cisplatin-based doublets are being used in the United States in the adjuvant setting. This is clear from the preliminary data from the Eastern Cooperative Group 1505 trial, which is currently underway to investigate the value in the adjuvant setting of the antivascular endothelial growth factor receptor monoclonal antibody bevacizumab. Preliminary data from the study indicate that trial oncologists (primarily in the United States) are choosing from all of the combinations of treatment available on the trial, which include cisplatin with gemcitabine, docetaxel, vinorelbine, or pemetrexed (25). In the first 636 patients (of a planned 1500) enrolled in the trial, 27% received cisplatin/vinorelbine, 33% received cisplatin/docetaxel, 25% received cisplatin/gemcitabine, and 16% received cisplatin/pemetrexed (which was added for only nonsquamous histology after enrollment had already begun). Data with these regimens, other than cisplatin/vinorelbine, in the adjuvant setting is very limited. For cisplatin/pemetrexed the TREAT (randomized Phase II trial on refinement of early-stage NSCLC adjuvant chemotherapy with cisplatin and pemetrexed versus cisplatin and vinorelbine preliminary results were presented at American Society of Clinical Oncology (ASCO) in 2011 and demonstrated feasibility of and high drug delivery with cisplatin/pemetrexed regimen (26). Efficacy from this trial will be difficult to interpret though as 38% of patients have Stage IB and 45% of patients in the study have squamous histology, which will likely reduce pemetrexed efficacy. Despite limited data with other regimens, many oncologists are now substituting other doublets for cisplatin–vinorelbine, and we await further data from ongoing trials of these regimens as adjuvant therapy.

■ NONPLATINUM REGIMENS

As an alternative to platinum-based treatment, investigators in Japan developed an oral antimetabolite, Uracil–tegafur (UFT), composed of a fixed ratio of uracil and tegafur. This compound has been studied extensively in Japan for adjuvant treatment after complete resection, and the treatment has demonstrated beneficial effects with the addition of UFT.

The West Japan Study Group for Lung Cancer Surgery conducted two studies, the second of which was the first trial to confirm a survival benefit of UFT in the adjuvant setting. Three arms consisting of 323 patients with resected Stage I to III NSCLC were randomly assigned to surgery alone, UFT alone, or cisplatin plus vindesine followed by UFT group (CVUft) (27). The overall 5-year survival rates were 60.6% for the CVUft group, 64.1% for the UFT group, and 49% for the control group (P = .044). A larger study comparing UFT versus observation was performed by the Japan Lung cancer Research Group (JLCRG) (28). In this study, Kato et al. randomized 979 patients with Stage I disease to observation alone or 2 years of postoperative UFT (250 mg/m^2/day). At a median follow-up of 73 months, adjuvant UFT was associated with a small (3%) but statistically significant improvement in 5-year survival. Subgroup analysis suggested that the magnitude of benefit was for patients with T2N0 carcinomas 84.9% versus 73.5% in the control group (HR 0.48, 95% CI: 0.29–0.81) and for patients with T1 disease with tumor sizes greater than 2 cm in diameter (P = .05). The benefit of UFT has been replicated in several other smaller studies in Japan. Meta-analyses of these additional studies included over 2,000 patients and revealed a reduction in mortality for adjuvant chemotherapy with UFT relative to treatment with surgery alone with a pooled HR of 0.77 (P = .15), results of which are similar to those of cisplatin-based doublet therapy in the adjuvant setting. UFT, therefore, has been used in Japan in lieu of cisplatin-based therapy and may be a possible option for patients in other countries as well.

■ ADJUVANT CHEMOTHERAPY IN THE ELDERLY

The role of adjuvant therapy in the elderly is a research question of particular significance given that the median age of diagnosis of NSCLC is among the elderly population at 70 years of age. Although elderly patients receive less adjuvant therapy due to toxicities and hospitalizations from treatment, recent studies indicate that the survival benefits seen with adjuvant chemotherapy may also extend to the elderly patient population despite the side effects of therapy, The JBR.10 trial showed a prolonged overall survival among 155 patients age 65 years and older (HR 0.61; 95% CI: 0.38–0.98; P = .04) (JBR.10). The LACE meta-analysis, which also included JBR.10, demonstrated a similar trend toward overall survival benefit for this patient population in a pooled analysis of patients aged 70 years and older. (HR 0.90, 95% CI: 0.70–1.16; P = .29) (29). Recent data presented at the ASCO annual meeting in 2011 demonstrate that these findings have increased chemotherapy administration for the elderly in the United States and Canada. One abstract demonstrated that out of a population-based study in Ontario, Canada, that administration of adjuvant therapy in patients over 70 years increased from 3% to 16% over the years of 2001 to 2006 and correlated with an overall survival improvement from 47% to 50% (30). Despite concerns of toxicity from chemotherapy, more patients were treated with cisplatin than with carboplatin (70% of elderly were treated with cisplatin and 28% treated with carboplatin). The other abstract examined SEER data from 1992 to 2005 and demonstrated that in the United States, 19% of patients greater than 65 years received chemotherapy in the adjuvant setting (31), but the use of carboplatin was more extensive than cisplatin, unlike what was seen in Canada. The evidence of benefit of adjuvant therapy for elderly patients has therefore been demonstrated and should be considered for patients with good performance status, regardless of age.

■ IMPROVING PATIENT SELECTION AND FUTURE OUTCOMES

The research from the past decade has clearly indicated the role of chemotherapy in the adjuvant setting for NSCLC. However, the lack of benefit in certain subsets such as stage IB tumors and the small benefit provided to other patients indicate the need to better understand who will benefit most from adjuvant therapy. Recently, investigation of predictive biomarkers help to select which patients are most at risk for recurrence and help determine which chemotherapy is the most efficacious for individual patients. The excision repair cross-complementation group 1 (ERCC1) for instance is a protein that is required for proper repair of DNA damage after insults such as from cisplatin. This protein functions in the nucleotide excision repair pathway and was one of the first proteins to be studied in the International Adjuvant Lung Trial. The patients low expression of ERCC1 in tumors showed prolonged survival (HR 0.65, 95% CI: 0.50–0.86; P = .002) with chemotherapy compared with observation, however this was not true among patients with tumors with higher ERCC1 expression (HR 1.14, 95% CI: 0.84–1.55; P = .40)

(32). This result, which was updated at ESMO in 2011, further indicated the benefit of adjuvant cisplatin-based chemotherapy in completely resected ERCC-1 negative tumors. Validation of these results are underway with multiple trials ongoing in the United States and Europe including SWOG 0720, which evaluated adjuvant therapy with cisplatin/gemcitabine for Stage 1 (tumors >2 cm) in patients with low tumor expression of ERCC1 and RRM1. The tailored postsurgical therapy in early-stage NSCLC trial and the international tailored chemotherapy adjuvant trial are Phase III trials evaluating the use of different chemotherapy possibilities based on expression levels of ERCC1 and other markers.

Other studies, such as the Spanish Customized Adjuvant Trial, are looking at BRCA1 mRNA levels to customize therapy in patients with resected early-stage (1–IIIA) disease. The trial is evaluating the rationale that patients with low BRCA1 mRNA levels have longer survival when treated with cisplatin-based chemotherapy, whereas patients with high BRCA1 mRNA levels have longer survival when treated with taxane-based therapy. Patients with high levels of BRCA1 mRNA receive docetaxel, intermediate levels receive docetaxel/cisplatin, and low-level expressions of BRCA1 mRNA receive cisplatin/gemcitabine.

Targeted pathways are also of extreme importance and have already lead to focused treatment in the metastatic setting for patients whose tumors express particular gene mutations. The epidermal growth factor receptor (EGFR) gene mutations are one example. Studies of EGFR-targeted drugs in earlier stages of disease have been ongoing. Although the negative results from the NCIC CTG BR.19 trial, which evaluated the EGFR targeted agent gefitinib in completely resected stage IB–IIIA NSCLC (only a small number of whom had EGFR mutations), raised questions regarding the efficacy of gefitinib; the trial was halted early and the small numbers make the interpretations difficult. The current randomized double-blinded trial in Adjuvant NSCLC with Tarceva trial is evaluating the role of EGFR-TKI erlotinib in the adjuvant treatment of patients with resected Stage IB–IIIA NSCLC. The double-blinded, placebo-controlled study randomized 945 patients with EGFR expression detected by either FISH or immunohistochemistry to either two years of daily erlotinib at 150 mg/day or placebo. This trial has completed accrual and full EGFR and other molecular analyses are being completed.

Inhibition of angiogenesis is also an area of study. Two trials, the ECOG4599 trial and Avastin in Lung cancer trial, have demonstrated the improvement of outcomes for patients with advanced NSCLC when combining bevacizumab, a monoclonal antibody that targets angiogenesis, with first-line doublet chemotherapy (33,34). Based on these positive results, the ongoing randomized ECOG 1505 trial evaluates four cycles of cisplatin-based doublet chemotherapy with or without bevacizumab (15 mg/kg) every 3 weeks.

The MAGE-A3 antigen-specific cancer immunotherapeutics is being evaluated by the MAGRIT (MAGE-A3 as adjuvant, non-small cell lung cancer immunotherapy) trial in the adjuvant setting. This trial is expected to help establish the role of vaccinations as adjuvant therapy for patient populations. Gene expression patterns are also an area investigated by multiple groups to both prognosticate and guide therapy.

■ CONCLUSION

The importance of adjuvant cisplatin-based therapy has been clearly demonstrated for patients with resected Stage II to IIIA and selected Stage IB NSCLC. The results of three large Phase III trials, the IALT, JBR.10, and ANITA, are largely responsible for standardizing adjuvant chemotherapy for NSCLC. Although the best regimen is still under evaluation, the data so far show a trend favoring cisplatin–vinorelbine, but there are many other cisplatin doublets that may be equally efficacious. The most definitive data exists in the metastatic setting and indicates that cisplatin–pemetrexed, cisplatin–docetaxel, or cisplatin–gemcitabine are equivalent and may be reasonable alternatives to cisplatin–vinorelbine. There are other alternatives as well including the use of UFT in Japan. Better understanding of how to predict which patients need adjuvant therapy and which therapy is optimal for a given patient is critical. Current studies are examining chemotherapy regimens in the adjuvant setting paired with evaluation of specific biomarkers in prospective randomized controlled clinical trials. Other studies are examining novel adjuvant treatments with non-chemotherapy agents. The results of these future studies will hopefully improve our understanding of NSCLC and improve the survival of patients with resected disease.

REFERENCES

1. Siegel R. Cancer Statistics: The impact on eliminating socioeconomic and racial disparities on premature cancer deaths. *Cancer J Clin.* 2011;61:212–36.
2. Kohler BA, Ward E, McCarthy BJ, et al. Annual report to the nation on the status of cancer, 1975–2007, featuring tumors of the brain and other nervous system. *J Natl Cancer Inst.* 2011;103:1–23.
3. Holmes EC, Gail M. Surgical adjuvant therapy for stage II and stage III adenocarcinoma and large cell undifferentiated carcinoma. *J Clin Oncol.* 1986;4:710–715.
4. Lad T, Rubenstein L, Sadeghi A. The Lung Cancer Study Group: The benefit of adjuvant treatment for resected local advanced non-small cell lung cancer. *J Clin Oncol.* 1998;6:125–207.
5. Niiranen A, Niitamo-Korbonen S, Kouri M, et al. Adjuvant chemotherapy after radical surgery for non-small cell lung cancer: A randomized study. *J Clin Oncol.* 1992;10:1927–1932.
6. Non-Small Cell Lung Cancer Collaborative Group: Chemotherapy in non-small cell lung cancer: A meta-analysis using updated data on individual patients from 52 randomized clinical trials. *BMJ.* 1995;311:899–909.
7. Non-Small Cell Lung Cancer Collaborative Group. Adjuvant chemotherapy, with or without postoperative radiotherapy, in operable non-small cell lung cancer: Two meta-analyses of individual patient data. *Lancet.* 2010;375:1267–1277.
8. Keller SM, Adak S, Wagner H, et al. A randomized trial of postoperative adjuvant therapy in patients with completely resected stage II or IIIA non-small cell lung cancer. *NEJM.* 2000;343:1217–1222.
9. Scagliotti GV, Roldano F, Torri V, et al. Randomized study of adjuvant chemotherapy for completely resected stage I, II, or IIIA non-small cell lung cancer. *J Natl Cancer Inst.* 2003;95:1453–1461.
10. Waller D, Peake RJ, Stephens RJ, et al. Chemotherapy for patients with non-small cell lung cancer: The surgical setting of the Big Lung Trial. *Eur J Cardiothorac Surg.* 2004;26:173–182.
11. The International Adjuvant Lung Cancer Trial Collaborative Group: Cisplatin-based adjuvant chemotherapy in patients with completely resected non-small cell lung cancer. *NEJM.* 2004;350: 351–360.
12. Arriagada R, Dunant A, Pignon JP, et al. Long-term results of the International Adjuvant Lung Cancer Trial (IALT) evaluating adjuvant cisplatin-based chemotherapy in resected non-small cell lung cancer. *J Clin Oncol.* 2010;28:35–42.
13. Winton T, Livingston R, Johnson D, et al. Vinorelbine plus cisplatin versus observation in resected non-small cell lung cancer. *NEJM.* 2005;352:2689–2597.
14. Douillard JY, Rosell R, De Lena M, et al. Adjuvant vinorelbine plus cisplatin versus observation in patients with completely resected stage IB-IIIA non-small cell lung cancer (Adjuvant Navelbine International Trialist Association [ANITA]: A randomized controlled trial. *Lancet Oncol.* 2006;7:719–727.
15. Pignon JP, Tribodet H, Scagliott GV, et al. Lung adjuvant cisplatin evaluation: A pooled analysis by the LACE collaborative group. *J Clin Oncol.* 2008;26:3552–3559.
16. Strauss GM, Herndon JE, Maddaus MA, et al. Randomized Clinical Trial of adjuvant chemotherapy with paclitaxel and carboplatin following resection in stage IB non-small cell lung cancer (NSCLC): Report of the Cancer and Leukemia Group B (CALGB) Protocol 9633. *J Clin Oncol.* 2004;22(621s):suppl; abstr 7019.
17. Strauss GM, Herndon JE, Maddaus MA, et al. Adjuvant paclitaxel plus carboplatin compared with observation in stage IB non-small cell lung cancer.

CALGB9633 with the Cancer and Leukemia Group B, Radiation Therapy Oncology Group, and the North Central Cancer Treatment Group Study Groups. *J Clin Oncol.* 2008;26:5043–5051.
18. Vincent MD, Butts C, Seymour L, et al. Updated survival analysis of JBR.10: A randomized phase III trial of vinorelbine/cisplatin versus observation in completely resected stage IB and II non-small cell lung cancer (NSCLC). *J Clin Oncol.* 2009;27(15s):suppl; abstr 7501.
19. Schiller JH, Harrington D, Belani CP, et al. Comparison of four chemotherapy regimens for advanced non-small-cell lung cancer. *NEJM.* 2002; 346:92–98.
20. Kelly K, Crowley J, Bunn PA Jr, et al. Randomized phase III trial of paclitaxel plus carboplatin versus vinorelbine plus cisplatin in the treatment of patients with advanced non-small-cell lung cancer: A Southwest Oncology Group trial. *J Clin Oncol.* 2001;19:3210–3218.
21. Ardizonni A, Boni L, Tiseo M, et al. Cisplatin versus carboplatin-based chemotherapy in first-line treatment of advanced non-small cell lung cancer: An individual patient data meta-analysis. *J Natl Cancer Inst.* 2007;99:847–857.
22. Jelic S, Mitrovic L, Radosavljevic D, et al. Survival advantage for carboplatin substituting cisplatin in combination with vindesine and mitomycin C for stage IIIB and IV squamous-cell bronchogenic carcinoma: A randomized phase III study. *Lung Cancer.* 2001;34:1–13.
23. David Ferry, Lucinda Billingham, Hugh Jarrett, et al. British Thoracic Oncology Group Trial, BROG2: Randomised phase III clinical trial of gemcitabine combined with cisplatin 50 mg/m2 (GC50) versus cisplatin 80 mg/m2 (GC80) versus carboplatin AUC 6 (GCB6) in Advanced NSCLC. *Journal of Thoracic Oncology.* 2011;6s (Suppl 2):S274 (Abstr#O01.03).
24. Ettinger DS, Akerley W, Bepler G, et al. "Non Small Cell Lung Cancer. *J Natl Compr Canc Netw.* 2010;8:740–801.
25. Wakelee HA, Dahlberg SE, Keller SM, et al. *Interim report of on-study demographics and toxicity from E1505, a phase III randomized trial of adjuvant chemotherapy with or without bevacizumab for completely resected early-stage non-small cell lung cancer.* Abstract presented at: the American Society of Clinical Oncology; June 2–4, 2011, Chicago, IL.
26. Kreuter M, Vansteenkiste J, Griesinger F, et al. *Trial on the refinement of early non-small cell lung cancer. Adjuvant chemotherapy with pemetrexed and cisplatin versus vinorelbine and cisplatin: The TREAT protocol.* Abstract presented at: the American Society of Clinical Oncology, June 2–4, 2011, Chicago, IL.
27. Wada H, Hitomi S, Teramatsu T. Adjuvant chemotherapy after complete resection in non-small cell lung cancer. West Japan Study Group for Lung Cancer Surgery. *J Clin Oncol.* 1996;14:1048–1054.
28. Kato H, Ichinose Y, Ohta M, et al. A randomized trial of adjuvant chemotherapy with uracil-tegafur for adenocarcinoma of the lung. *NEJM.* 2004;350:1713–1721.
29. Fruh M, Rolland E, Pignon P, et al. Pooled analysis of the effect of age on adjuvant cisplatin-based chemotherapy for completely resected non-small cell lung cancer. *J Clin Oncol.* 2008;26:3573–3581.
30. Cuffe S, Booth CM, Peng Y, et al. Adoption of adjuvant chemotherapy for non-small cell lung cancer in the elderly: A population-based outcomes study. *J Clin Oncol.* 2011;29(suppl), abstr 7012.
31. Gu F, Strauss GM, Wisnivesky, et al. *Platinum-based adjuvant chemotherapy in elderly patients with non-small cell lung cancer in the SEER-Medicare database: Comparison between carboplatin and cisplatin-based regimens.* Abstract presented at: the American Society of Clinical Oncology; June 2–4, 2011, Chicago, IL .
32. Olaussen KA, Dunant A, Fouret P, et al. 2006. DNA repair by ERCC1 in non-small-cell lung cancer and cisplatin-based adjuvant chemotherapy. *N Engl J Med.* 2006;355:983–91.
33. Sandler A, Gray R, Perry MC, et al. Paclitaxel-Carboplatin alone or with bevacizumab for non-small cell lung cancer. *NEJM.* 2006;355: 2542–2550.
34. Reck M, von Pawal J, Zatloukal P, et al. Overall survival with cisplatin-gemcitabine and bevacizumab or placebo as first-line therapy for non-squamous non-small cell lung cancer: Results from a randomized phase III trial (AVAiL). *Ann Oncol.* 2010;21:1804–1809.

Advancements in Radiotherapy for Lung Cancer

Neha P. Amin, David Raben, and Laurie E. Gaspar*

Department of Radiation Oncology, University of Colorado, Aurora, CO

ABSTRACT

Lung cancer remains the leading cause of cancer death for both men and women in the United States. Advancements in technology have enabled radiation oncologists to achieve highly conformal treatment plans that allow for safer dose escalation while sparing greater amounts of critical organs within the thorax. Positron emission tomography–computed tomography (CT) and four-dimensional CT are now incorporated into the planning armamentarium in an effort to better delineate tumor volume and take into consideration the movement of cancers in the various planes during radiation treatments. Advancements in treatment planning, delivery, and patient immobilization have contributed greatly to our recent ability to safely and effectively treat early-stage non-small cell lung cancer (NSCLC) with short course, high-intensity stereotactic body radiation therapy. The goals of therapy have remained constant over the years: improve patient outcomes while minimizing side effects from radiation therapy. Overall survival (OS) rates still remain disappointing for locally advanced NSCLC and small cell lung cancer (SCLC) patients. Over the past several decades, randomized trials within the United States and Europe have explored important questions designed to improve locoregional control and OS including evaluation of concurrent or induction chemoradiation, dose escalation, and targeted high-dose stereotactic radiation for NSCLC; accelerated versus conventional fractionated radiation for SCLC as well as the role of consolidative radiation in this disease.

Keywords: lung, NSCLC, SCLC, SBRT, IMRT, 4D-CT

*Corresponding author, Department of Radiation Oncology, University of Colorado, MS F-706, 1665 Aurora CT, STE 1032, Aurora, CO 80045

E-mail address: Laurie.Gaspar@ucdenver.edu

Emerging Cancer Therapeutics 3:1 (2012) 141–166.

DOI: 10.5003/2151–4194.3.1.141

demosmedpub.com/ecat

■ INTRODUCTION

Lung cancer is the leading cause of cancer death in the United States and in men worldwide (1,2). To reduce the incidence of this disease, great effort has been put forth by governments and cancer societies to educate the general public about environmental factors that increase an individual's risk of developing lung cancer, which primarily include smoking and second-hand smoke exposure, and, to a lesser extent, exposure to radon gas and asbestos (3–6). Despite these efforts, the United States population will have an estimated 221,130 new cases of lung cancer and 156,940 estimated deaths from lung cancer in 2011 (7). Global estimates from 2008 reported 1,608,800 new cases and 1,378,400 deaths from lung cancer (2).

Surgery, chemotherapy, and radiation therapy all play a role in the curative treatment or palliation of both non-small cell lung cancer (NSCLC) and small cell lung cancer (SCLC). This chapter highlights some of the more recent studies in lung cancer and advancements in the technical aspects of radiation therapy to the lung. Included in this discussion will be reflections on the recent advancements in technological innovations and treatment-planning systems that have allowed for delivery of highly conformal radiation therapy (CRT) plans with reduced treatment times and greater sparing of organs such as the esophagus, lungs, and heart.

■ TECHNICAL ASPECTS OF RADIATION THERAPY FOR LUNG CANCER

There have been advancements in radiation planning and delivery that have been applied to both conventional radiotherapy (RT) and stereotactic body radiation therapy (SBRT) used to treat NSCLC and SCLC patients.

In particular, SBRT has become more popular in the past decade. SBRT is a form of external beam radiation therapy that uses multiple highly focused radiation beams to deliver large doses of radiation in one to five treatments to extracranial tumors (8). Techniques for SBRT in the liver and lungs were pioneered at the Swedish Karolinska University hospital in the early 1990s (9) around the same time Japan was developing a method for lung SBRT which was clinically introduced in the mid-1990s. The biggest surge in adopting SBRT techniques in the United States began around 2008, with lung being the most common disease site treated with SBRT (10). Practice guidelines have been published pertaining to the conduct and technical requirements of SBRT (11). A recent survey of SBRT use in the United States revealed that the lung was the most common disease site treated with SBRT, and most physicians use a three-fraction regimen, with either 20 or 18 Gy per fraction, for peripheral lung lesions (10). As compared with conventional radiation for early-stage inoperable NSCLC patients, this approach has shown improved local control as well as significantly reducing overall treatment times with acceptable acute and late morbidities (12). The usage of SBRT will likely continue to grow in the upcoming years.

The technologic advancements that have made SBRT a possibility, and have also been applied when delivering conventional radiation treatment schedules (1.8–2 Gy per fraction), will be discussed in detail below as they have addressed three major reasons thought to contribute to local failure after radiation: geographic misses due to respiratory motion during treatment delivery, inadequacy and inaccuracy of radiologic scans for cancer staging and RT planning, and the inability to delivery adequate dose or escalate dose due to normal tissue complications.

Treatment Planning

Simulation: Two-Dimensional to Three-Dimensional to Four-Dimensional

The radiation treatment process begins with a simulation where images of the patient in a reproducible treatment position are obtained and used for planning. There has been a natural progression of simulation for radiation planning from two-dimensional (2D) to three-dimensional (3D) computed tomography (CT) to four-dimensional (4D) CT planning. When the 2D plain films were used from the 1980s to the mid-1990s, simple anterior–posterior/posterior–anterior beam arrangements were used with 2 to 3 cm margins around the gross tumor volume (GTV) to create the planning target volume (PTV) (13). Due to these generous margins and volumes, and limited beam arrangements, it was difficult to escalate the radiation dose to the tumor without increasing dose to normal tissues, thus increasing the chances of normal tissue complications (14). With the transition to 3D-CT-planning in the mid-1990, it was possible for more accurate localization of both the tumor and normal structures and an accurate body contour. This allowed for increased dose to the tumor while either maintaining or decreasing dose to normal structures, since an increased number of non-coplanar beams could be used for more conformal treatments. The CT also allowed for inhomogeneity corrections to achieve improved dosimetric accuracy. When 2D thorax radiation plans were compared with 3D plans, the 2D proposed treatment volumes had to be adjusted in about 30% of cases due to inadequate tumor coverage or to reduce the tumor volume after CT visualization (15). The use of 3D planning is currently the minimum standard of care (16).

While 3D-CT scans allowed for better delineation of the tumor volumes than 2D, they lacked the ability to incorporate the motion of the tumor obtained in 4D scans, which in some cases may have led to inadequate tumor coverage (17). 4D-CTs enable the respiratory-induced movement of the tumor and lymph nodes to be incorporated into treatment volumes to decrease geographic miss (18). Prior to 4D-CTs, fluoroscopy and slow CT scans had been used to try to capture the tumor movement during the radiation treatment. Fluoroscopy had been used widely but lung tumors were poorly visualized, and the mobility could not be accurately translated to the margins used in the planning CT scans (19). Slow CT scans (4 seconds per slice) also allowed for the intrafractional motion of the tumor to be captured (20,21).

4D-CT scans became commercially available in the mid-2000s and are being used more frequently for conventional RT and SBRT planning in lung cancer. When using the 4D-CT, one full respiratory cycle is captured and the respiratory waveform is recorded. The patient's anatomy at each specific phase of the respiratory cycle can be used to create multiple 3D sets that can be displayed in movie loops to visualize motion of the tumor, lymph nodes, and normal organs during a breathing cycle (22). One of the potential downsides to using 4D-CT scans to account for breathing-related tumor movement is that it could lead to an enlarged PTV which could increase chances of radiation pneumonitis, esophagitis, or chest wall pain depending on where the lesion is located (23). Abdominal compression plates (ACP) and respiratory-gating techniques have been used to limit the diaphragmatic movement with the goal of decreasing target volumes. These topics will be discussed below in more detail.

Lung tumors and mediastinal lymph nodes are both subject to respiratory-related movement, but there is no correlation of their respective amount of motion to each other. The majority of displacement occurs near the diaphragm (24,25). Maxim et al. evaluated 20 patients with lung tumors in various locations within the lung and described the motion of these tumors during normal breathing. No breathing coaching or abdominal compression was used to limit diaphragm movement. All of the tumors had the greatest displacement in the superior–inferior (SI) direction (compared with anterior–posterior and right–left directions), with tumors in the upper thorax moving less than those in the lower thorax. Surprisingly, centrally located tumors near the carina and hilum had more movement than initially expected. The mean and range SI movements included: carina 6.9 mm [3–19 mm], left hilum 5.7 mm (2.4–14.8 mm), right hilum 6.6 mm (2–13.2 mm), upper lung 3.7 mm (0.5–6.5 mm), and lower lung 10.4 (4.9–23 mm).

It can be assumed that tumors adjacent to the diaphragm would move the most, since this study reported SI displacements of the left and right diaphragms to be 20 mm (8.8–47.4 mm) and 16.9 mm (2.9–47.5 mm), respectively (26). The motion of mediastinal lymph nodes is also greatest in the lower mediastinum due to the diaphragmatic contraction and relaxation. An analysis of 100 mediastinal lymph nodes on 4D scan revealed the average nodal motion during quiet breathing was 0.68 cm (range, 0.17–1.64 cm), 77% moved greater than 0.5 cm, and 10% moved greater than 1.0 cm (27). Therefore, it is important to incorporate the movement of target lesions during radiation planning to decrease changes of underdosing the lesion.

Lung Motion Control

In addition to patient immobilization with a wing board, t-bar, alpha-cradle or its equivalent, it is also important to try to reduce the motion of the lung. Lung motion can compromise treatment outcomes due to either inadequate tumor coverage or by increasing the normal tissue complication rates when larger margins are needed. Abdominal compression and breath holding can be used starting at the time of simulation to help minimize target volumes, and then continued usage during treatment delivery to replicate the reduced tumor motion obtained at simulation. Respiratory gating and real-time tumor tracking (RTRT) can be used during treatment delivery and will be discussed later. In the United States, about 55% of physicians use abdominal compression or respiratory gating, while only about 15% use breath-hold techniques or RTRT (10). All of these techniques have been used to try to overcome the issue of lung motion during treatment delivery.

Abdominal Compression

Breathing-induced motion of the tumor can be reduced by applying external pressure near the diaphragm to decrease the diaphragm's motion. ACP are often placed 3 to 4 cm below the costal margin of the ribs and inferior to the xiphoid process. The force of the ACP can be measured and adjusted. Heinzerling et al. (28) reported on 10 patients, of which 4 patients had lower lobe lung tumors and 6 had liver tumors, and he observed that the mean SI movement without abdominal compression of 12 mm was reduced to 7.5 and 6.1 mm with medium and high levels of compression, respectively. This study did not observe the extent of tumor movement that has been previously reported (26); however, it did show the benefit of abdominal compression. Since the amount of pressure placed on the abdominal compression affects tumor movements, and the location of the tumor may dictate the amount of movement with or without abdominal compression, an individualized examination of the benefit of compression on patients should be performed.

Other variations of immobilization devices that apply abdominal compression include the BodyFIX® system, Elekta Stereotactic Body Frame® system (Elekta, Norcross, GA), or the Couch Integrated Immobilization System (Indiana University, Department of Radiation Oncology, Indianapolis, IN). Some potential disadvantages of abdominal compression include patient discomfort and difficulty with reproducing the setup (28).

Breathing Control

Active breathing control or other breath-hold techniques have been used to try to minimize the effects of breathing motion by trying to achieve the same breath-hold position during treatment delivery (29–31). Breath-hold techniques have been shown to improve the therapeutic ratio by allowing for decreased radiation to the volume of normal lung surrounding the tumor (32,33). A breath-hold can either be voluntary or assisted with an occlusion valve, and most methods use a spirometer to measure airflow. After monitoring several cycles of normal breathing, a reproducible baseline, usually at end exhalation, is established so that one can monitor if reproducible breath holds are achieved. Another variation of breath hold includes deep inspiration breath hold (34,35). These methods necessitate patient coaching prior to its use. The provider must consider patient comfort, cooperation, and the ability to reproduce the breath hold, especially in patients with compromised respiratory status (35,36).

Target Delineation

Being able to correctly define the tumor for treatment planning is important for treatment outcomes and for minimizing normal tissue complications. Target location and accounting for respiratory-induced target motion are especially crucial in SBRT accuracy due to the high dose per fraction delivered (37). It may be difficult to differentiate the tumor from atelectasis, effusions, or to identify the active components of the disease on a CT scan. However, the use of maximum intensity projection (MIP) scans, intravenous (IV) contrast, barium contrast, and positron emission tomography/CT (PET/CT) scans may help to better identify the normal structures and target volume.

Target Definitions

The following volumes are often drawn on planning CT scans during radiation planning. The GTV outlines the visible disease. The clinical target volume (CTV) incorporates microscopic disease. The internal target volume (ITV) is the volume that incorporates both the GTV/CTV and the internal margin (IM). The IM includes internal variations due to physiologic changes, like movements due to respiration. The PTV includes margins needed for anticipated setup error or patient movement during therapy.

When planning for SBRT, the GTV or ITV should be contoured using lung windows and IV contrast should be used for central lesions. The CTV is identical to the GTV for SBRT planning (38). The microscopic disease is assumed to be well covered by the surrounding penumbra dose. For example, if 54 to 60 Gy in three fractions is prescribed to the GTV, the dose falloff delivers 40 to 45 Gy to area 6 to 8 mm from GTV, which is sufficient to cover the usual extent of microscopic disease. The only difference in volumes when planning for conventional radiation treatments is that the CTV is created by volumetrically expanding the GTV or ITV by 0.5 to 1 cm.

Margins placed on the GTV or CTV to create the PTV or ITV during SBRT and conventional treatments should reflect the estimated tumor motion and setup error depending on the devices used to limit tumor and patient motion during treatment. If helical scanning with abdominal compression is used, a 0.5-cm axial and 1.0-cm craniocaudal margin should be added to the GTV to create the PTV. If a 4D-CT scan with compression is used, the ITV can be contoured on the MIP and expanded uniformly 5 mm to create the PTV.

Maximum Intensity Projection

If a 4D-CT is being used for the CT simulation, the MIP scan is a reliable clinical tool to delineate the ITV. The MIP scan combines the voxels with maximum intensity from each phase of the breathing scan, therefore capturing the motion of the tumor throughout the breathing cycle and delineating the ITV. The MIP is ideal when contouring parenchymal lesions, since these lung tumors often surrounded by normal lung and therefore will have the maximum intensity voxel. The MIP is more difficult to use and less useful when trying to distinguish a target volume near a normal structure of equal or greater density; for example, a tumor that is adherent to the diaphragm. MIP has been shown to be superior to averaged intensity 4D-CT and to 3D helical images when delineating the extent of tumor motion from breathing during SBRT (39). The ratio between ITVs generated from all 10 phases and those from MIP scans is about 1.04 (40). This ITV needs to be copied to the free-breathing scan for treatment planning, since MIP scans do not have the correct lung or electron densities needed for planning. The ITV may also need to be expanded after it is copied to the free-breathing scan if the free-breathing tumor movements exceed the ITV contours created using the MIP.

Intravenous Contrast

Multidetector CT scans of the thorax now allow for acquisition of large numbers of thin (3–5 mm) contiguous images that provide more detailed images than those provided by older CT technology that used nonhelical or single helical scanning, and thick slices of about 10 mm. However, assessment of the abnormal mediastinal and hilar lymph nodes continues to be a challenging aspect of thoracic imaging. Previous studies have analyzed if intravenous (IV) contrast administration prior to CT scans aids in assessing nodal stage and found that the contrast did not significantly aid in detecting mediastinal nodes; however, it was beneficial for detecting hilar nodes (41–43). In general, the mediastinal lymph nodes are more detectable than hilar nodes without contrast because they are surrounded by fatty tissue. The hilar nodes are near hilar vessels and lymphatic tissue with little fat between them, making them more difficult to detect without the aid of contrast (44). IV contrast may also be beneficial for centrally located tumor contiguous with vessels with the same density. Tumors surrounded by lung parenchyma can easily be detected without IV contrast.

While IV contrast can be beneficial in RT planning, it is not always necessary. It is likely that a lung cancer patient would have already had a staging diagnostic CT scan with IV contrast to identify abnormal lymph nodes. This patient may have also had a mediastinoscopy to obtain pathologic staging. It would be possible to fuse the IV contrast diagnostic scan or the PET/CT to the planning CT scan, especially if that patient has a contraindication for IV contrast. Therefore, it is not essential to administer IV contrast at the time of simulation unless the patient had pathologically enlarged hilar nodes.

If IV contrast is necessary for RT planning, it is important to get both a scan with and without IV contrast. The radiation planning will take place on the noncontrast scan, so that the changes in densities from the IV contrast will not affect the dose distributions.

Barium Oral Contrast

The use of esophageal oral contrast can help to identify the esophagus; however, oral contrast is not always necessary unless there is gross tumor surrounding the esophagus. The esophagus is sometimes difficult to track if there is no air in it. The esophagus can also move with normal breathing. Since the contrast could affect the dose computation due to its higher density, the esophagus with contrast should be assigned the density of soft tissue, so that it does not interfere the dose distribution. The ability to better define the esophagus may not result in less toxicity since it may be surrounded by involved lymph nodes, but does allow for overall improved accuracy of defining organs at risk (OAR) and being able to calculate a more accurate dose–volume histogram (45).

Positron Emission Tomography

Fluorodeoxyglucose (FDG) PET–CT scans can aid in delineating tumor volumes that can help to decrease geographic misses while also reducing RT volumes. PET reduces GTV volumes by enabling the differentiation between tumor and collapsed lung (or atelectasis) and identifying involved lymph node stations (46–49). These decreased target volumes enable dose escalation (48,50) and reduction of dose to normal structures (51).

Sensitivity and Specificity of PET

Many studies have evaluated the sensitivity and specificity of FDG PET scans for indeterminate lung lesions and mediastinal lymph node staging (52,53). In the evaluation of indeterminate lung lesions, the sensitivity and specificity range from 79% to 96% and from 40% to 83%, respectively (52). The specificity is often reduced in areas of inflammation.

Mediastinal staging and accurate identification of nodal metastases are clinically relevant for planning radiation in NSCLC patients since routine elective nodal irradiation (ENI) is no longer recommended in NSCLC (16). A CT scan offers a sensitivity and specificity of 56% and 81%, respectively. The current gold standard mediastinoscopy has a specificity of 100%, but a lower sensitivity of 78% for all stages, 82% when the CT scan shows enlarged lymph nodes, and 42% for normal-sized lymph nodes. PET has a well-established role in mediastinal lymph node staging: sensitivity and specificity are 83% and 89% for all stages, 91% and 70% when the CT scan shows enlarged lymph nodes, and 70% and 94% for normal-sized lymph nodes. Despite PET/CT scans reported high sensitivity rates, the mediastinoscopy remains the gold standard and the addition of endosonography can further improve sensitivity for mediastinal nodal metastases (54). Of note, chemotherapy can markedly reduce the accuracy of PET scans (55). The main clinical advantage of using PET is that it has a very high negative predictive value (>90%) for the detection of mediastinal lymph nodes.

Outcomes Using PET-Defined Volumes

There have not been any randomized studies that show that patient outcomes are better when using FDG PET-defined volumes; however, the outcomes have shown good local control. PET-based selective irradiation of involved lymph nodes in NSCLC patients has resulted in isolated nodal failures (INF) in less than 5% of patients (50,56). Fleckenstein et al. (57) reported on a prospective pilot trial on NSCLC patients that confined the target volume to only PET-positive areas using an autocontour-derived technique. Elective nodal stations were not irradiated. Patients were treated with concurrent chemoradiation therapy. This method allowed dose escalation in almost half of the treated patients, was associated with a low risk of isolated nodal recurrences (INR), and yielded favorable results with respect to survival and locoregional tumor control. Similarly, in a prospective trial of 60 patients with limited stage SCLC (LS-SCLC), selective nodal irradiation based on PET scans resulted in a low rate of INR of 3% versus a higher rate of INR of 11% when CT-based selective nodal irradiation was used (58).

Weaknesses of PET

Some weaknesses of using FDG PET images include the fact that the acquisition of the image is not respiration-gated, and the current 4 to 6-mm spatial resolution of PET scans is much lower than the 1-mm resolution that modern CT scanners can obtain (59,60). There are also variations in scanning protocols, patient position, immobilization devices, image reconstruction, and data analysis software that need standardization to compare between patients. One way to improve the fusion of the PET scan and planning CT is to obtain the PET scan in the treatment position, including immobilization device and a flat top table (61,62). A respiratory-gated PET combined with 4D-CT may reduce the blurring from free-breathing images, better define the extent of moving tumors, and improve radiation treatment planning for lung tumors (63).

FDG PET-Based Adaptive Radiation Therapy

FDG PET-based adaptive radiation therapy (ART) may help to further customize treatments to allow for tumor escalation and reduced NTCP. Additionally, it may be possible to align the distribution of PET activity within a tumor to the distribution of radiation doses within the tumor, that is, pushing hot spots or adding boosts to areas of higher standard uptake value (SUV) (52). PET is more sensitive in assessing therapeutic response than CT alone, and the metabolic activity of a tumor has been seen to change after 40 to 50 Gy (64). This response to treatment can be incorporated into ART if a mid-RT PET volume is used to adjust a plan midtreatment course. Patient outcomes after ART are currently being evaluated (65). The Radiation Therapy Oncology Group (RTOG) is planning a study that is assessing the value of ART based on an FDG PET scan done after 4 to 5 weeks of concurrent chemoradiation therapy for Stage III NSCLC.

Dosimetry

Inhomogeneity Correction

During radiation therapy to a lung lesion, the beam must transverse multiple tissues with varying densities, including fat, bone, muscle, and lung. These tissue inhomogeneities change the amount of radiation delivered to the target volume and normal tissues due to differences in the absorption of the primary beam, scatter of the photons, and the secondary electron fluence. The lower density of lung compared with other tissues causes higher dose within and beyond the lung (66). Radiation treatment planning to the lung requires tissue heterogeneity corrections for accurate dose computation for both conventional treatment (67,68) and SBRT (69). Accurate dose calculations are necessary to prevent large discrepancies between planned and actually delivered doses to individual patients.

The extent of the deviation of calculated dose depends on the algorithms and irradiation techniques investigated. The calculated differences in tumor dose with and without heterogeneity corrections range between 5% and 10% in both SBRT and conventionally fractionated treatment plans (69–73). Monte Carlo simulations are considered to be the gold standard in the presence of inhomogeneities (74). However, the collapsed cone algorithm, a type of convolution/superposition-based algorithm, has an accuracy of 2% to 5% and can be considered as a reasonably accurate representation of the actual dose given to the patient (75,76). Many past lung protocols did not require lung corrections in the dose prescription; however, current cooperative group lung protocols do require inhomogeneity corrections.

3D-Conformal Versus IMRT

3D-CRT and intensity-modulated radiotherapy (IMRT) are two techniques used in planning radiation therapy. IMRT uses inverse-planning to provide more conformal plans than 3D-CRT which could allow for about 10% to 15% dose escalation to the target volume while minimizing dose to the surrounding normal tissues, like lung and spinal cord (77–79). A nine-, seven- and five-field IMRT plan improved the therapeutic ratio of the PTV coverage to the lung V20 when compared with a three-field 3D conformal plan; however, this benefit was reduced when using five-field 3D conformal plans (77).

IMRT plans require more resources than 3D and should be viewed with some caution. The steeper dose gradient around the target volume in IMRT plans could result in higher chances of geometric miss, especially with the component of lung motion. IMRT should not be used when the target motion exceeds 1 cm. There is also more normal tissue receiving a lower radiation dose, which could contribute to toxicities, especially in the setting of concurrent chemoradiation (80). With an appropriate margin to account for lung motion and setup error, IMRT plans are equivalent to 3D plans in terms of tumor coverage and outcomes (81,82). IMRT requires increased time and effort in planning, quality assurance checks, and to a lesser extent time and resources on the machine. When a 3D plan cannot provide an acceptable plan in terms of dose to PTV or excessive radiation to normal tissues, then a five- to seven-field IMRT plan may offer a balance between a more conformal plan that also allows for practical plan delivery.

Commercial treatment-planning systems that are used for conventional RT planning are also used for SBRT planning. IMRT or 3D-conformal planning can be used. SBRT plans use about 10 to 12 nonopposing highly collimated beams or rotational arcs to produce a plan that has rapid dose falloff in all directions from the target (83–85). Multileaf collimators help to shape the beams and are preferred over customized blocks due to the ability to rapidly and accurately transfer treatment fields from the planning computer to the treatment machine, quicker treatment delivery, and superior geometric accuracy over alloy-blocked fields (86,87). The beam angles may be limited by potential collisions between the accelerator head and the patient or couch. Accurate beam modeling, including profiles and depth doses, is important for the smaller field sizes used in SBRT. Treatments should be planned as if to be delivered in less than 30 minutes to reduce patient motion during the lengthy time on the treatment table.

Protons

Proton therapy is an old modality that has been used more recently for the treatment of lung cancer patients. Compared with IMRT, protons may allow further dose escalation, and reduce dose to normal tissues. The same concerns in IMRT plans about tumor motion apply when using protons; however, while IMRT only treats a portion of the target volume at a particular time, the proton beam treats the entire volume. Also, protons deliver less integral dose to the patient, meaning that there is a smaller volume of normal tissues receiving low-dose radiation as compared with IMRT plans (88).

In summary, the use of IMRT and protons may reduce the volume of irradiated lung but may be of minimal benefit unless a patient has a very large tumor for which a 3D plan cannot meet the prescription dose to the PTV or stay under the dose constraints for OAR.

Treatment Delivery

As the planning software has developed to allow for more sophisticated plans, radiation treatment machines have also advanced to be able in deliver these sophisticated plans in a timely and precise manner. Both respiratory-gating and image-guidance capabilities on the machines help to improve accuracy of radiation treatments to allow for more conformal plans while minimizing radiation to normal tissues. Volumetric-modulated arc therapy (VMAT) has also recently emerged allowing for reduction in the time needed to deliver sophisticated RT plans.

Respiratory-Gated Radiation Therapy

In respiratory-gated treatment, the delivery of radiation only occurs during certain time intervals that are synchronous with the patient's respiratory cycle. This "duty-cycle" or "gated-treatment" is often near end expiration. End expiration is a more reproducible anatomic position than end inspiration since it is a passive action resulting from the relaxation of inspiratory muscles, while end inspiration could vary based on the patient's effort. Since the beam delivery time is inversely proportional to the duty cycle, the choice of gate width is usually between 20% and 40% of the tidal volume (with 0% being end expiration) (89). This allows for reduced tumor motion while treatments can be completed in a reasonable amount of time. During respiratory gating, it has been found that breath-hold technique may be more difficult for some patients, but when compared with using a free-breathing technique, it is more reproducible, there is less movement of lungs, and it is more efficient during CT simulation and treatment delivery (30).

Respiratory gating systems include both internal gating and external gating systems based on the location of the surrogates used to generate the gating signals. Internal gating uses implanted fiducial markers in the tumor as the surrogates for RTRT. External gating uses markers on the surface of the patient's abdomen, so that the abdominal surface motion is the surrogate signal for the lung movement. This is the system used by most gated therapy treatments like the Varian Real-Time Position Management™ system. Since the relationship between the tumor motion and the surrogate external signal from abdominal movement may be inconsistent both inter- and intrafractionally, it is important that the appropriate quality assurance checks are performed to ensure a clinically acceptable accuracy (37). In the United States, only about 30% of physicians used internal fiducial markers, and mostly in the private practice setting (10).

Respiratory gating has been shown to add an additional layer of improvement in reducing the PTV needed to cover the target volume. Underberg et al. (90) retrospectively evaluated 15 patients with Stage III lung cancer to assess the reduction in PTV, mean lung dose (MLD), and lung V20 when using a 4D-CT scan and respiratory gating to plan and deliver radiation. The PTV using a 4D scan was significantly reduced from a conventional PTV created using 1.5 to 2 cm margins; the PTV was further reduced when using a gating window of treatment. Overall, the use of a PTV created with both 4D and gating allowed for a statistically significant mean absolute reduction in MLD and V20 of 2.8 Gy (relative 14.2%) and 4.6% (relative 16.2%) respectively. Similarly, Underberg et al. (91) studied the differences in PTV when planning for SBRT in Stage I lung cancer patients and observed that PTV was reduced by approximately 50% when using an ITV created from the GTV contoured from 10 phases of the respiratory cycle + 3 mm margin compared with using the GTV from the mid-three phases of the respiratory cycle + 1 cm margin. This PTV was further reduced by approximately 70% when gating was used to create a PTV with a duty cycle of 20% to 40% of respiration. In summary, respiratory gating does allow for reduced volume of PTV needed for tumor coverage; however, treatments can be prolonged and patients may not tolerate the gating.

Image-Guided Radiation Therapy

The availability of on-board imaging has allowed for image-guided radiation therapy (IGRT), which allows for daily image guidance to more accurately position the target volume. IGRT may result in less chance of target miss, smaller setup margins, less normal tissue exposed to high-radiation doses, and the possibility for adapting plans based on the changes in a patient's anatomy and organ motion during and/or between (intra- and/or inter-) treatment fractions (92). Some form of geometric verification should especially be used prior to each SBRT treatment since misalignment of just one high-dose fraction can lead to geographic miss, resulting in decreased tumor control and increased normal tissue complication probabilities.

Many treatment machines have on-board imaging capabilities with either kilovoltage- or megavoltage (MV) based imaging. Although there has been concern raised regarding the image quality from MVCT, there are studies indicating that it is adequate for IGRT of lung targets. The preferred method is to use an in-room CT scan prior to each treatment, like a cone-beam CT scan, to obtain volumetric data on the target. Other less favorable options include portal films compared with the digitally reconstructed radiograph or electronic portal imaging devices (EPID). The majority of physicians use in-room volumetric imaging, followed by in-room planar imaging, for target localization (93,94).

An additional aspect to IGRT that is more experimental at the moment and not widely used in clinical practice includes the capability to create 3D "volumetric" imaging that provides complete volumetric and anatomic information based on the daily treatment room coordinates. This scan can then reconstruct dose distributions based on the planning CT scan. This capability could allow for image-guided ART where the treating physician could modify treatment parameters according to changes in the patient's anatomy before each treatment or at specific time points during the course of RT (95,96).

Volumetric-Modulated Arc Therapy

VMAT is a new method of operating the linear accelerator that can deliver highly conformal dose distributions similar to those created by other forms of IMRT; however, VMAT provides the widest range of beam orientations and can deliver sophisticated RT plans in the shortest time possible (97). VMAT is able to achieve these goals using one or more gantry arcs with a continuously varying beam aperture, gantry rotation speed, and dose rate (98). At the moment, VMAT plans have their greatest margin of benefit in SBRT delivery due to the ability to shorten treatment time during high-dose fractions. Figure 1 displays a VMAT plan used to deliver an SBRT treatment to a patient with a centrally located tumor. VMAT allowed for the dose to be reduced to the nearby trachea and esophagus. Less time on the table is more comfortable to patients and may reduce patient movement during treatments.

■ NON-SMALL CELL LUNG CANCER

Radiation therapy has an established role in both locally advanced and medically inoperable early-stage NSCLC lung cancer. Technical

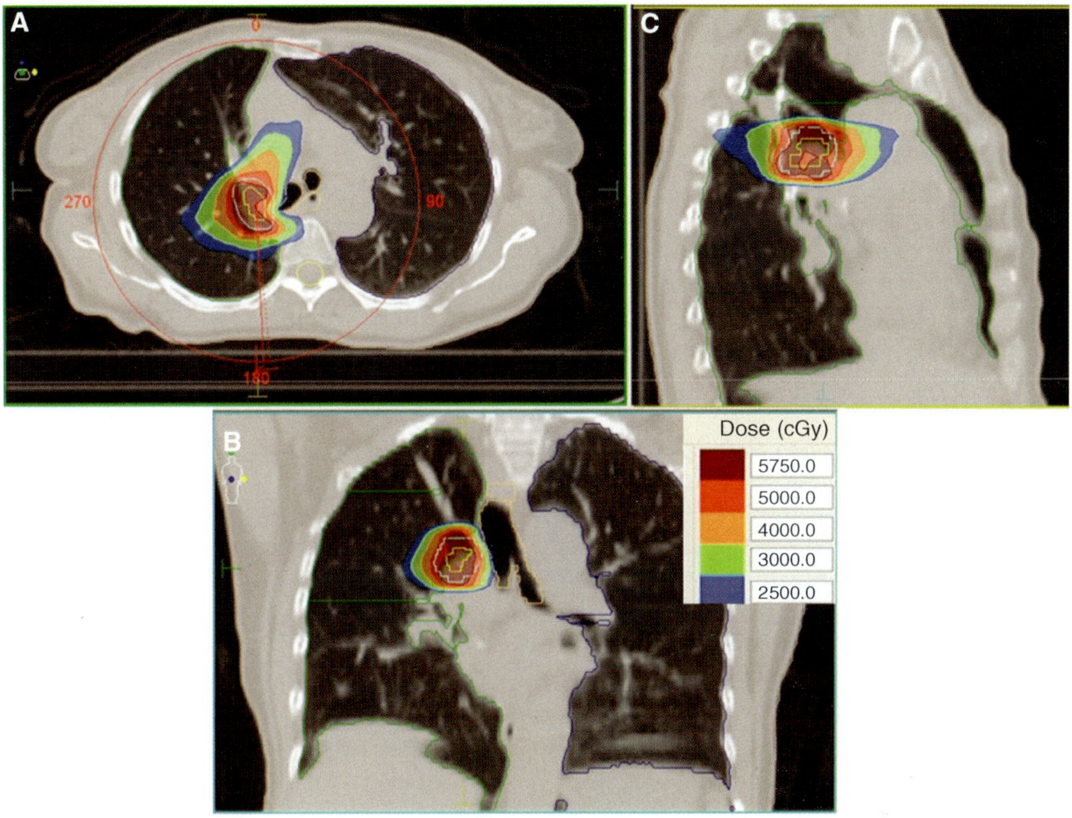

FIGURE 1
Radiation plan for a patient with a right hilar lesion in the (A) axial, (B) coronal, and (C) sagittal planes. The internal target volume (yellow) was expanded 5 mm radially and 7 mm in the superior–inferior direction to create the planning target volume (PTV) (white). A 360 degree VMAT arc was used for treatment delivery. The PTV was treated to 50 Gy in 5 fractions. The max dose to the PTV = 67.74 Gy, and 95.3% of the PTV received 50 Gy. Delivery time for each fraction was 10.8 minutes. The lung (total lung minus ITV) V20 = 2.32% and V10 = 10%. The trachea V18 = 12%. The esophagus mean dose = 8.3% and V30 = 0.07%.

advancements have permitted an increased therapeutic ratio, that is, increased dose to the tumor and reduced dose to normal tissues. Controversies still remain in regards to optimal primary target volumes, elective nodal coverage, and the benefit of dose escalation.

Early-Stage NSCLC

The treatment of choice for medically operable Stage I (T1–2, N0) NSCLC patients has traditionally been surgical resection, which results in high local control and 5-year OS rates ranging from 60% to 70% (99,100). However, there is a cohort of patients who are medically inoperable secondary to comorbidities whose options in the past were limited to either no treatment or conventional radiation therapy. Patients who do not receive any therapy for their early-stage lung cancer have a very low 5-year OS rate ranging from about 0% to 20%, and over 50% of them die from their lung cancer (99,101). Conventional radiation to 45 to 66 Gy in 1.8 to 2.0 Gy per fraction offer only minimal improvement with reported 5-year OS rates ranging from 10% to 30% (102–104). Recent technical and imaging advancements have allowed us to steer a different course—that of SBRT to the primary parenchymal lesion. Since elective nodal failure rates are low in early-stage lung cancer, involved field-only radiation therapy is routine (105). SBRT is a newer option that shows very promising results within single- and multi-institutional trials to observation and conventional therapy.

Stereotactic Body Radiation Therapy

SBRT has been accepted as first-line therapy for medically inoperable early-stage NSCLC patients; however, the optimal dose fractionation is still in debate (10,12). The recently reported RTOG 0236 trial was the first North American multicenter, cooperative group study to test SBRT in treating medically inoperable patients with early-stage NSCLC (12). The results revealed that SBRT, delivered in three fractions to a corrected dose of 54 Gy, was safe for peripheral tumors and provided excellent 3-year local control and OS rates of about 98% and 56%, respectively (12). Nagata et al. (106) also reported excellent local control rates of 100% on early-stage NSCLC patients using a dose fractionation of 48 Gy in four fractions. RTOG 0915 (107) is a Phase II trial that accrued 88 medically inoperable patients, with peripheral T1–2N0 tumors, who were randomized to 34 Gy/1 fraction versus 48 Gy/4 fractions. This trial closed in March 2011 with the primary objective to evaluate Grade 3 or higher toxicities at 1 year and secondary objectives of local control and OS. The arm that is found to be superior from this study will likely be compared with the standard 54 Gy/3 fractions regimen established by RTOG 0236. These studies will all help to establish safe and effective treatment regimens when using SBRT to treat early-stage lung cancer.

There have been acceptable levels of toxicity from SBRT thus far. Most of the complications are less than Grade 2 according to National Cancer Institute common terminology criteria. In RTOG 0236, Grade 3 and 4 pulmonary adverse events were observed in eight (14.5%) and one (2%) patient, respectively. Ideally, the amount of total lung minus GTV/ITV that receives ≥20 Gy (V20) should remain below 10% to reduce changes of radiation pneumonitis (108–110). Rib fractures or chest wall pain is a possibility when treating tumors adjacent to the chest wall; however, this can be minimized by restricting the amount of volume of chest wall that receives 30 Gy to less than 30 cm^3 (111,112). Conservative treatments with antiinflammatory medications are effective in reducing chest wall pain. In RTOG 0236, only 5% of patients experienced Grade 3 musculoskeletal side effects. While RTOG 0236 did not observe any Grade 5 side effects, there have been a few serious Grade 5 complications reported from Japan, and these morbidities were often associated with interstitial pneumonitis (113). Other OAR include the spine and brachial plexus (114). It is important to try to minimize normal tissue complications by following dose constraints to normal tissues. As the experience with SBRT continues to mature, we will get a better understanding of late toxicities from this treatment regimen (115).

It is still unclear if SBRT's excellent local control rates translate into OS advantages over surgery in medically operable patients. The local control rates with SBRT appear comparable with local control rates reported when using surgery (116,117), RTOG 0618 is a Phase II trial, that is now closed, that treated 33 medically operable Stage I or II NSCLC patients with SBRT to 60 Gy in three fractions without heterogeneity corrections. The aim of this study is to determine whether SBRT achieves primary tumor control ≥90% at 2 years. JCOG 0403 is another closed Phase II study for T1N0M0 NSCLC patients, 65 operable and 100 inoperable, treated with 48 Gy/4 fractions. Patient accrual was completed in 2008, so the 3-year OS for the operable patients should be coming out shortly. The ongoing ACOSOG/RTOG 1021 (118) study is currently evaluating the 3-year OS rate in patients at high risk for surgery treated with sublobar resection versus SBRT. All of these studies will help to compare SBRT with surgery for early-stage NSCLC patients.

SBRT local control rates appear to be far superior to local control rates obtained when using conventional RT alone; however, it has not been directly compared (119). TROG 0902 is an ongoing Phase III trial comparing 3D-CRT with 60 to 66 Gy at 2 Gy per fraction versus SBRT 54 Gy in three fractions (18 Gy per fraction) in inoperable Stage I NSCLC patients. Similarly, the Scandinavian SPACE trial is a Phase II randomized trial of 3D-CRT 70 Gy in 35 fractions versus SBRT 45 Gy in three fractions. These trials will evaluate the safety and efficacy of SBRT compared with standard fractionation.

Most of the published reports and ongoing studies are in peripheral NSCLC but an active area of research, and the aim of RTOG 0813, will determine if SBRT can safely treat centrally located tumors, defined as located within a 2-cm radius around the main tracheo-bronchial tree. These centrally located tumors became a topic of concern after results from a single-institution Phase II study on early-stage inoperable NSCLC with 60 Gy in three fractions for T1 and 66 Gy in three fractions for T2 revealed that hilar or pericentral tumors had an 11-fold increased risk in Grade 3 to 5 adverse events and a 2-year freedom from severe adverse events of 54% compared with 83% of more peripheral tumors (120). RTOG 0813 has been designed to deliver SBRT in five fractions on alternating days over 1.5 to 2 weeks. The first cohort will receive 50 Gy in five fractions and will either escalate or reduce the dose by 0.5 Gy per fraction as dictated by resulting toxicities. Figure 1 is an example of an SBRT plan for a centrally located tumor. The highest dose fractionation will be 60 Gy at 12 Gy per fraction. The dose-limiting toxicity in this study is defined as any treatment-related Grade 3 or worse toxicity (per CTCAE, v. 4, MedDRA, v. 12.0), that occurs within 1 year from the start of SBRT including, but not limited to, pericarditis, pneumonitis, pulmonary hemorrhage, or fistula.

Locally Advanced NSCLC

The current accepted "standard of care" for patients with locally advanced, unresectable NSCLC is platin-based chemotherapy concurrent with thoracic radiation therapy (TRT) to 60 to 66 Gy at 2 Gy per fraction. Recent investigations have focused on trying to optimize radiation therapy by dose escalation to the tumor while minimizing the dose received by surrounding normal tissue. A movement away from elective nodal coverage and investigations in ART may help in achieving safe dose escalation.

Dose Escalation

For more than 30 years, the accepted standard radiation prescription dose for treating locally advanced NSCLC has been 60 to 66 Gy, as established by RTOG 73–01 (121). This was not enough dose to achieve acceptable local control; pathologic local–regional failure rates were shown to be as high as 80% when using posttherapy bronchoscopic biopsies (122). Thankfully, the actual clinically detected local failure rates were lower, but OS still remained low. This dose was established in an era where 2D planning was primarily used, lymph nodes were being treated prophylactically, and the resulting large volumes of normal tissue in the treatment field limited the safety of escalating dose. There have been many technologic advances since RTOG 73–01 that now allow for dose escalation, including 3D- and 4D-CT-based treatment planning, CRT, and PET, which better delineates gross disease.

One could hypothesize that increased radiation doses will kill more cancer cells, which may result in better local control and survival. Single-institution Phase I/II prospective studies from University of North Carolina (123), RTOG 0117 (124), and NCCTG 0028 (125) showed that dose escalation to 74 Gy could be given safely with concurrent chemotherapy. The results from RTOG 0117 revealed a 25.9-month median survival in patients receiving 74 Gy, which is much improved from the 17-month median survival reported in

RTOG 9410 (126) and other trials where patients received the standard 60 Gy dose (127,128). Unfortunately, this improvement in median survival could not be reproduced in the RTOG 0617 (129) study, a randomized Phase III study comparing 60 with 74 Gy. In June 2011, the 74 Gy dose escalation arm of the RTOG 0617 study was closed to accrual after an interim analysis revealed that 74 Gy did not result in an improved median survival compared with 60 Gy. Therefore, 60 Gy remains the standard RT dose with concurrent chemotherapy. It is unclear if this question of dose escalation will be studied again in the near future.

Elective Nodal Irradiation

Until recent years, ENI was standard treatment in North America. This was born out of studies such as RTOG 73–01 in which patients with radiographically negative lymph nodes had a higher survival rate if they had adequate coverage of the hilar and mediastinal lymph nodes, although the increased survival rate was not statistically significant (130). However, there has been a definite trend, particularly in NSCLC, to eliminate ENI. This is primarily due to the observed low rates of ENI INF.

Evidence from a number of studies suggests that there is only a low (<10%) chance of elective nodal failure when involved field radiation therapy (IFRT) volumes are used in Stage III NSCLC patients (131). RTOG 9311 (132) was the first cooperative group study to omit ENI in its prospective radiation dose escalation study for patients with Stages I to III NSCLC, and isolated elective nodal failures occurred in <8% of patients. A randomized trial from China of inoperable Stage III NSCLC patients compared IFRT versus ENI and found that only 7% of patients in the IFRT group developed elective nodal failures in untreated lymph nodes (133). It is likely that these low-elective nodal failure rates are due to the use of chemotherapy and incidental 40 to 50 Gy doses that cover the ipsilateral hilum, paratracheal, and subcarinal nodes, especially when the primary tumor is located adjacent to these areas. Also, these patients may die of other comorbidities, distant metastases, or local failures prior to clinical or radiographic evidence of elective nodal failure. The main advantage of omitting ENI is the reduction of radiation to normal tissue, particularly the lung. In the randomized trial from China (133), the rates of radiation pneumonitis for the ENI group compared with the IFRT were 39% and 17% ($P < .05$), respectively.

ENI has not been used in recent NSCLC dose escalation studies that use modern technology. Radiation planning for the lung has evolved from 2D- to 3D-CRT, and FDG PET scans are being increasingly relied upon to improve treatment accuracy (53). FDG PET scans have an 83% sensitivity, 89% specificity, and >90% negative predictive value for the detection of involved mediastinal lymph nodes (52). In the 2D treatment-planning era, 40 to 50 Gy was often delivered to the elective regional nodal areas followed by a cone-down boost of an additional 20 Gy to the primary tumor site (13). Elective nodal regions included the ipsilateral and contralateral, hilum, mediastinal, and supraclavicular areas. However, prophylactically irradiating clinically uninvolved nodal areas seemed unnecessary when the gross tumor was not controlled by the inability to dose escalate due to larger volumes when including ENI.

Adaptive Radiotherapy for NSCLC Lung Cancer

Another method that has been used to improve the therapeutic ratio is ART. The shape, size, and location of tumors and normal tissues can change during the standard 5 to 7 week radiation course used to treat NSCLC. For example, as patients respond to their NSCLC treatments, there can be changes in tumor size, which may allow for dose escalation. Additionally, some lung cancer patients also have fluctuating pleural effusions, atelectasis, and infections. For example, it is possible that the collapsed portions of the lungs may reexpand as the tumor responds. This reexpansion could affect the spatial relationship of the tumor to the normal lung, as well as the breathing-related movement of the tumor. Since these changes are impossible to predict for individual patients, imaging during the course of treatment can help determine if an adaptive RT plan could benefit the patient.

ART is generally most useful when tumors show an early response to treatment. NSCLC tumors have been observed to regress between 0.6% and 2.4% per day, as measured by EPID, or CT or PET–CT scans (65,134–137). Guckenberger et al. retrospectively analyzed 13 NSCLC patients who showed an average continuous tumor regression of 1.2% per day, which resulted in an average 49% ± 15% volume reduction of GTV after 6 weeks of treatment (138). Woodford et al. (139) analyzed GTV changes in 17 patients who received daily MVCT during 30 fractions of lung RT and found that while changes in GTV were difficult to predict based on the patient's initial tumor characteristics, that ART may be beneficial if the GTV decreased by more than 30% within the first 20 fractions of treatment. There is reportedly no difference in tumor regression when radiation therapy is used alone compared with when it is used concurrently with chemoradiation (137). Multiple adaptations of volumes during a treatment course may allow for dose escalation and lung sparing, but it would be time-consuming to perform. A single-plan adaptation after 3 weeks, a single-plan adaptation after 5 weeks, and a twice-plan adaptation after 3 and 5 weeks reduced the MLD by 5.0% ± 4.4%, 5.6% ± 2.9%, and 7.9% ± 4.8%, respectively. The amount of lung sparing with the twice ART allowed an iso-MLD escalation of the GTV dose from 66.8 ± 0.8 Gy to 73.6 ± 3.8 Gy.

In contrast to studies showing that ART may be beneficial for treating NSCLC tumors, other studies did not report that a reduction in tumor volume allowed for dose escalation. Gillham et al. (140) analyzed 10 NSCLC patients by performing a PET–CT prior to initiation of therapy, and again performed PET–CT after a dose of 50 Gy had been administered over 5 weeks. Despite a median PTV reduction of 20%, only 4 of 10 patients could safely be dose escalated to 78 Gy. This was mostly because the normal tissue had already received 50 Gy, therefore surpassing many dose thresholds for normal tissue toxicities. It is possible that if the PET–CT scan had been performed earlier, after the second or third week, there may have been greater success in adapting the RT plan to allow for dose escalation.

A careful analysis of the regression patterns of the tumor and surrounding lung is required before adaptive plan modifications can be safely applied, since microscopic disease may be undertreated otherwise. A reduction in GTV does not imply that the CTV, which incorporates areas of potential microscopic disease, will likewise be reduced. A tumor could either push normal tissue away or infiltrate into the surrounding tissue. For example, if a tumor is pushing on the lung, then the healthy lung tissue that is being pushed on will likely move in the same direction as the tumor when it regresses. Monitoring such movements of the surrounding healthy lung tissue would allow for a safe adaptive RT plan with reduction in target volumes, since the lung with potential microscopic spread would remain within the target volume. Additionally, normal lung tissue that was not previously part of the target volume could be spared radiation that is meant to target only the high-dose region. In contrast, if a tumor is infiltrative and the normal lung remains in its original location as the tumor regresses, then the CTV and PTV should not be altered since that would compromise the dose to microscopic disease (141). Supporters of ART claim that this method does not compromise dose coverage nor the probability of tumor control in areas of potential microscopic disease (142). Such an approach would still allow for sufficient doses to control the microscopic disease from the dose received during the 3 or 5 weeks of treatment prior to adaptation of the RT plan and from the distributions of dose falloff when using either 3D-CRT or IMRT plans.

ART still needs to be studied on a larger scale and in a prospective fashion. With the recent interim analysis of RTOG 0617 (129) establishing that dose escalation to 74 Gy does not offer a survival benefit compared with 60 Gy, ART would probably only add a marginal benefit if the goal is simply dose escalation. However, ART would still probably be beneficial in many applications, and most beneficial in patients with centrally obstructive lesions causing atelectasis.

■ SMALL CELL LUNG CANCER

SCLC makes up approximately 20% of lung cancer diagnoses with a majority of these patients (60%–70%) presenting with extensive disease or Stage IV disease. Concurrent chemotherapy with thoracic radiation and prophylactic cranial irradiation (PCI) are established standard-of-care treatments for LS-SCLC (143,144). PCI has also been investigated in patients with extensive stage SCLC (ES-SCLC) patients (145). Recent trials in LS-SCLC have investigated dose escalation in both PCI (RTOG 0212) and in thoracic radiation (RTOG 0538/CALGB 30610) (146,147). In the hopes of improving overall outcome in ES-SCLC patients who demonstrate a partial or complete response (CR) to platinum-based systemic chemotherapy, the ongoing RTOG 0937 trial for ES-SCLC patients is evaluating the potential benefits of administering consolidative thoracic radiation to the primary site as well as to residual oligometastatic disease (148).

Limited Stage Small Cell Lung Cancer

Prescription and Dose Fractionation

The addition of TRT to chemotherapy for the treatment of LS-SCLC was shown to significantly improve long-term survival in patients with LS-SCLC, and has been established as the current standard of care (149,150). Concurrent chemoradiation has been shown to have superior outcomes to sequential therapy in terms of locoregional control and survival, however, at the expense of added acute toxicity (151). Initially, it was believed that 45 to 50 Gy using daily treatments was sufficient to control SCLC due to its radiosensitivity (152); however, the duration of clinical response was deemed low (144). The Intergroup trial 0096 (INT 0096) randomized LS-SCLC patients to TRT with the first cycle of etoposide/cisplatin with either 45 Gy in daily 180 cGy per fraction or an accelerated regimen of 45 Gy in twice a day treatments (BID) of 1.5 Gy per fraction (144). The accelerated TRT significantly improved OS; however, this regimen has not been well accepted in practice as noted in a 2003 pattern of care study (153). It is possible that the increased esophageal toxicity or the logistical issues with twice per day treatments make the 45 Gy/1.5 Gy BID unattractive. Another valid concern with INT 0096 is that the standard arm of 45 Gy did not offer an equivalent biologic effective dose (BED) to 45 Gy BID, and its biologic efficacy would be much lower than giving a total dose of 60 Gy in daily fractions.

CALGB 30610 (146) is currently enrolling LS-SCLC patients on their Phase III study to compare TRT regimens with concurrent cisplatin and etoposide starting day 1 of chemotherapy cycle 1 or 2. The two high-dose arms, including 70 Gy (2 Gy once daily over 7 weeks) or 61.2 Gy (1.8 Gy once daily for 16 days followed by 1.8 Gy twice daily for 9 days), will be compared with 45 Gy (1.5 Gy twice daily over 3 weeks) to evaluate if higher doses improve median and 2-year survival in patients with LS-SCLC. The BEDs of the 45, 63, and 70 Gy arms are estimated at 43, 63, and 57 Gy, respectively. These arms will also be compared in terms of side effect profile, response rates, local relapse, distant metastases, and brain metastases. Concurrent Once-daily Verses twice daily RadioTherapy (CONVERT) (154) is another ongoing Phase III trial in Europe and Canada that is studying 45 Gy in 30 fx BID versus 66 Gy in 33 fractions. All patients receive concurrent radiation starting on day 1 of cycle 2 of chemotherapy, therefore allowing for after one cycle of induction chemotherapy. Tumor volume reduction with chemotherapy may allow for sparing of normal tissue and better radiation therapy tolerance. Both of these trials will help to determine the best radiation regimen for LS-SCLC patients.

Elective Nodal Irradiation

ENI is still considered acceptable for SCLC treatment; however, some feel that the role of ENI is unresolved (155). The extent of ENI often differs; some physicians may routinely electively cover the hilar and subcarinal nodes, but not extend elective coverage up to the supraclavicular lymph nodes. An earlier Phase II trial from the Netherlands on 27 patients with LS-SCLC disease treated with concurrent cisplatin–etoposide and TRT to the primary disease and only involved lymph nodes had seven (26%) patients with INF in the ipsilateral supraclavicular region (156). In contrast, when the same institutions in Netherlands performed a prospective study of 60 patients using FDG PET-based selective nodal irradiation, there was only a 3% rate of INF (58).

The ongoing studies in SCLC are evaluating dose escalation. It is difficult to include both ENI and dose escalation due to excessive normal tissue toxicities. The CONVERT study does not use ENI, and the CALGB 30610 study includes ENI to the ipsilateral hilum only. The results of these studies will add to the understanding of necessary volumes for ENI in SCLC patients.

Adaptive Radiation Therapy

ART has not been evaluated extensively in SCLC. There is potential benefit it patients who present with bulky disease necessitating a large volume of normal tissue. In the CALGB 30610 study, a reduction in PTV is permitted in the 70 Gy arm after 44 Gy (2 Gy daily) and in the 61.2 Gy arm after 28.8 Gy (1.8 Gy daily) has been delivered which is when the twice daily treatments begin.

Prophylactic Cranial Irradiation

About 10% to 15% of SCLC patients present with brain metastases, and the remaining patients have a 50% to 80% chance of metastasizing to the brain within 2 years of diagnosis (157,158). The meta-analysis by Auperin et al. (143) established PCI as standard of care in LS-SCLC patients due to its findings of reduction in intracranial relapse at 3 years from 58.6% to 33.3% and improvement in 3-year OS rates from 15.3% to 20.7%. Various dose fractionation schedules were used to treat PCI, including total doses of 8 Gy, 24 to 25 Gy, 30 Gy, and 36 to 40 Gy. While larger doses led to greater decreases in the risk of brain metastasis, there was no difference in OS.

The question of PCI dose fractionation was studied in an international cooperative group setting. Le Pechoux et al. (147) compared the standard 25 Gy in 10 fractions with 36 Gy in 18 fractions and with 36 Gy in 24 fractions twice per day (1.5 Gy per fraction) in 720 LS-SCLC patients with CR after chemoradiation. There was no observed difference in quality of life, and few patients had severe deterioration of neuropsychological and cognitive functions over the first 3 years (159). While there was not a difference in the total incidence of brain metastases between the two groups, there was an unexpected significantly worse survival in the higher PCI dose arm at 2 years (42% in the standard arm vs. 37% in the higher dose arm, $P = .05$). In conclusion, 25 Gy in 10 fractions remains the standard of care for PCI in LS-SCLC patients.

Extensive Stage Small Cell Lung Cancer

The role of radiation therapy in ES-SCLC patients has traditionally been reserved for palliative treatment to bulky symptomatic disease and brain metastases. However, if a patient has a CR or near CR, it was not uncommon for some physicians to give consolidative TRT and PCI (160). With platinum-based multiagent chemotherapy, the estimated overall response rate and CR rate is 40% to 70% and 10% to 20%, respectively (161). Most patients will recur despite excellent initial responses. In an effort to improve outcomes with initial therapy, the use of TRT and radiation to oligometastatic disease is currently being tested. Radiation can help to maximize control of macroscopic disease that has been hypothesized to improve survival and quality of life.

A previous study did show the benefit of radiation therapy in select ES-SCLC patients. Jeremic et al. (160) reported results of a Phase III trial of patients with ES-SCLC who achieved CR or PR after three cycles of cisplatin and etoposide and were then randomized to two cycles of carboplatin and etoposide ± concurrent hyperfractionated radiation therapy (54 Gy in 36 fractions BID) to the thorax. Patients with brain metastases were excluded and all patients received PCI. The radiation therapy group had a statistically significant improvement in median survival and 5-year OS.

PCI in ES-SCLC patients is supported by the findings of an EORTC Phase III trial reported by Slotman et al. (145) ES-SCLC patients who responded to four to six cycles of chemotherapy and did not have CT or MRI evidence of brain metastases were randomized to PCI versus no PCI. PCI significantly reduced the incidence of brain metastases at 1 year from 40% to 15% and improved OS at 1 year from 13% to 27% in these ES-SCLC patients.

RTOG 0937 (148) is currently investigating the outcomes benefit of consolidative thoracic radiation to prechemotherapy primary thoracic disease and radiation therapy to residual one to four extracranial oligometastatic diseases in patients with ES-SCLC who achieve a CR or PR with platinum-based systemic chemotherapy. This randomized Phase II study will treat all patients with PCI to 25 Gy in 10 fractions starting on day 1 of TRT concurrently and other sites of metastatic sites if possible. The patients randomized to TRT will receive radiation to the site of the original intrathoracic prechemotherapy primary disease, including involved regional lymphatics, to 45 Gy in 15 fractions of 3 Gy daily. The one to four sites of postchemotherapy residual extracranial metastatic sites will also receive 45 Gy in 15 fractions (estimated to be biologically similar to 60 Gy in 30 fractions). The investigators hope to show that radiation can offer better early control in ES-SCLC patients that will hopefully result in improved OS.

■ REFERENCES

1. Ferlay J, Shin HR, Bray F, Forman D, Mathers C, Parkin DM. Estimates of worldwide burden of cancer in 2008: GLOBOCAN 2008. *Int J Cancer.* 2010;127:12:2893–2917.
2. Jemal A, Bray F, Center MM, Ferlay J, Ward E, Forman D. Global cancer statistics. *CA Cancer J Clin.* 2011;61:69–90.
3. Lubin JH, Richter BS, Blot WJ. Lung cancer risk with cigar and pipe use. *J Natl Cancer Inst.* 1984;73:377–381.
4. Saracci R. Asbestos and lung cancer: an analysis of the epidemiological evidence on the asbestos-smoking interaction. *Int J Cancer.* 1977;20: 323–331.
5. Samet JM, Nero AV Jr. Indoor radon and lung cancer. *N Engl J Med.* 1989;320:591–594.
6. Taylor R, Cumming R, Woodward A, Black M. Passive smoking and lung cancer: a cumulative meta-analysis. *Aust N Z J Public Health.* 2001;25: 203–211.
7. Siegel R, Ward E, Brawley O, Jemal A. Cancer statistics, 2011: the impact of eliminating socioeconomic and racial disparities on premature cancer deaths. *CA Cancer J Clin.* 2011;61:212–236.
8. Timmerman RD, Kavanagh BD, Cho LC, Papiez L, Xing L. Stereotactic body radiation therapy in multiple organ sites. *J Clin Oncol.* 2007;25: 947–952.
9. Lax I, Blomgren H, Naslund I, Svanstrom R. Stereotactic radiotherapy of malignancies in the abdomen. Methodological aspects. *Acta Oncol.* 1994;33:677–683.
10. Pan H, Simpson DR, Mell LK, Mundt AJ, Lawson JD. A survey of stereotactic body radiotherapy use in the United States. *Cancer.* 2011;117: 4566–4572.
11. Potters L, Kavanagh B, Galvin JM, et al. American Society for Therapeutic Radiology and Oncology (ASTRO) and American College of Radiology (ACR) practice guideline for the performance of stereotactic body radiation therapy. *Int J Radiat Oncol Biol Phys.* 2009;76:326–332.
12. Timmerman R, Paulus R, Galvin J, et al. Stereotactic body radiation therapy for inoperable early stage lung cancer. *JAMA.* 2010;303:1070–1076.
13. Movsas B, Langer CJ. RTOG 9801: a phase III study of amifostine mucosal protection for patients with favorable prognosis inoperable stage IIIIIA/B nonsmall cell lung cancer (NSCLC) receiving

sequential induction and concurrent hyperfractionated radiotherapy with paclitaxel and carboplatin. 1998–2002:55.

14. McGibney C, Holmberg O, McClean B, et al. Dose escalation of chart in non-small cell lung cancer: is three-dimensional conformal radiation therapy really necessary? *Int J Radiat Oncol Biol Phys.* 1999;45:339–350.
15. Dobbs HJ, Parker RP, Hodson NJ, Hobday P, Husband JE. The use of CT in radiotherapy treatment planning. *Radiother Oncol.* 1983;1: 133–141.
16. Senan S, De Ruysscher D, Giraud P, Mirimanoff R, Budach V. Literature-based recommendations for treatment planning and execution in high-dose radiotherapy for lung cancer. *Radiother Oncol.* 2004;71:139–146.
17. Starkschall G, Britton K, McAleer MF, et al. Potential dosimetric benefits of four-dimensional radiation treatment planning. *Int J Radiat Oncol Biol Phys.* 2009;73:1560–1565.
18. Haasbeek CJ, Slotman BJ, Senan S. Radiotherapy for lung cancer: clinical impact of recent technical advances. *Lung Cancer.* 2009;64:1–8.
19. Stevens CW, Munden RF, Forster KM, et al. Respiratory-driven lung tumor motion is independent of tumor size, tumor location, and pulmonary function. *Int J Radiat Oncol Biol Phys.* 2001;51:62–68.
20. Lagerwaard FJ, Van Sornsen de Koste JR, Nijssen-Visser MR, et al. Multiple "slow" CT scans for incorporating lung tumor mobility in radiotherapy planning. *Int J Radiat Oncol Biol Phys.* 2001;51:932–937.
21. de Koste JR, Lagerwaard FJ, de Boer HC, Nijssen-Visser MR, Senan S. Are multiple CT scans required for planning curative radiotherapy in lung tumors of the lower lobe? *Int J Radiat Oncol Biol Phys.* 2003;55:1394–1399.
22. Keall P. 4-Dimensional computed tomography imaging and treatment planning. *Semin Radiat Oncol.* 2004;14:81–90.
23. Wolthaus JW, Sonke JJ, van Herk M, et al. Comparison of different strategies to use four-dimensional computed tomography in treatment planning for lung cancer patients. *Int J Radiat Oncol Biol Phys.* 2008;70:1229–1238.
24. Weiss E, Wijesooriya K, Dill SV, Keall PJ. Tumor and normal tissue motion in the thorax during respiration: analysis of volumetric and positional variations using 4D CT. *Int J Radiat Oncol Biol Phys.* 2007;67:296–307.
25. Donnelly ED, Parikh PJ, Lu W, et al. Assessment of intrafraction mediastinal and hilar lymph node movement and comparison to lung tumor motion using four-dimensional CT. *Int J Radiat Oncol Biol Phys.* 2007;69:580–588.
26. Maxim PG, Loo BW Jr, Shirazi H, Thorndyke B, Luxton G, Le QT. Quantification of motion of different thoracic locations using four-dimensional computed tomography: implications for radiotherapy planning. *Int J Radiat Oncol Biol Phys.* 2007;69:1395–1401.
27. Pantarotto JR, Piet AH, Vincent A, van Sornsen de Koste JR, Senan S. Motion analysis of 100 mediastinal lymph nodes: potential pitfalls in treatment planning and adaptive strategies. *Int J Radiat Oncol Biol Phys.* 2009;74:1092–1099.
28. Heinzerling JH, Anderson JF, Papiez L, et al. Four-dimensional computed tomography scan analysis of tumor and organ motion at varying levels of abdominal compression during stereotactic treatment of lung and liver. *Int J Radiat Oncol Biol Phys.* 2008;70:1571–1578.
29. Wong JW, Sharpe MB, Jaffray DA, et al. The use of active breathing control (ABC) to reduce margin for breathing motion. *Int J Radiat Oncol Biol Phys.* 1999;44:911–919.
30. Berson AM, Emery R, Rodriguez L, et al. Clinical experience using respiratory gated radiation therapy: comparison of free-breathing and breath-hold techniques. *Int J Radiat Oncol Biol Phys.* 2004;60:419–426.
31. McNair HA, Brock J, Symonds-Tayler JR, et al. Feasibility of the use of the Active Breathing Coordinator (ABC) in patients receiving radical radiotherapy for non-small cell lung cancer (NSCLC). *Radiother Oncol.* 2009;93:424–429.
32. Burnett SS, Sixel KE, Cheung PC, Hoisak JD. A study of tumor motion management in the conformal radiotherapy of lung cancer. *Radiother Oncol.* 2008;86:77–85.
33. Panakis N, McNair HA, Christian JA, et al. Defining the margins in the radical radiotherapy

of non-small cell lung cancer (NSCLC) with active breathing control (ABC) and the effect on physical lung parameters. *Radiother Oncol.* 2008;87:65–73.

34. Hanley J, Debois MM, Mah D, et al. Deep inspiration breath-hold technique for lung tumors: the potential value of target immobilization and reduced lung density in dose escalation. *Int J Radiat Oncol Biol Phys.* 1999;45:603–611.
35. Rosenzweig KE, Hanley J, Mah D, et al. The deep inspiration breath-hold technique in the treatment of inoperable non-small-cell lung cancer. *Int J Radiat Oncol Biol Phys.* 2000;48:81–87.
36. Nelson C, Starkschall G, Balter P, et al. Respiration-correlated treatment delivery using feedback-guided breath hold: a technical study. *Med Phys.* 2005;32:175–181.
37. Jiang SB, Wolfgang J, Mageras GS. Quality assurance challenges for motion-adaptive radiation therapy: gating, breath holding, and four-dimensional computed tomography. *Int J Radiat Oncol Biol Phys.* 2008;71:S103–S107.
38. Bezjak A, Bradley J, Gaspar LE, Timmerman RD. Seamless phase I/II study of stereotactic lung radiotherapy (SBRT) for early stage, centrally located, non-small cell lung cancer (NSCLC) in medically inoperable patients (RTOG 0813). Trial started February 2, 2009.
39. Bradley JD, Nofal AN, El Naqa IM, et al. Comparison of helical, maximum intensity projection (MIP), and averaged intensity (AI) 4D CT imaging for stereotactic body radiation therapy (SBRT) planning in lung cancer. *Radiother Oncol.* 2006;81:264–268.
40. Underberg RW, Lagerwaard FJ, Slotman BJ, Cuijpers JP, Senan S. Use of maximum intensity projections (MIP) for target volume generation in 4DCT scans for lung cancer. *Int J Radiat Oncol Biol Phys.* 2005;63:253–260.
41. Cascade PN, Gross BH, Kazerooni EA, et al. Variability in the detection of enlarged mediastinal lymph nodes in staging lung cancer: a comparison of contrast-enhanced and unenhanced CT. *AJR Am J Roentgenol.* 1998;170:927–931.
42. Patz EF Jr, Erasmus JJ, McAdams HP, et al. Lung cancer staging and management: comparison of contrast-enhanced and nonenhanced helical CT of the thorax. *Radiology.* 1999;212:56–60.
43. Detterbeck F, Puchalski J, Rubinowitz A, Cheng D. Classification of the thoroughness of mediastinal staging of lung cancer. *Chest.* 2010;137:436–442.
44. Takahashi M, Nitta N, Takazakura R, Nagatani Y, Ushio N, Murata K. Detection of mediastinal and hilar lymph nodes by 16-row MDCT: is contrast material needed? *Eur J Radiol.* 2008;66:287–291.
45. Kong FM, Ritter T, Quint DJ, et al. Consideration of dose limits for organs at risk of thoracic radiotherapy: atlas for lung, proximal bronchial tree, esophagus, spinal cord, ribs, and brachial plexus. *Int J Radiat Oncol Biol Phys.* 2011;81:1442–1457.
46. Nestle U, Kremp S, Grosu AL. Practical integration of [18F]-FDG-PET and PET-CT in the planning of radiotherapy for non-small cell lung cancer (NSCLC): the technical basis, ICRU-target volumes, problems, perspectives. *Radiother Oncol.* 2006;81:209–225.
47. Nestle U, Schaefer-Schuler A, Kremp S, et al. Target volume definition for 18F-FDG PET-positive lymph nodes in radiotherapy of patients with non-small cell lung cancer. *Eur J Nucl Med Mol Imaging.* 2007;34:453–462.
48. van Der Wel A, Nijsten S, Hochstenbag M, et al. Increased therapeutic ratio by 18FDG-PET CT planning in patients with clinical CT stage N2-N3M0 non-small-cell lung cancer: a modeling study. *Int J Radiat Oncol Biol Phys.* 2005;61:649–655.
49. De Ruysscher D, Wanders S, Minken A, et al. Effects of radiotherapy planning with a dedicated combined PET-CT-simulator of patients with non-small cell lung cancer on dose limiting normal tissues and radiation dose-escalation: a planning study. *Radiother Oncol.* 2005;77:5–10.
50. De Ruysscher D, Wanders S, van Haren E, et al. Selective mediastinal node irradiation based on FDG-PET scan data in patients with non-small-cell lung cancer: a prospective clinical study. *Int J Radiat Oncol Biol Phys.* 2005;62:988–994.
51. van Loon J, van Baardwijk A, Boersma L, Ollers M, Lambin P, De Ruysscher D. Therapeutic implications of molecular imaging with PET in

the combined modality treatment of lung cancer. *Cancer Treat Rev*. 2011;37:331–343.

52. Hellwig D, Baum RP, Kirsch C. FDG-PET, PET/CT and conventional nuclear medicine procedures in the evaluation of lung cancer: a systematic review. *Nuklearmedizin*. 2009;48:59–69, quiz N8–9.
53. De Ruysscher D, Kirsch CM. PET scans in radiotherapy planning of lung cancer. *Radiother Oncol*. 2010;96:335–338.
54. Annema JT, van Meerbeeck JP, Rintoul RC, et al. Mediastinoscopy vs endosonography for mediastinal nodal staging of lung cancer: a randomized trial. *JAMA*. 2010;304:2245–2252.
55. Dooms C, Verbeken E, Stroobants S, Nackaerts K, De Leyn P, Vansteenkiste J. Prognostic stratification of stage IIIA-N2 non-small-cell lung cancer after induction chemotherapy: a model based on the combination of morphometric-pathologic response in mediastinal nodes and primary tumor response on serial 18-fluoro-2-deoxy-glucose positron emission tomography. *J Clin Oncol*. 2008;26:1128–1134.
56. Sulman EP, Komaki R, Klopp AH, Cox JD, Chang JY. Exclusion of elective nodal irradiation is associated with minimal elective nodal failure in non-small cell lung cancer. *Radiat Oncol*. 2009;4:5.
57. Fleckenstein J, Hellwig D, Kremp S, et al. F-18-FDG-PET Confined radiotherapy of locally advanced NSCLC with concomitant chemotherapy: results of the PET-PLAN pilot trial. *Int J Radiat Oncol Biol Phys*. 2011;81:e283–e289.
58. van Loon J, De Ruysscher D, Wanders R, et al. Selective nodal irradiation on basis of (18)FDG-PET scans in limited-disease small-cell lung cancer: a prospective study. *Int J Radiat Oncol Biol Phys*. 2010;77:329–336.
59. Wu K, Ung YC, Hornby J, et al. PET CT thresholds for radiotherapy target definition in non-small-cell lung cancer: how close are we to the pathologic findings? *Int J Radiat Oncol Biol Phys*. 2010;77:699–706.
60. Nestle U, Weber W, Hentschel M, Grosu AL. Biological imaging in radiation therapy: role of positron emission tomography. *Phys Med Biol*. 2009;54:R1–R25.
61. Grgic A, Nestle U, Schaefer-Schuler A, Kremp S, Kirsch CM, Hellwig D. FDG-PET-based radiotherapy planning in lung cancer: optimum breathing protocol and patient positioning--an intraindividual comparison. *Int J Radiat Oncol Biol Phys*. 2009;73:103–111.
62. Ollers M, Bosmans G, van Baardwijk A, et al. The integration of PET-CT scans from different hospitals into radiotherapy treatment planning. *Radiother Oncol*. 2008;87:142–146.
63. Aristophanous M, Berbeco RI, Killoran JH, et al. Clinical utility of 4D FDG-PET/CT scans in radiation treatment planning. *Int J Radiat Oncol Biol Phys*. 2011;82(1):e99–e105.
64. Wong CY, Schmidt J, Bong JS, et al. Correlating metabolic and anatomic responses of primary lung cancers to radiotherapy by combined F-18 FDG PET-CT imaging. *Radiat Oncol*. 2007;2:18.
65. Feng M, Kong FM, Gross M, Fernando S, Hayman JA, Ten Haken RK. Using fluorodeoxyglucose positron emission tomography to assess tumor volume during radiotherapy for non-small-cell lung cancer and its potential impact on adaptive dose escalation and normal tissue sparing. *Int J Radiat Oncol Biol Phys*. 2009;73:1228–1234.
66. Khan FM. *The Physics of Radiation Therapy*. 4th ed. Philadelphia, PA: Lippincott Williams and Wilkens; 2010.
67. Klein EE, Morrison A, Purdy JA, Graham MV, Matthews J. A volumetric study of measurements and calculations of lung density corrections for 6 and 18 MV photons. *Int J Radiat Oncol Biol Phys*. 1997;37:1163–1170.
68. Orton CG, Chungbin S, Klein EE, Gillin MT, Schultheiss TE, Sause WT. Study of lung density corrections in a clinical trial (RTOG 88–08). Radiation Therapy Oncology Group. *Int J Radiat Oncol Biol Phys*. 1998;41:787–794.
69. Herman Tde L, Gabrish H, Herman TS, Vlachaki MT, Ahmad S. Impact of tissue heterogeneity corrections in stereotactic body radiation therapy treatment plans for lung cancer. *J Med Phys*. 2010;35:170–173.
70. Xiao Y, Papiez L, Paulus R, et al. Dosimetric evaluation of heterogeneity corrections for RTOG 0236: stereotactic body radiotherapy of inoperable stage

I-II non-small-cell lung cancer. *Int J Radiat Oncol Biol Phys.* 2009;73:1235–1242.

71. Mizuno H, Okamoto H, Fukuoka M, et al. Multi-institutional retrospective analysis of the inhomogeneity correction for radiation therapy of lung cancer. *J Radiat Res. (Tokyo)* 2011;52: 69–74.
72. Chang D, Liu C, Dempsey JF, et al. Predicting changes in dose distribution to tumor and normal tissue when correcting for heterogeneity in radiotherapy for lung cancer. *Am J Clin Oncol.* 2007;30:57–62.
73. Ding GX, Duggan DM, Lu B, et al. Impact of inhomogeneity corrections on dose coverage in the treatment of lung cancer using stereotactic body radiation therapy. *Med Phys.* 2007;34: 2985–2994.
74. Schuring D, Hurkmans CW. Developing and evaluating stereotactic lung RT trials: what we should know about the influence of inhomogeneity corrections on dose. *Radiat Oncol.* 2008;3:21.
75. Fogliata A, Nicolini G, Vanetti E, Clivio A, Winkler P, Cozzi L. The impact of photon dose calculation algorithms on expected dose distributions in lungs under different respiratory phases. *Phys Med Biol.* 2008;53:2375–2390.
76. Vanderstraeten B, Reynaert N, Paelinck L, et al. Accuracy of patient dose calculation for lung IMRT: a comparison of Monte Carlo, convolution/superposition, and pencil beam computations. *Med Phys.* 2006;33:3149–3158.
77. Christian JA, Bedford JL, Webb S, Brada M. Comparison of inverse-planned three-dimensional conformal radiotherapy and intensity-modulated radiotherapy for non-small-cell lung cancer. *Int J Radiat Oncol Biol Phys.* 2007;67:735–741.
78. Schwarz M, Alber M, Lebesque JV, Mijnheer BJ, Damen EM. Dose heterogeneity in the target volume and intensity-modulated radiotherapy to escalate the dose in the treatment of non-small-cell lung cancer. *Int J Radiat Oncol Biol Phys.* 2005;62:561–570.
79. Lievens Y, Nulens A, Gaber MA, et al. Intensity-modulated radiotherapy for locally advanced non-small-cell lung cancer: a dose-escalation planning study. *Int J Radiat Oncol Biol Phys.* 2010;80:306–313.
80. Vogelius IR, Westerly DC, Aznar MC, et al. Estimated radiation pneumonitis risk after photon versus proton therapy alone or combined with chemotherapy for lung cancer. *Acta Oncol* 2011;50:772–776.
81. Schwarz M, Van der Geer J, Van Herk M, Lebesque JV, Mijnheer BJ, Damen EM. Impact of geometrical uncertainties on 3D CRT and IMRT dose distributions for lung cancer treatment. *Int J Radiat Oncol Biol Phys.* 2006;65:1260–1269.
82. Sura S, Gupta V, Yorke E, Jackson A, Amols H, Rosenzweig KE. Intensity-modulated radiation therapy (IMRT) for inoperable non-small cell lung cancer: the Memorial Sloan-Kettering Cancer Center (MSKCC) experience. *Radiother Oncol.* 2008;87:17–23.
83. Cardinale RM, Wu Q, Benedict SH, Kavanagh BD, Bump E, Mohan R. Determining the optimal block margin on the planning target volume for extracranial stereotactic radiotherapy. *Int J Radiat Oncol Biol Phys.* 1999;45:515–520.
84. Papiez L, Timmerman R, DesRosiers C, Randall M. Extracranial stereotactic radioablation: physical principles. *Acta Oncol.* 2003;42:882–894.
85. Liu R, Wagner TH, Buatti JM, Modrick J, Dill J, Meeks SL. Geometrically based optimization for extracranial radiosurgery. *Phys Med Biol.* 2004;49:987–996.
86. De Meerleer GO, Derie CM, Vakaet L, Fortan LG, Mersseman BK Jr, De Neve WJ. Execution of a single-isocenter three-field technique, using a multileaf collimator or tray-mounted cerrobend blocks: effect on treatment time. *Int J Radiat Oncol Biol Phys.* 1997;39:255–259.
87. LoSasso T, Kutcher GJ. Multileaf collimation versus alloy blocks: analysis of geometric accuracy. *Int J Radiat Oncol Biol Phys.* 1995;32:499–506.
88. Chang JY, Zhang X, Wang X, et al. Significant reduction of normal tissue dose by proton radiotherapy compared with three-dimensional conformal or intensity-modulated radiation therapy in Stage I or Stage III non-small-cell lung cancer. *Int J Radiat Oncol Biol Phys.* 2006;65:1087–1096.
89. Mageras GS, Yorke E. Deep inspiration breath hold and respiratory gating strategies for reducing organ motion in radiation treatment. *Semin Radiat Oncol.* 2004;14:65–75.

90. Underberg RW, van Sornsen de Koste JR, Lagerwaard FJ, Vincent A, Slotman BJ, Senan S. A dosimetric analysis of respiration-gated radiotherapy in patients with stage III lung cancer. *Radiat Oncol.* 2006;1:8.
91. Underberg RW, Lagerwaard FJ, Slotman BJ, Cuijpers JP, Senan S. Benefit of respiration-gated stereotactic radiotherapy for stage I lung cancer: an analysis of 4DCT datasets. *Int J Radiat Oncol Biol Phys.* 2005;62:554–560.
92. Hong TS, Welsh JS, Ritter MA, et al. Megavoltage computed tomography: an emerging tool for image-guided radiotherapy. *Am J Clin Oncol.* 2007;30:617–623.
93. Simpson DR, Lawson JD, Nath SK, Rose BS, Mundt AJ, Mell LK. Utilization of advanced imaging technologies for target delineation in radiation oncology. *J Am Coll Radiol.* 2009;6:876–883.
94. Simpson DR, Lawson JD, Nath SK, Rose BS, Mundt AJ, Mell LK. A survey of image-guided radiation therapy use in the United States. *Cancer.* 2010;116:3953–3960.
95. Mohan R, Zhang X, Wang H, et al. Use of deformed intensity distributions for on-line modification of image-guided IMRT to account for interfractional anatomic changes. *Int J Radiat Oncol Biol Phys.* 2005;61:1258–1266.
96. Ma CM, Paskalev K. In-room CT techniques for image-guided radiation therapy. *Med Dosim.* 2006;31:30–39.
97. Bedford JL, Warrington AP. Commissioning of volumetric modulated arc therapy (VMAT). *Int J Radiat Oncol Biol Phys.* 2009;73:537–545.
98. Otto K. Volumetric modulated arc therapy: IMRT in a single gantry arc. *Med Phys.* 2008;35:310–317.
99. Flehinger BJ, Kimmel M, Melamed MR. The effect of surgical treatment on survival from early lung cancer. Implications for screening. *Chest.* 1992;101:1013–1018.
100. Ginsberg RJ, Rubinstein LV. Randomized trial of lobectomy versus limited resection for T1 N0 non-small cell lung cancer. Lung Cancer Study Group. *Ann Thorac Surg.* 1995;60:615–622; discussion 22–23.
101. McGarry RC, Song G, des Rosiers P, Timmerman R. Observation-only management of early stage, medically inoperable lung cancer: poor outcome. *Chest.* 2002;121:1155–1158.
102. Kaskowitz L, Graham MV, Emami B, Halverson KJ, Rush C. Radiation therapy alone for stage I non-small cell lung cancer. *Int J Radiat Oncol Biol Phys.* 1993;27:517–523.
103. Dosoretz DE, Katin MJ, Blitzer PH, et al. Radiation therapy in the management of medically inoperable carcinoma of the lung: results and implications for future treatment strategies. *Int J Radiat Oncol Biol Phys.* 1992;24:3–9.
104. Sibley GS, Jamieson TA, Marks LB, Anscher MS, Prosnitz LR. Radiotherapy alone for medically inoperable stage I non-small-cell lung cancer: the Duke experience. *Int J Radiat Oncol Biol Phys.* 1998;40:149–154.
105. Bradley JD, Wahab S, Lockett MA, Perez CA, Purdy JA. Elective nodal failures are uncommon in medically inoperable patients with Stage I non-small-cell lung carcinoma treated with limited radiotherapy fields. *Int J Radiat Oncol Biol Phys.* 2003;56:342–347.
106. Nagata Y, Takayama K, Matsuo Y, et al. Clinical outcomes of a phase I/II study of 48 Gy of stereotactic body radiotherapy in 4 fractions for primary lung cancer using a stereotactic body frame. *Int J Radiat Oncol Biol Phys.* 2005;63: 1427–1431.
107. Videtic G. A randomized phase II study comparing 2 stereotactic body radiation therapy (SBRT) schedules for medically inoperable patients with stage I peripheral non-small cell lung cancer (RTOG 0915). Trial started March 22, 2011.
108. Kimura T, Matsuura K, Murakami Y, et al. CT appearance of radiation injury of the lung and clinical symptoms after stereotactic body radiation therapy (SBRT) for lung cancers: are patients with pulmonary emphysema also candidates for SBRT for lung cancers? *Int J Radiat Oncol Biol Phys.* 2006;66:483–491.
109. Wu J, Li H, Shekhar R, Suntharalingam M, D'Souza W. An evaluation of planning techniques for stereotactic body radiation therapy in lung tumors. *Radiother Oncol.* 2008;87:35–43.
110. Okunieff P, Petersen AL, Philip A, et al. Stereotactic Body Radiation Therapy (SBRT) for lung metastases. *Acta Oncol.* 2006;45:808–817.

111. Stephans KL, Djemil T, Tendulkar RD, Robinson CG, Reddy CA, Videtic GM. Prediction of chest wall toxicity from lung stereotactic body radiotherapy (SBRT). *Int J Radiat Oncol Biol Phys.* 2012;82:974–980.
112. Dunlap NE, Cai J, Biedermann GB, et al. Chest wall volume receiving >30 Gy predicts risk of severe pain and/or rib fracture after lung stereotactic body radiotherapy. *Int J Radiat Oncol Biol Phys.* 2010;76:796–801.
113. Nagata Y, Hiraoka M, Mizowaki T, et al. Survey of stereotactic body radiation therapy in Japan by the Japan 3-D Conformal External Beam Radiotherapy Group. *Int J Radiat Oncol Biol Phys.* 2009;75:343–347.
114. Forquer JA, Fakiris AJ, Timmerman RD, et al. Brachial plexopathy from stereotactic body radiotherapy in early-stage NSCLC: dose-limiting toxicity in apical tumor sites. *Radiother Oncol.* 2009;93:408–413.
115. Marks LB, Bentzen SM, Deasy JO, et al. Radiation dose-volume effects in the lung. *Int J Radiat Oncol Biol Phys.* 2010;76:S70–S76.
116. Onishi H, Shirato H, Nagata Y, et al. Stereotactic Body Radiotherapy (SBRT) for operable stage I non-small-cell lung cancer: can SBRT be comparable to surgery? *Int J Radiat Oncol Biol Phys.* 2011;81(5):1352–1358.
117. Grills IS, Mangona VS, Welsh R, et al. Outcomes after stereotactic lung radiotherapy or wedge resection for stage I non-small-cell lung cancer. *J Clin Oncol.* 2010;28:928–935.
118. Timmerman R. A randomized phase III study of sublobar resection (+/- brachytherapy) versus stereotactic body radiation therapy in high risk patients with stage I non-small cell lung cancer (NSCLC). Trial started May 9, 2011.
119. Qiao X, Tullgren O, Lax I, Sirzen F, Lewensohn R. The role of radiotherapy in treatment of stage I non-small cell lung cancer. *Lung Cancer.* 2003;41:1–11.
120. Timmerman R, McGarry R, Yiannoutsos C, et al. Excessive toxicity when treating central tumors in a phase II study of stereotactic body radiation therapy for medically inoperable early-stage lung cancer. *J Clin Oncol.* 2006;24:4833–4839.
121. Perez CA, Stanley K, Rubin P, et al. A prospective randomized study of various irradiation doses and fractionation schedules in the treatment of inoperable non-oat-cell carcinoma of the lung. Preliminary report by the Radiation Therapy Oncology Group. *Cancer.* 1980;45:2744–2753.
122. Le Chevalier T, Arriagada R, Tarayre M, et al. Significant effect of adjuvant chemotherapy on survival in locally advanced non-small-cell lung carcinoma. *J Natl Cancer Inst.* 1992;84:58.
123. Kong FM, Ten Haken RK, Schipper MJ, et al. High-dose radiation improved local tumor control and overall survival in patients with inoperable/unresectable non-small-cell lung cancer: long-term results of a radiation dose escalation study. *Int J Radiat Oncol Biol Phys.* 2005;63:324–333.
124. Bradley JD, Bae K, Graham MV, et al. Primary analysis of the phase II component of a phase I/II dose intensification study using three-dimensional conformal radiation therapy and concurrent chemotherapy for patients with inoperable non-small-cell lung cancer: RTOG 0117. *J Clin Oncol.* 2010;28:2475–2480.
125. Schild SE, McGinnis WL, Graham D, et al. Results of a Phase I trial of concurrent chemotherapy and escalating doses of radiation for unresectable non-small-cell lung cancer. *Int J Radiat Oncol Biol Phys.* 2006;65:1106–1111.
126. Curran WJ Jr, Paulus R, Langer CJ, et al. Sequential vs. concurrent chemoradiation for stage III non-small cell lung cancer: randomized phase III trial RTOG 9410. *J Natl Cancer Inst.* 2011;103:1452–1460.
127. Furuse K, Fukuoka M, Kawahara M, et al. Phase III study of concurrent versus sequential thoracic radiotherapy in combination with mitomycin, vindesine, and cisplatin in unresectable stage III non-small-cell lung cancer. *J Clin Oncol.* 1999;17:2692–2699.
128. Zatloukal P, Petruzelka L, Zemanova M, et al. Concurrent versus sequential chemoradiotherapy with cisplatin and vinorelbine in locally advanced non-small cell lung cancer: a randomized study. *Lung Cancer.* 2004;46:87–98.
129. Bradley J. A randomized phase III comparison of standard-dose (60 Gy) versus highdose (74 Gy) conformal radiotherapy with concurrent and

consolidation carboplatin/paclitaxel +/- cetuximab (IND #103444) in patients with stage IIIA/IIIB non-small cell lung cancer. Trial started November 27, 2007.

130. Perez CA, Stanley K, Grundy G, et al. Impact of irradiation technique and tumor extent in tumor control and survival of patients with unresectable non-oat cell carcinoma of the lung: report by the Radiation Therapy Oncology Group. *Cancer.* 1982;50:1091–1099.
131. Rosenzweig KE, Sim SE, Mychalczak B, Braban LE, Schindelheim R, Leibel SA. Elective nodal irradiation in the treatment of non-small-cell lung cancer with three-dimensional conformal radiation therapy. *Int J Radiat Oncol Biol Phys.* 2001;50:681–685.
132. Bradley J, Graham MV, Winter K, et al. Toxicity and outcome results of RTOG 9311: a phase I-II dose-escalation study using three-dimensional conformal radiotherapy in patients with inoperable non-small-cell lung carcinoma. *Int J Radiat Oncol Biol Phys.* 2005;61:318–328.
133. Yu JM, Sun XD, Li MH, et al. [Involved-field three-dimensional conformal radiation treatment for stage III non-small-cell lung]. *Zhonghua Zhong Liu Za Zhi.* 2006;28:526–529.
134. Siker ML, Tome WA, Mehta MP. Tumor volume changes on serial imaging with megavoltage CT for non-small-cell lung cancer during intensity-modulated radiotherapy: how reliable, consistent, and meaningful is the effect? *Int J Radiat Oncol Biol Phys.* 2006;66:135–141.
135. Erridge SC, Seppenwoolde Y, Muller SH, et al. Portal imaging to assess set-up errors, tumor motion and tumor shrinkage during conformal radiotherapy of non-small cell lung cancer. *Radiother Oncol.* 2003;66:75–85.
136. Kupelian PA, Ramsey C, Meeks SL, et al. Serial megavoltage CT imaging during external beam radiotherapy for non-small-cell lung cancer: observations on tumor regression during treatment. *Int J Radiat Oncol Biol Phys.* 2005;63:1024–1028.
137. Fox J, Ford E, Redmond K, Zhou J, Wong J, Song DY. Quantification of tumor volume changes during radiotherapy for non-small-cell lung cancer. *Int J Radiat Oncol Biol Phys.* 2009;74: 341–348.
138. Guckenberger M, Wilbert J, Richter A, Baier K, Flentje M. Potential of adaptive radiotherapy to escalate the radiation dose in combined radiochemotherapy for locally advanced non-small cell lung cancer. *Int J Radiat Oncol Biol Phys.* 2011;79:901–908.
139. Woodford C, Yartsev S, Dar AR, Bauman G, Van Dyk J. Adaptive radiotherapy planning on decreasing gross tumor volumes as seen on megavoltage computed tomography images. *Int J Radiat Oncol Biol Phys.* 2007;69:1316–1322.
140. Gillham C, Zips D, Ponisch F, et al. Additional PET/CT in week 5–6 of radiotherapy for patients with stage III non-small cell lung cancer as a means of dose escalation planning? *Radiother Oncol.* 2008;88:335–341.
141. Sonke JJ, Belderbos J. Adaptive radiotherapy for lung cancer. *Semin Radiat Oncol.* 2010;20: 94–106.
142. Guckenberger M, Richter A, Wilbert J, Flentje M, Partridge M. Adaptive radiotherapy for locally advanced non-small-cell lung cancer does not underdose the microscopic disease and has the potential to increase tumor control. *Int J Radiat Oncol Biol Phys.* 2011;81:e275–e282.
143. Auperin A, Arriagada R, Pignon JP, et al. Prophylactic cranial irradiation for patients with small-cell lung cancer in complete remission. Prophylactic Cranial Irradiation Overview Collaborative Group. *N Engl J Med.* 1999;341:476–484.
144. Turrisi AT 3rd, Kim K, Blum R, et al. Twice-daily compared with once-daily thoracic radiotherapy in limited small-cell lung cancer treated concurrently with cisplatin and etoposide. *N Engl J Med.* 1999;340:265–271.
145. Slotman B, Faivre-Finn C, Kramer G, et al. Prophylactic cranial irradiation in extensive small-cell lung cancer. *N Engl J Med.* 2007;357: 664–672.
146. Bogart J, Komaki R. Phase III randomized study of three different thoracic radiotherapy regimens in patients with limited-stage small cell lung cancer receiving cisplatin and etoposide (RTOG 0538/ CALGB 30610). Trial started March 15, 2008.
147. Le Pechoux C, Dunant A, Senan S, et al. Standard-dose versus higher-dose prophylactic cranial irradiation (PCI) in patients with limited-stage

small-cell lung cancer in complete remission after chemotherapy and thoracic radiotherapy (PCI 99-01, EORTC 22003-08004, RTOG 0212, and IFCT 99-01): a randomised clinical trial. *Lancet Oncol.* 2009;10:467–474.

148. Gore E, Sun A, Ramalingam S. Randomized phase II study comparing prophylactic cranial irradiation alone to prophylactic cranial irradiation and consolidative extra-cranial irradiation for extensive disease small cell lung cancer (ED-SCLC) (RTOG 0937). Trial started March 18, 2010.
149. Pignon JP, Arriagada R, Ihde DC, et al. A meta-analysis of thoracic radiotherapy for small-cell lung cancer. *N Engl J Med.* 1992;327:1618–1624.
150. Warde P, Payne D. Does thoracic irradiation improve survival and local control in limited-stage small-cell carcinoma of the lung? A meta-analysis. *J Clin Oncol.* 1992;10:890–895.
151. Jeremic B, Shibamoto Y, Acimovic L, Milisavljevic S. Initial versus delayed accelerated hyperfractionated radiation therapy and concurrent chemotherapy in limited small-cell lung cancer: a randomized study. *J Clin Oncol.* 1997;15: 893–900.
152. Carney DN, Mitchell JB, Kinsella TJ. In vitro radiation and chemotherapy sensitivity of established cell lines of human small cell lung cancer and its large cell morphological variants. *Cancer Res.* 1983;43:2806–2811.
153. Movsas B, Moughan J, Komaki R, et al. Radiotherapy patterns of care study in lung carcinoma. *J Clin Oncol.* 2003;21:4553–4559.
154. Faivre-Finn C. CONVERT - Concurrent ONce-daily VErsus twice-daily RadioTherapy. Trial started April 2008.
155. Sorensen M, Felip E. Small-cell lung cancer: ESMO clinical recommendations for diagnosis, treatment and follow-up. *Ann Oncol.* 2009;20(suppl 4):71–72.
156. De Ruysscher D, Bremer RH, Koppe F, et al. Omission of elective node irradiation on basis of CT-scans in patients with limited disease small cell lung cancer: a phase II trial. *Radiother Oncol.* 2006;80:307–312.
157. Hirsch FR, Paulson OB, Hansen HH, Vraa-Jensen J. Intracranial metastases in small cell carcinoma of the lung: correlation of clinical and autopsy findings. *Cancer.* 1982;50:2433–2437.
158. Arriagada R, Le Chevalier T, Borie F, et al. Prophylactic cranial irradiation for patients with small-cell lung cancer in complete remission. *J Natl Cancer Inst.* 1995;87:183–190.
159. Le Pechoux C, Laplanche A, Faivre-Finn C, et al. Clinical neurological outcome and quality of life among patients with limited small-cell cancer treated with two different doses of prophylactic cranial irradiation in the intergroup phase III trial (PCI99-01, EORTC 22003-08004, RTOG 0212 and IFCT 99-01). *Ann Oncol.* 2011;22:1154–1163.
160. Jeremic B, Shibamoto Y, Nikolic N, et al. Role of radiation therapy in the combined-modality treatment of patients with extensive disease small-cell lung cancer: a randomized study. *J Clin Oncol.* 1999;17:2092–2099.
161. Hanna N, Bunn PA Jr, Langer C, et al. Randomized phase III trial comparing irinotecan/cisplatin with etoposide/cisplatin in patients with previously untreated extensive-stage disease small-cell lung cancer. *J Clin Oncol.* 2006;24: 2038–2043.

Emerging Concepts in the Treatment of Epidermal Growth Factor Receptor Mutation-Positive Lung Cancer

Dustin A. Deming[1,2] and Anne M. Traynor[1,2]*

[1]*Division of Hematology/Oncology, Department of Medicine, University of Wisconsin, Madison, WI*

[2]*University of Wisconsin Carbone Cancer Center, Madison, WI*

ABSTRACT

Lung cancer is the most common cause of cancer-related mortality in the United States. The standard platinum-doublet chemotherapy regimens have demonstrated limited efficacy for the treatment of non-small cell lung cancer (NSCLC). Over the past 5 years, the clinical importance of epidermal growth factor receptor (EGFR) mutations has been discovered, including as a marker of response to the tyrosine kinase inhibitors (TKIs) erlotinib and gefitinib. Here, we review multiple clinical trials evaluating the use of erlotinib and gefitinib in the setting of EGFR mutations. These studies have led to recommendations that all patients with NSCLC who are being considered for EGFR TKI therapy should have their tumor tested for EGFR mutations to determine whether an EGFR TKI therapy is appropriate. This is a major advance in the treatment of NSCLC as it provides patients the option of a treatment with an improved response rate, progression-free survival, and toxicity profile.

Keywords: epidermal growth factor receptor, lung cancer, erlotinib, gefitinib

*Corresponding author, 3103 WI Institute Medical Research, 1111 Highland Ave, Madison, WI 53705

E-mail address: amt@medicine.wisc.edu

Emerging Cancer Therapeutics 3:1 (2012) 167–184.

DOI: 10.5003/2151–4194.3.1.167

demosmedpub.com/ecat

■ INTRODUCTION

Lung cancer is the leading cause of cancer-related death with an estimated 221,130 new cases and 156,940 deaths in 2011 in the United States (1). Non-small cell lung cancer (NSCLC) accounts for the majority of lung cancer cases, and unfortunately, most patients present at a stage of disease not amenable to curative approaches. Conventional chemotherapy, consisting of platinum-doublet therapy, for NSCLC has been investigated over the past decade with limited effectiveness (2). The benefit from these agents has reached a plateau, suggesting that another approach to therapy design is needed. Recent advances in understanding the biology of NSCLC have led to an improvement in therapies, most notably the use of targeted therapies directed at the epidermal growth factor receptor (EGFR). Tyrosine kinase inhibitors (TKIs) directed at the kinase domain of mutant EGFR have been developed, including erlotinib and gefitinib. The proper targeting of these agents has led to an advance in the treatment of patients with improved response rates (RRs), progression-free survival (PFS), and decreased toxicities. In this chapter, we discuss the biology behind EGFR mutations and the clinical trials that have supplanted EGFR TKIs as a standard treatment for patients with EGFR-mutant lung cancer.

■ EGFR SIGNALING PATHWAYS AND MUTATIONS

The EGFR is a receptor tyrosine kinase that is normally expressed on many cell types, including cells of epithelial, neural, and mesenchymal origin. It is part of a family of receptor tyrosine kinases and consists of three regions: an extracellular ligand-binding domain, a single transmembrane helix domain, and a cytoplasmic kinase domain (3). As a receptor tyrosine kinase, EGFR activation occurs in response to ligand binding. This causes dimerization of the receptors, resulting in intrinsic protein tyrosine kinase activation via intermolecular phosphorylation within its cytoplasmic domain. Tyrosine kinase activation then leads to propagation of downstream signaling. It activates essential signaling pathways in solid tumors, including the RAS/RAF/MEK/ERK, STAT, and PI3K/AKT/mammalian target of rapamycin (mTOR) cascades. These signaling pathways are implicated in vital cellular functions in cancer cells, such as cell growth, local invasion, angiogenesis, metastasis, protein translation, and cell metabolism.

Mutation of the EGFR oncogene is found in 10% to 40%, or more, of lung carcinomas, depending on the patient population (4). These mutations are more frequently found in women, patients with adenocarcinomas, those who had never smoked, and Asians (5). Activating mutations of the tyrosine kinase domain of the EGFR gene result in activation of downstream signaling pathways independent of ligand binding. Nearly 90% of lung cancer-specific EGFR mutations comprise a leucine-to-arginine substitution at position 858 (L858R) on exon 21 and small inframe deletions in exon 19 around the conserved LREA motif (6). These mutations cause constitutive activation of the tyrosine kinase of the EGFR. The TKIs targeting mutant EGFR, erlotinib and gefitinib, are reversible inhibitors at the adenosine triphosphate (ATP) binding site of the EGFR kinase domain, inhibiting downstream signaling. The EGFR mutation has been shown to predict response to EGFR TKIs, but has also demonstrated to be a marker of improved prognosis regardless of the therapy given (7).

Clinical characteristics have not been reliable in predicting response to EGFR TKIs, and EGFR mutations can be seen in some unexpected clinical settings, even rarely in patients with squamous cell carcinomas (8). In a recent analysis, 19% of tumors from men with NSCLC had EGFR mutations, as did 40% of tumors from former or current smokers (9). The American Society of Clinical Oncology (ASCO), on the basis of the results presented below, recommends that all patients with NSCLC who are being considered for first-line therapy with an EGFR TKI have their tumor tested for EGFR mutations to determine whether an EGFR TKI or chemotherapy is the appropriate first-line therapy (10). Similarly, the National Comprehensive Cancer Network (NCCN) and the European Society for Medical Oncology (ESMO) recommend EGFR mutation analysis in all patients with metastatic nonsquamous NSCLC prior to EGFR TKI use (11,12).

■ AGENTS TARGETING MUTANT EGFR

Erlotinib

Erlotinib (Tarceva, OSI-774, Genentech/Roche/OSI Pharmaceuticals) is an oral anilinoquinazoline that can reversibly inhibit the EGFR tyrosine kinase with an IC_{50} of 2 nmol/L (13). Erlotinib is 1,000-fold more potent against the EGFR tyrosine kinase than most other kinases (14). The optimal dose and schedule of erlotinib were investigated in a Phase I trial including 40 patients (15). The incidence of severe diarrhea and cutaneous toxicities was quite high at doses greater than 150 mg orally daily. The recommended dose for further clinical studies is 150 mg daily. However, the optimal dose of erlotinib required in the setting of EGFR mutations is unknown. Patients with EGFR-mutant NSCLC have responded to therapy at doses as low as 25 mg orally daily (16). Erlotinib is the only EGFR TKI approved by the U.S. Food and Drug Administration (FDA) for use in the United States.

Gefitinib

Gefitinib (Iressa, ZD1839, Astra Zeneca) is also an oral anilinoquinazoline derivative that can reversibly inhibit the EGFR tyrosine kinase with an IC_{50} of 20 nmol/L (17). The optimal dose and schedule of gefitinib were investigated in multiple Phase I trials (18–21). Intermittent and continuous dose schedules were assessed ranging from 50 to 1000 mg/day. The main dose-limiting toxicities were diarrhea and cutaneous toxicity, which occurred at doses ranging from 700 to 1000 mg/day. Pharmacodynamic studies revealed that gefitinib daily doses greater than 150 mg were associated with target inhibition. The most common side effects were nausea, rash, and diarrhea. Dosing was tolerated up to 600 mg per day. The continuous 250 and 500 mg per day regimens were chosen to be studied further, though doses even lower have shown efficacy in the setting of sensitizing mutations of the EGFR gene (22).

■ EGFR TARGETING IN TREATMENT OF REFRACTORY ADVANCED NSCLC

The EGFR TKIs erlotinib and gefitinib have been investigated in treatment refractory NSCLC patients in multiple clinical trials (Table 1). In two Phase II studies (Iressa dose evaluation in advanced lung cancer [IDEAL-1] and IDEAL-2), improved RRs with limited toxicities from gefitinib were observed in the setting of treatment refractory advanced NSCLC (23,24). The subsequent Phase III Iressa Survival Evaluation in Lung Cancer (ISEL) and Iressa NSCLC Trial Evaluating Response and Survival Versus Taxotere (INTEREST) studies demonstrated improved RR and PFS with EGFR TKIs, but no prolongation of OS (25–28).

The pivotal Phase III National Cancer Institute of Canada Clinical Trials Group (NCIC-CTG) BR.21 trial randomized 731 advanced unselected NSCLC patients to either erlotinib or placebo in the second- or third-line setting (29). Antitumor response (8.9% vs. <1%), PFS (2.2 vs. 1.8 months), and median overall survival (OS) (6.7 vs. 4.7 months) all favored erlotinib over placebo ($P < .001$ for all measures). Improvement in quality of life measures was also seen with erlotinib. This study demonstrated that EGFR TKI therapy prolonged survival in patients with NSCLC refractory to prior chemotherapy, and led to the FDA approval of erlotinib.

The largest prospective study to date evaluating the EGFR mutation status in patients with

TABLE 1 Selected clinical trials of EGFR TKI for patients with treatment refractory NSCLC

	Agent	Patient Population	Number of Patients	RR (%)	PFS (months)	Median OS (months)
Phase II						
IDEAL-1 (23)	Gefitinib (250 and 500 mg/day)	Unselected advanced treatment refractory NSCLC	210	18.4 vs. 19	2.7 vs. 2.8	7.6 vs. 8.0
IDEAL-2 (24)	Gefitinib (250 and 500 mg/day)	Caucasian unselected advanced treatment refractory NSCLC	221	12 vs. 9	Not available	7 vs. 6
Spanish Lung Cancer Group (30)	Erlotinib (150 mg/day)	EGFR-mutant advanced NSCLC	350	70.6	13	27
Phase III						
BR.21 (29)	Erlotinib (150 mg/day) vs. placebo	Unselected advanced treatment refractory NSCLC	731	8.9 vs. <1 ($P < .001$)	2.2 vs. 1.8 ($P < .001$)	6.7 vs. 4.7 ($P < .001$)
ISEL (25)	Gefitinib (250 mg/day) vs. placebo	Unselected advanced treatment refractory NSCLC	1,692	8 vs. 1.3	3.0 vs. 2.6 ($P < .001$)	5.6 and 5.1 ($P = .089$)
INTEREST (27)	Gefitinib (250 mg/day) vs. docetaxel	Unselected advanced treatment refractory NSCLC	1,466	9.1 vs. 7.6 ($P = .33$)	2.2 vs. 2.7 (P = NS)	7.6 vs. 8.0 (P = NS)

NS = not statistically significant.

advanced NSCLC was conducted by the Spanish Lung Cancer Group which screened 2,105 patients with untreated or relapsed advanced NSCLC for EGFR mutations (30). A total of 350 patients (16.6%) carried EGFR mutations, which included deletions in exon 19 (62.2%) and exon 21 (37.8%). The RR in 217 mutation-positive patients who received erlotinib as first-, second-, or third-line therapy was 70.5%, while PFS measured 14 months and median OS was 27 months. OS was similar when examining those who received erlotinib as first- or second-line therapy. Similar to prior reports, mutations were more frequent in women, never smokers, and in those with adenocarcinoma histology.

■ EGFR TARGETING IN FIRST-LINE TREATMENT OF ADVANCED NSCLC

In addition to the pretreated advanced setting, the use of erlotinib and gefitinib in first-line treatment has been examined. The European TOPICAL study compared erlotinib with placebo in an unselected, untreated population of 670 NSCLC patients (adenocarcinoma and squamous cell carcinoma) whose performance status was too poor for standard chemotherapy (31). In this nonenriched population, erlotinib did not improve OS (HR was 0.98 [95% CI 0.82–1.15; $P = .77$]), but a trend for prolonged PFS was detected (HR was 0.86 [95% CI 0.74–1.01, $P = .07$]).

In terms of examining EGFR TKI activity in EGFR-positive patients, the multicenter iTARGET trial prospectively investigated a clinically enriched population of chemo-naive patients with nonsquamous histology (32). Thirty-four (35%) of 98 patients had tumors harboring EGFR mutations. Treatment with gefitinib at 250 mg daily in 31 of these patients yielded a RR of 55%, PFS of 9.2 months, and OS of 17.5 months. A combined analysis of 7 prospective Japanese studies examining 148 patients with EGFR mutations who received gefitinib showed a RR of 76%, median PFS of 9.7 months, and OS of 24.3 months (33). These encouraging results prompted the comparison of first-line EGFR TKIs to chemotherapy in untreated EGFR mutation-positive patients.

■ EGFR TARGETING IN FIRST-LINE TREATMENT OF ADVANCED NSCLC IN PATIENTS WITH EGFR MUTATIONS

Six randomized Phase III studies have been conducted, including IPASS, First-SIGNAL, WTOG3405, NEJ002, OPTIMAL, and EURTAC (Table 2), evaluating EGFR TKIs in preselected populations. These studies have made EGFR TKIs the standard of care for the first-line treatment of advanced NSCLC possessing EGFR mutations.

The IPASS study was a randomized, multicenter Phase III clinical trial examining gefitinib (250 mg oral daily) versus carboplatin (AUC 5 or 6) and paclitaxel (200 mg/m^2) as first-line therapy in nonsmokers or former light smokers with advanced NSCLC in East Asia (34). It evaluated the appropriateness of patient selection for first-line EGFR TKI therapy based on predictive clinical and demographic factors. A total of 1,217 patients from 87 centers with Stage IIIB or IV lung adenocarcinoma who had no prior systemic therapy enrolled. Noninferiority for PFS for the two arms was the primary endpoint. The median PFS was 5.7 months in the gefitinib group and 5.8 months in the chemotherapy group for the population as a whole. Of the 1,217 patients enrolled, 437 patients had tumor samples that were evaluated for EGFR mutation status. Two hundred and sixty one (21.4% of the enrolling population) patients were positive for EGFR mutations, with 140 (53.6%) exon 19 deletions and 111 (42.5%) mutations in exon 21. Clinical and demographic predictors did not correlate with the mutation profile in many cases. The RR and PFS were improved for patients with *EGFR* mutations who received gefitinib (71.2% and 9.5 months), compared with chemotherapy (47.3% and 6.3 months [PFS: HR 0.48; 95% CI 0.36–0.64; $P < .001$]). In contrast, RR and PFS

TABLE 2 Prospective randomized Phase III studies of EGFR TKIs in the first-line setting

	Agent	Patient Population	Number of Patients	RR (%)	Median PFS (months)	Median OS (months)
IPASS (10,34,35)	Gefitinib vs. carboplatin/ paclitaxel	All	1,217	43 vs. 32.2 ($P < .001$)	5.7 vs. 5.8 ($P < .001$)	18.8 vs. 17.4 (P = NS)
		EGFR-mutant	261	71.2 vs. 47.3 ($P < .001$)	9.5 vs. 6.3 ($P < .001$)	21.6 vs. 21.9 (P = NS)
		EGFR WT	176	1.1 vs. 23.5 ($P = .0013$)	1.5 vs. 5.5 ($P < .001$)	11.2 vs. 12.7 (P = NS)
OPTIMAL (44)	Erlotinib vs. carboplatin/ gemcitabine	First-line EGFR-mutant advanced NSCLC	154	83 vs. 36 ($P < .001$)	13.1 vs. 4.6 ($P = .16$)	Not available
First SIGNAL (40)	Gefitinib vs. cisplatin/ gemcitabine	All	306	53.5 vs. 45.3 ($P = .1533$)	6.1 vs. 6.6 ($P = .044$)	21.3 vs. 23.3 ($P = .428$)
		EGFR-mutant	42	84.6 vs. 37.5 ($P = .002$)	6.1 vs. 6.6 ($P = .084$)	30.6 vs. 26.5 ($P = .648$)
		EGFR WT	54	25.9 vs. 51.9 ($P = .051$)	2.1 vs. 6.4 ($P = .071$)	18.4 vs. 23.3 ($P = .632$)
NEJ002 (42)	Gefitinib vs. carboplatin/ paclitaxel	Japanese EGFR mutation-positive advanced NSCLC	224	73.7 vs. 30.7 ($P < .001$)	10.8 vs. 5.4 ($P < .001$)	30.5 vs. 23.6 ($P = .31$)
WJTOG3405 (43)	Gefitinib vs. cisplatin/ docetaxel	Japanese EGFR-mutant first-line advanced NSCLC	172	62.1 vs. 32.2 ($P < .001$)	9.2 vs. 6.3 ($P < .001$)	30.9 vs. not reached ($P = .211$)
EURTAC (45)	Erlotinib vs. platinum-based chemo	Caucasian EGFR-mutant first-line advanced NSCLC	153	54.5 vs. 10.5 ($P < .001$)	9.4 vs. 5.2 ($P < .001$)	22.9 vs. 18.8 ($P = .42$)

were superior for those in the carboplatin and paclitaxel arm (23.5% and 5.5 months) compared with those in the gefitinib arm (1.1% and 1.5 months) in patients with wild-type (WT) EGFR (PFS: HR 2.85; 95% CI 2.05–3.98; $P < .001$). At final OS analysis and data cutoff, results showed that OS for gefitinib was 18.8 months (21.6 months for EGFR mutation positive and 11.2 months for EGFR mutation negative) and 17.4 months (21.9 months for EGFR mutation positive and 12.7 months for EGFR mutation negative) for the combination of carboplatin and paclitaxel, which were not significantly different (HR 0.90, 95% CI 0.79–1.02; $P = .109$) (10,35). Over half (60%) of patients on the gefitinib arm subsequently received second-line platinum-based chemotherapy, while 52% of patients who received initial carboplatin and paclitaxel went on to receive second-line EGFR TKI therapy. This cross-over likely diminished the ability of the trial to detect an OS benefit. In a subsequent biomarker analysis, EGFR mutations were found to be the strongest predictive biomarker for PFS and tumor response (36).

Efficacy outcomes from IPASS confirmed that patients with EGFR mutations have a better prognosis regardless of the type of therapy given. For example, RR and OS were superior in EGFR mutation-positive patients who received either gefitinib or chemotherapy in IPASS, compared with contemporary outcomes seen in unselected patients treated with first-line carboplatin and paclitaxel (37–39). The positive prognostic effect of the presence of the EGFR mutation was previously described in a subgroup analysis of the TRIBUTE trial where patients with EGFR mutations demonstrated improved RR, TTP, and OS compared with those with WT EGFR (7). Importantly, IPASS also demonstrated that clinical and demographic predictors are inadequate for selecting patients for first-line EGFR TKI therapy, and that such treatment is most appropriate for patients whose tumors harbor EGFR-sensitizing mutations, while patients with WT EGFR tumors will gain more benefit from standard chemotherapy.

In the First-Line Single Agent Iressa Versus Gemcitabine and Cisplatin Trial in Never-smokers with Adenocarcinoma of the Lung (First-SIGNAL), first-line gefitinib was compared with gemcitabine and cisplatin in 313 Korean patients with advanced adenocarcinoma of the lung who had never smoked (40). In the overall population, the RR was 53.5% in the gefitinib arm and 45.3% with chemotherapy ($P = .1533$) (41). Mutations in the EGFR gene were found in 42 patients (13.4% of the study population). The RR in EGFR-mutant patients for gefitinib was 84.6% compared with 37.5% with chemotherapy ($P = .002$). In patients with WT EGFR tumors, the RR to gefitinib was 25.9% versus 51.9% with chemotherapy ($P = .051$). There was a trend for improvement in PFS and OS in patients with EGFR mutations treated with gefitinib, but this was not statistically significant. There was also a trend for decreased PFS and OS for patients with EGFR WT tumors treated with gefitinib compared with chemotherapy. Generalizations from this trial are limited by the small number of patients with EGFR mutations.

The NEJ002 Phase III trial, conducted by the North-East Japan Study Group, randomized the first-line use of gefitinib (250 mg orally daily) to carboplatin (AUC 6) and paclitaxel (200 mg/m^2) in 230 patients with advanced NSCLC and known mutant EGFR (42). The RR and PFS were superior in the gefitinib arm (73.7% and 10.8 months), compared with the chemotherapy arm (30.7% and 5.4 months; HR for PFS 0.30, 95% CI 0.51–0.92; $P = .01$). As expected, gefitinib was better tolerated than chemotherapy in this population.

The West Japan Thoracic Oncology Group also found that RR and PFS were statistically superior in 177 EGFR mutation-positive first-line patients randomized to gefitinib (62.1% and 9.2 months), compared with treatment with cisplatin and docetaxel (32.2% and 6.3 months), in their prospective, multicenter trial (43). Cross-over in subsequent lines of treatment again limited the ability to detect an OS improvement with gefitinib in this population.

Two randomized Phase III trials have compared the efficacy of erlotinib with standard chemotherapy in the EGFR mutation-positive population in the first-line setting of advanced NSCLC. First, the OPTIMAL study compared erlotinib with carboplatin and gemcitabine in 154 Chinese patients with sensitizing EGFR mutations (44). PFS was the primary endpoint. As with three of the four trials using gefitinib, both RR (83% vs. 36%) and PFS (13.1 vs. 4.6 months) were statistically significantly improved by the use of erlotinib, compared with chemotherapy, respectively.

Second, the European Randomized Trial of Tarceva Versus Chemotherapy (EURTAC) was conducted by the Spanish Lung Cancer Group. These investigators screened 1,227 treatment-naïve patients with advanced NSCLC for EGFR mutations, and randomized 174 patients (14.2%) found to have EGFR mutations to either erlotinib or to four cycles of a platinum-based doublet (45). In contrast to the five studies described above, the EURTAC population was primarily Caucasian. The primary endpoint was PFS. Interim analyses of the first 153 patients were presented at the ASCO 2011 Annual Meeting. The RR was 54.5% for the erlotinib arm and 10.5% for standard chemotherapy group ($P < .0001$), while PFS in the erlotinib arm was 9.4 versus 5.2 months in the chemotherapy group (HR 0.42; $P < .0001$). Median OS was 22.9 months in the erlotinib arm and 18.8 months in those given chemotherapy (HR 0.80; $P = .42$).

Multiple conclusions derive from analyses of these six prospective randomized trials. First, clinical and demographic patient characteristics are insufficient in determining which patients will benefit from EGFR TKI therapy. Testing for the presence of an EGFR mutation analysis is the best method to determine which patient will respond to gefitinib and erlotinib. Second, the clinical evidence to date rests upon the presence of an EGFR-sensitizing mutation and does not rely upon the presence or absence of other mutations, such as in the KRAS gene. Therefore, screening of patients with advanced nonsquamous NSCLC for EGFR mutations who are candidates for EGFR TKIs is recommended prior to first-line treatment by ASCO, ESMO, and the NCCN. Third, PFS is prolonged in the majority of these studies in EGFR mutation-positive patients who receive an EGFR TKI up front. OS is not consistently improved since it is likely confounded by subsequent cross-over treatment. Prolongation of PFS in the first-line setting of advanced NSCLC is highly clinically meaningful since every trial above describes fewer and less severe treatment-related toxicities associated with the use of EGFR TKIs, compared with the use of cytotoxic chemotherapies. Multiple trials also reported improvements in quality of life with the use of EGFR TKIs. The lower toxicity profile of EGFR TKIs requires that EGFR testing be done, so that patients are not denied these better tolerated therapies based upon clinical and demographic parameters alone. And fourth, first-line treatment with chemotherapy is strongly recommended, rather than EGFR TKIs, in EGFR mutation-negative patients who are fit for cytotoxic treatment.

■ EGFR-TARGETED THERAPY IN ADJUVANT SETTING OF ADVANCED NSCLC

Provocative single institution retrospective nonrandomized data raise the possibility of benefit from the use of peri-operative EGFR TKIs in early-stage patients with EGFR mutation-positive NSCLC. In a recent review from Memorial Sloan-Kettering Cancer Center, 167 patients with EGFR mutation expressing tumors who had completely resected Stage I to III NSCLC were reviewed following the use of either preoperative or postoperative EGFR TKI therapy (either erlotinib or gefitinib) (46). After controlling for use of peri-operative chemotherapy, a trend toward an improved disease-free survival was observed in patients receiving EGFR TKIs compared with those who did not: the 2-year disease-free interval was 89% for patients who received the EGFR TKI and 72% for those in the control group

(HR = 0.53; 95% CI 0.28–1.03; P = .06). Interestingly, those patients who stopped therapy and then recurred were still largely sensitive to the TKIs upon reinitiating (47).

Postoperative EGFR TKI therapy was evaluated in Phase III NCIC BR.19 trial that randomized unselected NSCLC patients to gefitinib 250 mg or placebo daily for 2 years following resection (48). No disease-free survival or OS advantage was observed with adjuvant gefitinib, even when examining those patients with sensitizing EGFR mutations. However, interpretation of these results is unclear due to the fact that this study was closed prematurely in 2005 and was underpowered.

Phase III RADIANT trial randomized 945 patients with Stage IB to IIIA NSCLC that was positive for the EGFR protein (by IHC) or gene amplification (by FISH) to either placebo or erlotinib (150 mg daily for 2 years) either immediately postoperatively or following four cycles of platinum-based adjuvant therapy (49). Accrual completed in April 2010, and subset analyses on EGFR mutation-positive patients are eagerly anticipated. In addition, a multicenter Phase II trial is accruing patients with resected Stage I to IIIA NSCLC that contains somatic *EGFR* mutations to investigate the safety and efficacy of postoperative erlotinib in this setting (50).

■ EGFR-TARGETED THERAPY IN LOCALLY ADVANCED NSCLC

The SWOG 0023 study demonstrated that unselected patients did not benefit from gefitinib therapy following the completion of chemoradiation for Stage III NSCLC (51). Data on the use of EGFR TKIs in patients with EGFR mutations and locally advanced NSCLC are sparse and preliminary (52,53). A single-institution retrospective analysis suggested that there was an association between lower local recurrence rates and the presence of an EGFR mutation in patients treated with chemoradiation for locally advanced NSCLC (54).

■ EGFR TARGETING AS MAINTENANCE THERAPY IN ADVANCED NSCLC

The addition of erlotinib to bevacizumab significantly prolonged PFS, when compared with bevacizumab alone (4.8 vs. 3.7 months, HR 0.72, 95% CI 0.59–0.88, P = .0012), in the maintenance setting of advanced NSCLC in 768 unselected patients (55). Erlotinib, alone, was assessed as maintenance therapy in the Sequential Tarceva in Unresectable NSCLC study (56). In this Phase III clinical trial, 889 unselected patients who had completed four cycles of chemotherapy for advanced NSCLC received either erlotinib (150 mg daily) or placebo. PFS was significantly prolonged with erlotinib compared with placebo for the population as a whole, 12.3 versus 11.1 weeks, respectively (HR 0.71, 95% CI 0.2–0.82; $P < .0001$). OS was also lengthened with erlotinib, 12 months versus placebo 11 months (HR 0.81, 95% CI 0.70–0.95; $P = .0088$). However, the greatest benefit with erlotinib was seen in patients with EGFR mutations (PFS for HR 0.10, 95% CI 0.04–0.25; $P < .0001$). Erlotinib maintenance therapy was well tolerated with only 17% of patients requiring a dose reduction secondary to an adverse event. This study suggests that erlotinib can be used as maintenance therapy for patients with NSCLC who do not progress after four cycles of standard chemotherapy, and these results led to the approval of erlotinib by the FDA for this indication.

■ EGFR TARGETING IN THE TREATMENT OF CENTRAL NERVOUS SYSTEM DISEASE

NSCLC has a high propensity to metastasize to the central nervous system (CNS) where metastatic disease can exert a profound detriment on a patient's performance status and quality of life. Standard cytotoxic chemotherapy has diminutive CNS penetration as these agents do not routinely cross the blood brain barrier. EGFR TKIs offer the advantage of being able to cross the blood brain barrier more consistently.

Prospective studies have demonstrated intracranial RRs of 10% to 30% in unselected NSCLC patients and up to 70% in Asian never smoking patients with adenocarcinomas and brain metastases (57–59). Heon et al. (60) investigated the risk of CNS progression in patients with EGFR mutation-positive advanced NSCLC treated with gefitinib or erlotinib as initial therapy for advanced NSCLC. They found that the incidence of CNS progression was 28% after a median follow-up of 42.2 months. This rate is significantly decreased compared with historical controls receiving standard systemic chemotherapy, suggesting a lower risk of CNS progression in patients with EGFR mutations treated with gefitinib or erlotinib. Further research in this area is highly warranted.

MECHANISMS OF RESISTANCE TO EGFR-DIRECTED THERAPIES

EGFR TKIs have significant efficacy and fewer and usually less severe side effects compared with standard platinum-doublet chemotherapy for the treatment of EGFR mutation-positive NSCLC. However, at some point, all tumors develop acquired resistance to EGFR TKIs. This occurs on average after 9 to 10 months of therapy, but can also be infrequently seen *de novo*. Tumors typically develop acquired resistance when downstream signaling cascades are reactivated despite EGFR TKI therapy. Some of the multiple mechanisms by which acquired resistance occurs and ways to overcome them are discussed here.

EGFR Resistance Mutations

While some EGFR mutations sensitize tumors to EGFR TKIs, others have been associated with resistance to erlotinib and gefitinib. The most commonly identified EGFR resistance mutation is a substitution of a threonine residue with methionine at position 790 (T790M) in exon 20. Erlotinib and gefitinib are reversible competitive inhibitors of the EGFR ATP-binding site. The T790M substitution results in an increased affinity of the receptor for ATP compared with the EGFR TKIs. This abrogates the ability of erlotinib and gefitinib to inhibit EGFR signaling (61). The T790M mutation can be found in up to 50% of tumors that have acquired EGFR TKI resistance (62). Other less common resistance mutations have also been described (63). Like the T790M mutation, these other resistance mutations also tend not to exist in patients lacking a sensitizing mutation of the EGFR gene. Interestingly, patients with T790M mutations have a relatively more favorable postprogression course, compared with those whose acquired resistance to EGFR TKIs is not mediated by the T790M mutation (64).

Multiple strategies are under investigation to overcome EGFR resistance mutations. Various irreversible pan-EGFR inhibitors are being developed, including BIBW2992, PF00299804, and HKI-272 (Table 3) (65). These agents are irreversible inhibitors of EGFR and have also demonstrated in vitro activity against cancer cells with T790M mutations. In addition, heat shock protein 90 (HSP90) inhibitors and Src kinase inhibitors are being investigated in this setting (66–68).

RAS/RAF/MEK Activation

The RAS/RAF/MEK/ERK pathway downstream of the EGFR is one of the most commonly investigated signaling cascades in cancer. This pathway has shown to be important for cell proliferation, differentiation, and growth, among others. Mutations of the KRAS gene are the most common abnormality of this signaling pathway in NSCLC, with 10% to 30% of tumors possessing mutations (69). These mutations have been associated with resistance to EGFR TKIs. In a meta-analysis, the objective RR was only 3% (6/210) in EGFR WT NSCLC patients possessing KRAS mutation (70). In NSCLC, KRAS mutations and

TABLE 3 Mechanisms of EGFR TKI resistance and potential therapies

Mechanisms of Resistance	Cellular Defects	Targeted Therapies		Ongoing NSCLC-Targeted Therapy Combination Clinical Trials
EGFR TKI resistance mutations	T790M EGFR mutation Other EGFR resistance mutations	*Pan-EGFR TKIs* BIBW2992 XL647 HKI-272 PF-00299804 BMS-690514 BMS-599626 AZD8931 Pazopanib Lapatinib Vandetanib *Src inhibitors* Dasatinib KX2–391 AZD0530 XL228 XL999	*HSP90 inhibitors* AUY922 STA-9090 AT13387 IPI-504 MPC-3100 SNX-5422 CNF-2024 XL888	• AUY922 + erlotinib • PF-00299804 + PF-02341066 • BIBW2992 + rapamycin • Dasatinib + erlotinib • Pazopanib + erlotinib
Ras/Raf/MEK signaling	KRAS mutations BRAF mutations	*BRAF inhibitors* PLX4032 GSK2118436 XL281 RO5212054	*MEK inhibitors* AZD6244 PD-325901 GDC-0973 TAK-733 AS703026 GSK11202212 RO4987655 RO5126766 MEK162 BAY86–9766	• MEK162 + BKM120 • AZD6244 + erlotinib • GSK11202212 + everolimus • GSK11202212 + erlotinib
PI3K/AKT/mTOR signaling	PIK3CA mutations AKT mutations Loss of PTEN (mutation/methylation)	*PI3K inhibitors* BEZ235 XL147 GDC-0941 BKM120 PX-866 BAY80–6946 SF1126 ZSTK474 PF-04691502 PF-05212384 Palomid 529 DS-7423 XL765 AMG 319 PKC412	*AKT inhibitors* MK2206 Perifosine GSK2141795 SR13668 GSK690693 *mTOR inhibitors* Rapamycin Temsirolimus Everolimus Ridaforolimus Deferolimus	• XL765 + erlotinib • XL147 + erlotinib • MK2206 + erlotinib • MK2206 + gefitinib • Everolimus + vatalanib • Everolimus + gefitinib • Rapamycin + sunitinib • Everolimus + erlotinib • Everolimus + sorafenib • Everolimus + BIBF 1120

(*Continued*)

TABLE 3 Mechanisms of EGFR TKI resistance and potential therapies (*Continued*)

Mechanisms of Resistance	Cellular Defects	Targeted Therapies		Ongoing NSCLC-Targeted Therapy Combination Clinical Trials
MET signaling	MET amplification/ mutation HGF	*Met antibodies* MetMab *HGF* AV-299	*MET TKIs* PF02341066 GSK1363089 ARQ197 XL880 XL184 SCH-900105 JNJ38877605 PF-02341066 INC280	• MetMab + erlotinib • ARQ197 + erlotinib • AV-299 + gefitinib
IGF-1/R signaling	IGF-1R overexpression IGF upregulation	*IGF1/R antibodies* CP-751 IMC-A12 AVE-1642 BMS 754807 BIIB022 AMG 479 CP-751,871 Figitumumab	*IGF1R TKIs* OSI-906 AXL1717 MK-0646 R1507 BMS 536924 AEW541	• IMC-A12 + temsirolimus • IMC-A12 + erlotinib • AMG 479 + everolimus
VEGF/R signaling	VEGFR Overexpression VEGF upregulation	*VEGF Antibodies* Bevacizumab AVE005	*Antiangiogenic TKIs* Sorafenib Sunitinib Vatalanib BIBF 1120 AMG706 Pazopanib Axitinib Cedirinib	• Bevacizumab + erlotinib • Sunitinib + erlotinib • Vatalanib + everolimus

Source: Ongoing combination clinical trials were identified from www.clinicaltrials.gov.

EGFR mutations are virtually mutually exclusive and, thus, KRAS does not lead to acquired EGFR TKI resistance in the setting of EGFR mutations. Mutations in the BRAF gene occur infrequently in NSCLC, in 2% to 3% of cases (71). Clinical trials targeting both the EGFR and the RAS/RAF/MEK pathways simultaneously are underway. The RAS/RAF/MEK pathway is being targeted primarily with BRAF and MEK inhibitors at present.

PI3K/AKT/mTOR Activation

Similar to the RAF/MEK/ERK signaling cascade, the PI3K/AKT/mTOR pathway is also involved in critical cellular functions. Mutations in the PIK3CA gene are identified in up to 17% of NSCLC (72). Mutations in the AKT gene are much less common (73). Many new agents are being developed that target this pathway including PI3K, AKT, and mTOR inhibitors. These agents are being studied individually, but also in combination with EGFR TKIs (74). The AKT pathway can also be activated by amplification of the IGF1R, particularly in response to EGFR inhibition (75). Monoclonal antibodies and TKIs targeting IGF1R are intense investigation in the treatment of NSCLC.

MET Amplification/Mutation

Amplifications and mutations of the MET oncogene encoding the receptor tyrosine kinase for hepatocyte growth factor (HGF) have been identified in approximately 20% of cases of acquired resistance to EGFR TKIs in NSCLC (76,77). Alterations of MET can result in persistent activation of the PI3K/AKT pathway in the setting of EGFR inhibition. Both monoclonal antibodies and TKIs targeting the receptor are under evaluation. The randomized OAM4558g Phase II study examined a monoclonal antibody targeting MET in combination with erlotinib versus erlotinib plus placebo in the second- or third-line setting in 128 patients with advanced NSCLC (78). Over half of the patients had elevated c-MET protein expression per IHC, and this was associated with a worse prognosis in the erlotinib plus placebo cohort. The addition of the MET targeting antibody to erlotinib significantly improved PFS and OS in patients with tumors demonstrating amplification of the MET gene or MET IHC positivity.

VEGFR Activation and Inhibitors of Angiogenesis

Angiogenesis is important in multiple malignancies and vascular endothelial growth factor (VEGF) inhibition has demonstrated improved clinical outcomes in colon cancer, ovarian cancer, renal cell carcinoma, and NSCLC. The pivotal ECOG 4599 trial demonstrated the benefit of bevacizumab, a monoclonal antibody against VEGF, in addition to carboplatin and paclitaxel (79). Multiple trials have examined the combination of erlotinib and bevacizumab in unselected patients in the pretreated setting of advanced NSCLC (80,81). Other antiangiogenic agents are also being investigated for the treatment of NSCLC in combination with EGFR TKIs, including sunitinib and sorafenib (82,83). However, clinical evidence supporting the use of VEGF inhibition as means to overcome acquired resistance to EGFR TKIs in patients with EGFR mutations is not yet available.

CONCLUSIONS

Testing advanced NSCLC tumors for the presence of EGFR mutations in the first-line setting is now recommended by multiple oncology societies since international clinical trials have yielded superior efficacy and quality of life outcomes when patients harboring tumors with EGFR mutations were treated with EGFR TKIs. It is apparent from this evidence that relying solely on clinical and demographic data is inadequate in determining which patients will benefit from these agents, which are usually better tolerated than chemotherapeutics. Subset analyses are eagerly awaited in determining the potential role for postoperative erlotinib in EGFR mutation-positive patients. And means to overcome acquired resistance to EGFR TKIs in EGFR mutation-positive patients, such as with inhibition of MET amplification, is a highly active area of research.

REFERENCES

1. American Cancer Society. *Cancer Facts & Figures 2011*. Atlanta, GA: American Cancer Society, 2011.
2. Schiller JH, Harrington D, Belani CP, et al. Comparison of four chemotherapy regimens for advanced non-small-cell lung cancer. *N Engl J Med*. 2002;346(2):92–98.
3. Ullrich A, Schlessinger J. Signal transduction by receptors with tyrosine kinase activity. *Cell*. 1990;61(2):203–212.

4. Lynch TJ, Bell DW, Sordella R, et al. Activating mutations in the epidermal growth factor receptor underlying responsiveness of non-small-cell lung cancer to gefitinib. *N Eng J Med.* 2004;350: 2129–2139.
5. Shigematsu H, Lin L, Takahashi T, et al. Clinical and biological features associated with epidermal growth factor receptor gene mutations in lung cancers. *J Natl Cancer Inst.* 2005;97(5):339–346.
6. Tsao MS, Sakurada A, Cutz JC, et al. Erlotinib in lung cancer – molecular and clinical predictors of outcome. *N Engl J Med.* 2005;353(2):133–144.
7. Eberhard DA, Johnson BE, Amler LC, et al. Mutations in the epidermal growth factor receptor and in KRAS are predictive and prognostic indicators in patients with non-small-cell lung cancer in combination with erlotinib. *J Clin Oncol.* 2005;23(25):5900–5909.
8. Tokumo M, Toyooka S, Kiura K, et al. The relationship between epidermal growth factor receptor mutations and clinicopathologic features in non-small cell lung cancers. *Clin Cancer Res.* 2005;11:1167–1173.
9. D'Angelo SP, Pietanza MC, Johnson ML, et al. Incidence of EGFR exon 19 deletions and L858R in tumor specimens from men and cigarette smokers with lung adenocarcinomas. *J Clin Oncol.* 2011;29(15):2066–2070.
10. Leigh Keedy L, Temin S, Somerfield MR, et al. American Society of Clinical Oncology provisional clinical opinion: epidermal growth factor receptor (EGFR) mutation testing for patients with advanced non-small-cell lung cancer considering first-line EGFR tyrosine kinase inhibitor therapy. *J Clin Oncol.* 2011;29:2121–2127.
11. National Comprehensive Cancer Network Lung Cancer Guidelines 2011. www.nccn.org
12. D'addario G, Fruh M, Reck M, et al. Metastatic non-small-cell lung cancer: ESMO clinical practice guidelines for diagnosis, treatment and follow-up. *Ann Oncol.* 2010;21(suppl 5):v116–v119.
13. Bos M, Mendelsohn J, Kim YM, et al. PD153035, a tyrosine kinase inhibitor, prevents epidermal growth factor receptor activation and also inhibits growth of cancer cells in a receptor number-dependent manner. *Clin Cancer Res.* 1997;3: 2099–2106.
14. Moyer JD, Barbacci EG, Iwata KK, et al. Induction of apoptosis and cell cycle arrest by OSI-774, an inhibitor of epidermal growth factor receptor tyrosine kinase. *Cancer Res.* 1997;57:4838–4848.
15. Hidalgo M, Siu LL, Nemunaitis J, et al. Phase I and pharmacologic study of OSI-774, an epidermal growth factor receptor tyrosine kinase inhibitor, in patients with advanced solid malignancies. *J Clin Oncol.* 2001;19(13):3267–3279.
16. Yeo WL, Riely GJ, Yeap BY, et al. Erlotinib at a dose of 25 mg daily for non-small cell lung cancers with EGFR mutations. *J Thorac Oncol.* 2010;5:1048–1053.
17. Woodburn JR, Barker AJ, Gibson KH, et al. ZD1839, an epidermal growth factor tyrosine kinase inhibitor selected for clinical development. *Proc Am Assoc Cancer Res.* 1997;38:633–634. Abstract.
18. Herbst RS, Maddox AM, Rothenberg ML, et al. Selective oral epidermal growth factor receptor tyrosine kinase inhibitor ZD1839 is generally well-tolerated and has activity in non-small-cell lung cancer and other solid tumors: results of a phase I trial. *J Clin Oncol.* 2002;20(18):3815–3825.
19. Nakagawa K, Tamura T, Negoro S, et al. Phase I pharmacokinetic trial of the selective oral epidermal growth factor receptor tyrosine kinase inhibitor gefitinib ('Iressa', ZD1839) in Japanese patients with solid malignant tumors. *Ann Oncol.* 2003;14(6):922–930.
20. Ranson M, Hammond LA, Ferry D, et al. ZD1839, a selective oral epidermal growth factor receptor-tyrosine kinase inhibitor, is well tolerated and active in patients with solid, malignant tumors: results of a phase I trial. *J Clin Oncol.* 2002;20(9):2240–2250.
21. Baselga D, Rischin D, Ranson M, et al. Phase I safety and pharmacokinetic, and pharmacodynamic trial of ZD1839, a selective oral epidermal growth factor receptor tyrosine kinase inhibitor, in patients with five selected solid tumor types. *J Clin Oncol.* 2002;20(21):4292–4302.
22. Satoh H, Inoue A, Kobayashi K, et al. Low-dose gefitinib treatment for patients with advanced non-small cell lung cancer harboring sensitive epidermal growth factor receptor mutations. *J Thorac Oncol.* 2011;6:1413–1417.

23. Kris MG, Natale RB, Herbst RS, et al. Efficacy of gefitinib, an inhibitor of the epidermal growth factor receptor tyrosine kinase, in symptomatic patients with non-small cell lung cancer. *JAMA*. 2003;290(6):2149–2158.
24. Fukuoka M, Yano S, Giaccone G, et al. Multi-institutional randomized phase II trial of gefitinib for previously treated patients with advanced non-small cell lung cancer. *J Clin Oncol*. 2003;21:2237–2246.
25. Thatcher N, Chang A, Parikh P, et al. Gefitinib plus best supportive care in previously treated patients with refractory advanced non-small-cell lung cancer: results from a randomized, placebo-controlled, multicentre study (Iressa Survival Evaluation in Lung Cancer). *Lancet*. 2005;366: 1527–1537.
26. Hirsch FR, Varella-Garcia M, Bunn Jr PA, et al. Molecular predictors of outcome with gefitinib in a phase III placebo-controlled study in advanced non-small cell lung cancer. *J Clin Oncol*. 2006;24:5034–5042.
27. Kim ES, Hirsch V, Mok T, et al. Gefitnib versus docetaxel in previously treated non-small-cell lung cancer (INTEREST): a randomized phase III trial. *Lancet*. 2008;372:1809–1818.
28. Douillard JY, Shepherd FA, Hirsh V, et al. Molecular predictors of outcome with gefitinib and docetaxel in previously treated non-small cell lung cancer: data from the randomized phase III INTEREST trial. *J Clin Oncol*. 2009;28(5):744–752.
29. Shepherd FA, Pereira JR, Ciuleanu T, et al. Erlotinib in previously treated non-small-cell lung cancer. *N Eng J Med*. 2005;353(2):123–126.
30. Rosell R, Moran T, Queralt C, et al. Screening for epidermal growth factor receptor mutations in lung cancer. *N Eng J Med*. 2009;361(10):958–967.
31. Lee S, Rudd R, Khan I, et al. TOPICAL: randomized phase III trial of erlotinib compared with placebo in chemotherapy-naïve patients with advanced non-small cell lung cancer (NSCLC) and unsuitable for first-line chemotherapy. *J Clin Oncol*. 2010;28(suppl):540s. Abstract 7504.
32. Sequist LV, Martins RG, Spigel D, et al. First-line gefitinib in patients with advanced non-small cell lung cancer harboring somatic EGFR mutations. *J Clin Oncol*. 2008;26(15):2442–2449.
33. Morita S, Okamoto I, Kobayashi K, et al. Combined survival analysis of prospective clinical trials of gefitinib for non-small cell lung cancer with EGFR mutations. *Clin Cancer Res*. 2009;15(13):4493–4498.
34. Mok TS, Wu YL, Thongprasert S, et al. Gefitinib or carboplatin-paclitaxel in pulmonary adenocarcinoma. *N Eng J Med*. 2009;361(10):947–957.
35. Yang CH, Fukuoka M, Mok TS, et al. Final overall survival (OS) results from a phase III, randomized, open-label, first-line study of gefitinib (G) v carboplatin/paclitaxel (C/P) in clinically selected patients with advanced nonsmall cell lung cancer (NSCLC) in Asia (IPASS). *Ann Oncol*. 2010;21(suppl 8):viii1–viii2.
36. Fukuoka M, Wu YL, Thongprasert S, et al. Biomarker analyses and final overall survival results from a phase III, randomized, open-label, first-line study of gefitinib versus carboplatin/paclitaxel in clinically selected patients with advanced non-small-cell lung cancer in Asia (IPASS). *J Clin Oncol*. 2011;29(21):2866–2874.
37. Scagliotti G, Novello S, von Pawel J, et al. Phase III study of carboplatin and paclitaxel alone or with sorafenib in advanced non-small cell lung cancer. *J Clin Oncol*. 2010;28(11):1835–1841.
38. Lara PN, Douillard JY, Nakagawa K, et al. Randomized phase III placebo-controlled trial of carboplatin and paclitaxel with or without the vascular disrupting agent vadimezan (ASA404) in advanced non-small-cell lung cancer. *J Clin Oncol*. 2011;29(22):2965–2971.
39. Hirsh V, Paz-Ares L, Boyer M, et al. Randomized phase III trial of paclitaxel/carboplatin with or without PF-3512676 (Toll-like receptor 9 agonist) as first-line treatment for advanced non-small cell lung cancer. *J Clin Oncol*. 2011;29(19):2667–2674.
40. Lee JS, Park K, Kim SW, et al. A randomized phase III study of gefitinib (IRESSATM) versus standard chemotherapy (gemcitabine plus cisplatin) as a first-line treatment for never-smokers with advanced or metastatic adenocarcinoma of the lung. 13th World Conference on Lung Cancer. *J Thorac Oncol*. 2009;4(9)(suppl 1):S283–S284.
41. Gridelli C, De Marinis F, Di Maio M, et al. Gefitinib as first-line treatment for patients with advanced non-small-cell lung cancer with activating

epidermal growth factor receptor mutation: review of the evidence. *Lung Cancer.* 2011;71:249–257.

42. Maemondo M, Inoue A, Kobayashi K, et al. Gefitinib or chemotherapy for non-small-cell lung cancer with mutated EGFR. *N Eng J Med.* 2010;362(25):2380–2388.
43. Mitsudomi T, Morita S, Yatabe Y, et al. Gefitinib versus cisplatin plus docetaxel in patients with non-small-cell lung cancer harboring mutations of the epidermal growth factor receptor (WJTOG3405): an open label, randomized phase 3 trial. *Lancet Oncol.* 2010;11:121–128.
44. Zhou C, Wu YL, Chen G, et al. Erlotinib versus chemotherapy as first-line treatment for patients with advanced EGFR mutation-positive non-small-cell lung cancer (OPTIMAL, CTONG-0802): a multicentre, open-label, randomized, phase 3 study. *Lancet Oncol.* 2011;12:735–742.
45. Rosell R, Gervais R, Vergnenegre A, et al. Erlotinib versus chemotherapy in advanced non-small cell lung cancer patients with epidermal growth factor receptor mutations: interim results of the European erlotinib versus chemotherapy (EURTAC) phase III randomized trial. *J Clin Oncol.* 2011;29(suppl). Abstract 7503.
46. Janjigan YY, Park BJ, Zakowski MF, et al. Impact on disease-free survival of adjuvant erlotinib or gefitinib in patients with resected lung adenocarcinomas that harbor EGFR mutations. *J Thorac Oncol.* 2011;6(3):569–575.
47. Oxnard GR, Janjigian YY, Arcila ME, et al. Maintained sensitivity to EGFR tyrosine kinase inhibitors in EGFR-mutant lung cancer recurring after adjuvant erlotinib or gefitinib. *Clin Cancer Res.* 2011;17(19):1–7.
48. Goss GD, Lorimer I, Tsao MS, et al. A phase III randomized, double-blind, placebo-controlled trial of the epidermal growth factor receptor inhibitor gefitinib in completely resected stage IB-IIIA non-small cell lung cancer (NSCLC): NCIC CTG BR.19. *J Clin Oncol.* 28(suppl):18s. Abstract LBA7005.
49. Richardson F, Richardson K, Senello G, et al. Biomarker analysis from completely resected NSCLC patients enrolled in an adjuvant erlotinib clinical trial (RADIANT). *J Clin Oncol.* 2009;27(suppl):15s. Abstract 7520.
50. Neal JW, Pennell NA, Goodgame BW, et al. A multicenter phase II trial of adjuvant erlotinib in patients with resected non-small cell lung cancer (NSCLC) and mutations in the epidermal growth factor receptor (EGFR): toxicity evaluation. *J Clin Oncol.* 2010;28(suppl):15s. Abstract 7078.
51. Kelly K, Chansky K, Gaspar LE, et al. Phase III trial of maintenance gefitinib or placebo after concurrent chemoradiotherapy and docetaxel consolidation in inoperable stage III non-small-cell lung cancer: SWOG S0023. *J Clin Oncol.* 2008;26(15):2450–2456.
52. Li F, Zhu GY, Li XN, et al. The role of EGFR mutation status in patients with stage III non-squamous non-small cell lung cancer treated with chemoradiotherapy. *J Clin Oncol.* 2011;29(suppl). Abstract 7032.
53. Ahn HK, Choi YL, Sun J, et al. The association of epidermal growth factor receptor (EGFR) mutation and survival in N2(+) non-small cell lung cancer patients treated with platinum-based neoadjuvant concurrent chemoradiotherapy. *J Clin Oncol.* 2011;29(suppl). Abstract 7034.
54. Mak RH, Doran E, Muzikansky A, et al. Outcomes after combined modality therapy for EGFR-mutant and wild-type locally advanced NSCLC. *Oncologist.* 2011;16(6):886–895.
55. Kabbinavar FF, Miller VA, Johnson BE, et al. Overall survival (OS) in ATLAS, a phase IIIb trial comparing bevacizumab (B) therapy with or without erlotinib (E) after completion of chemotherapy (chemo) with B for first-line treatment of locally advanced, recurrent, or metastatic non-small cell lung cancer (NSCLC). *J Clin Oncol.* 2010;28(suppl):15s. Abstract 7526.
56. Cappuzzo F, Ciuleanu T, Stelmakh L, et al. Erlotinib as maintenance treatment in advanced non-small cell lung cancer: a multicentre, randomized, placebo-controlled phase 3 study. *Lancet Oncol.* 2010;11:521–529.
57. Ceresoli GL, Cappuzzo F, Gregorc V, Bartolini S, Crino L, Villa E. Gefitinib in patients with brain metastases from non-small-cell lung cancer: a prospective trial. *Ann Oncol.* 2004;15: 1042–1047.
58. Wu C, Li YL, Wang ZM, Li Z, Zhang TX, Wei Z. Gefitinib as palliative therapy for lung

adenocarcinoma metastatic to the brain. *Lung Cancer.* 2007;57:359–364.
59. Kim JE, Lee DH, Choi Y, et al. Epidermal growth factor receptor tyrosine kinase inhibitors as a first-line therapy for never-smokers with adenocarcinoma of the lung having asymptomatic synchronous brain metastasis. *Lung Cancer.* 2009;65:351–354.
60. Heon S, Yeap BY, Britt GJ, et al. Development of central nervous system metastases in patients with advanced non-small-cell lung cancer and somatic EGFR mutations treated with gefitinib or erlotinib. *Clin Cancer Res.* 2010;16(23):5873–5882.
61. Kosaka T, Yatabe Y, Endoh H, et al. Analysis of epidermal growth factor receptor gene mutation in patients with non-small cell lung cancer and acquired resistance to gefitinib. *Clin Cancer Res.* 2006;12:5764–5769.
62. Balak MN, Gong Y, Reily GJ, et al. Novel D761Y and common secondary T790M mutations in epidermal growth factor receptor mutant lung adenocarcinomas with acquired resistance to kinase inhibitors. *Clin Cancer Res.* 2006;12: 6494–6501.
63. Nguyen KS, Kobayashi, Costa DB. Acquired resistance to epidermal growth factor receptor tyrosine kinase inhibitors in non-small-cell lung cancers dependent on the epidermal growth factor receptor pathway. *Clin Lung Cancer.* 2009;10(4): 281–289.
64. Oxnard GR, Arcilla ME, Sima CS, et al. Acquired resistance to EGFR tyrosine kinase inhibitors in EGFR-mutant lung cancer: distinct natural history of patients with tumors harboring the T790M mutation. *Clin Cancer Res.* 2011;17(6):1616–1622.
65. Pao W, Chielecki J. Rational, biologically based treatment of EGFR-mutant non-small-cell lung cancer. *Nat Rev.* 2010;10:760–774.
66. Johnson FM, Bekele BN, Feng L, et al. Phase II study of dasatinib in patients with advanced non-small cell lung cancer. *J Clin Oncol.* 2010;28(30):4609–4615.
67. Sequist LV, Gettinger S, Senzer NN, et al. Activity of IPI-504, a novel heat-shock protein 90 inhibitor, in patients with molecularly defined non-small-cell lung cancer. *J Clin Oncol.* 2010;28(33):4953–4960.
68. Pal SK, Figlin RA, Reckamp K. Targeted therapies for non-small cell lung cancer: an evolving landscape. *Mol Cancer Ther.* 2010;9:1931–1944.
69. Slebos RJ, Hruban RH, Dalesio O, et al. Relationship between K-ras oncogene activation and smoking in adenocarcinoma of the human lung. *J Natl Cancer Inst.* 1991;83:1024–1027.
70. Mao C, Qiu LX, Liao RY, et al. KRAS mutations and resistance to EGFR-TKIs treatment in patients with non-small cell lung cancer: a meta-analysis of 22 studies. *Lung Cancer.* 2010;69:272–278.
71. Davies H, Bignell GR, Cox C, et al. Mutations of the BRAF gene in human cancer. *Nature.* 2002;417(6892):949–954.
72. Okudela K, Suzuki M, Kageyama S, et al. PIK3CA mutation and amplification in human lung cancer. *Pathol Int.* 2007;57(10):664–671.
73. Lee SY, Kim MJ, Jin G, et al. Somatic mutations in epidermal growth factor receptor signaling pathway genes in non-small cell lung cancers. *J Thorac Oncol.* 2010;5(11):1734–1740.
74. Price KA, Azzoli CG, Krug LM, et al. Phase II trial of gefitinib and everolimus in advanced non-small cell lung cancer. *J Thorac Oncol.* 2010;5(10): 1623–1629.
75. Guix M, Faber AC, Wang SE, et al. Acquired resistance to EGFR tyrosine kinase inhibitors in cancer cells is mediated by loss of IGF-binding proteins. *J Clin Invest.* 2008;118:2609–2619.
76. Engelman JA, Zejnullahu K, Mitsudomi T, et al. MET amplification leads to gefitinib resistance in lung cancer by activating ERBB3 signaling. *Science.* 2007;316:1039–1043.
77. Bean J, Brennan C, Shih JY, et al. MET amplification occurs with or without T790M mutations in EGFR mutant lung tumors with acquired resistance to gefitinib or erlotinib. *Proc Natl Acad Sci U S A.* 2007;104:20932–20937.
78. Spigel DR, Ervin TJ, Ramlau R, et al. Final efficacy results from OAM4558g, a randomized phase II study evaluating MetMAb or placebo in combination with erlotinib in advanced NSCLC. *J Clin Oncol.* 2011;29(suppl): Abstract 7505.
79. Sandler A, Gray R, Perry MC, et al. Paclitaxel-carboplatin alone or with bevacizumab for non-small-cell lung cancer. *N Engl J Med.* 2006; 355(24):2542–2550.

80. Dingemans AM, de Langen AJ, van den Boogaart V, et al. First-line erlotinib and bevacizumab in patients with locally advanced and/or metastatic non-small-cell lung cancer: a phase II study including molecular imaging. *Ann Oncol.* 2011;22(3):559–566.
81. Herbst RS, Johnson DH, Mininberg E, et al. Phase I/II trial evaluating the anti-vascular endothelial growth factor monoclonal antibody bevacizumab in combination with the HER-1/epidermal growth factor receptor tyrosine kinase inhibitor erlotinib for patients with recurrent non-small-cell lung cancer. *J Clin Oncol.* 2005;23(11):2544–2555.
82. O'Mahar SE, Campbell TC, Hoang T, et al. Phase I study of sunitinib and erlotinib in advanced nonsquamous non-small cell lung cancer. *J Thorac Oncol.* 2011;6(5):951–953.
83. Lind JSW, Dingemans AMC, Groen HJM, et al. A multicenter phase II study of erlotinib and sorafenib in chemotherapy-naïve patients with advanced non-small cell lung cancer. *Clin Cancer Res.* 2010;16(11):3078–3087.

Index

Note: Page numbers followed by "*f*" and "*t*" denote figures and tables, respectively.